The Final FRCA Short Answer Questions

A Practical Study Guide

Elizabeth Combeer
Consultant Anaesthetist
Frimley Health NHS Foundation Trust

Illustrations by Paul Hatton

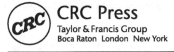

CRC Press
Taylor & Francis Group
Boca Raton London New York

CRC Press is an imprint of the
Taylor & Francis Group, an **informa** business

CRC Press
Taylor & Francis Group
6000 Broken Sound Parkway NW, Suite 300
Boca Raton, FL 33487-2742

© 2019 by Taylor & Francis Group, LLC
CRC Press is an imprint of Taylor & Francis Group, an Informa business

No claim to original U.S. Government works

Printed on acid-free paper

International Standard Book Number-13: 978-1-138-49932-4 (Paperback); 978-1-138-49939-3 (Hardcover)

**Visit the Taylor & Francis Web site at
http://www.taylorandfrancis.com**

**and the CRC Press Web site at
http://www.crcpress.com**

CONTENTS

LIST OF ABBREVIATIONS

2,3DPG	2,3 diphosphoglycerate
A-a	Alveolar-arterial
AAA	Abdominal aortic aneurysm
AAGBI	Association of Anaesthetists of Great Britain and Ireland
ABG	Arterial blood gas
ACE	Angiotensin converting enzyme
ADP	Adenosine diphosphate
ALS	Adult life support
ALT	Alanine transaminase
APL	Adjustable pressure limiting
ARDS	Acute respiratory distress syndrome
ASA	American Society of Anesthesiologists
ATP	Adenosine triphosphate
AVPU	Alert, voice, pain, unresponsive
BIS	Bispectral index
BJA	*British Journal of Anaesthesia*
BMI	Body mass index
BP	Blood pressure
bpm	Beats per minute
cAMP	Cyclic adenosine monophosphate
CBG	Capillary blood glucose
CCT	Certificate of Completion of Training
CEACCP	*Continuing Education in Anaesthesia, Critical Care & Pain*
CICO	Can't intubate, can't oxygenate
CK	Creatine kinase
CKD	Chronic kidney disease
CMV	Cytomegalovirus
CNS	Central nervous system
CO	Cardiac output
COETT	Cuffed oral endotracheal tube
COX	Cyclic oxygenase
CPAP	Continuous positive airway pressure
CRP	C-reactive protein
CSF	Cerebrospinal fluid
CT	Computed tomography
CVC	Central venous catheter
CVP	Central venous pressure
CXR	Chest radiograph
DAS	Difficult Airway Society
DIC	Disseminated intravascular coagulation
DVT	Deep vein thrombosis
EBV	Epstein–Barr virus

ECG	Electrocardiogram
Echo	Echocardiogram
ECMO	Extracorporeal membrane oxygenation
EEG	Electroencephalogram
eGFR	Estimated glomerular filtration rate
ENT	Ear, nose and throat
ERCP	Endoscopic retrograde cholangiopancreatography
ESR	Erythrocyte sedimentation rate
etCO$_2$	End-tidal carbon dioxide
ETT	Endotracheal tube
EVAR	Endovascular aneurysm repair
FEV$_1$	Forced expiratory volume in 1 second
FiO$_2$	Fraction of inspired oxygen
FRC	Functional residual capacity
GA	General anaesthetic
GCS	Glasgow Coma Scale
GGT	Gamma-glutamyl transferase
GMC	General Medical Council
HIV	Human immunodeficiency virus
HSV	Herpes simplex virus
IASP	International Association for the Study of Pain
ICP	Intracranial pressure
ICU	Intensive care unit
INR	International normalised ratio
IQ	Intelligence quotient
iv	Intravenous
IVC	Inferior vena cava
ivi	Intravenous infusion
JVP	Jugular venous pressure
LMA	Laryngeal mask airway
LSCS	Lower segment caesarean section
LVEDP	Left ventricular end-diastolic pressure
M&M	Morbidity and mortality
MAC	Minimum alveolar concentration
MAP	Mean arterial pressure
MDI	Metered dose inhaler
MEOWS	Modified Early Obstetric Warning Score
MRI	Magnetic resonance imaging
NHS	National Health Service
NICE	National Institute for Health and Care Excellence
NMBD	Neuromuscular blocking drug
NMDA	N-methyl-D-aspartate
NPSA	National Patient Safety Agency
NSAIDs	Non-steroidal anti-inflammatory drugs
OAA	Obstetric Anaesthetists' Association
ODP	Operating Department Practitioner
PaCO$_2$	Partial pressure of carbon dioxide in arterial blood
PACU	Post-anaesthetic care unit
PaO$_2$	Partial pressure of oxygen in arterial blood
PCA	Patient controlled analgesia
PCR	Polymerase chain reaction
PEA	Pulseless electrical activity

PEEP	Positive end-expiratory pressure
PEG	Percutaneous endoscopic gastrostomy
PEJ	Percutaneous endoscopic jejunostomy
PONV	Postoperative nausea and vomiting
RSI	Rapid sequence induction
S1Q3T3	S wave in lead 1, Q wave and inverted T wave in lead 3
SAD	Supraglottic airway device
SIRS	Systemic inflammatory response syndrome
SVR	Systemic vascular resistance
SVRI	Systemic vascular resistance index
TCI	Target controlled infusion
TENS	Transcutaneous electrical nerve stimulation
TIVA	Total intravenous anaesthesia
TNF	Tumour necrosis factor
VATER	Syndrome of vertebral, cardiac, renal and limb anomalies, tracheo-oesophageal fistula, and anal atresia
vCJD	Variant Creutzfeldt–Jakob disease
VF	Ventricular fibrillation
VRIII	Variable rate intravenous insulin infusion
VT	Ventricular tachycardia
V/Q	Ventilation:perfusion
WHO	World Health Organisation

PASSING THE FINAL SAQ

These are my top tips for approaching the Final SAQ. They are based on what I find myself saying repeatedly at weekly teaching with the trainees at Frimley.

Print Off a Copy of the Syllabus

Both basic and intermediate-level syllabi are tested in the Final. I know these are dauntingly large documents, but it really is important that you understand the breadth of what you need to learn, and looking at these helps you direct your reading. Revision for subspecialties such as burns, cardiothoracics, neuro, paediatrics and obstetrics can largely be covered by searching for *CEACCP/BJA Education* articles that relate to the specified learning objectives. In this way, you will be learning the College-approved facts on the subject. There is also a very strong link between topics addressed in the exam and topics that have been featured in these articles within the preceding two years. Every time you do some revision that relates to something in the syllabus, cross it off. Remember that a broad understanding is more important than learning a few topics in great detail.

Three Types of Questions

There are three main types of questions in the Final SAQ. Firstly, there are those that relate to new guidance or reports (such as National Audit Projects or National Institute for Health and Care Excellence guidance). Secondly, there are the questions that test knowledge of the manner of anaesthesia provision for specific operations or in particular situations. The third group assesses knowledge of how particular patient conditions impact on anaesthesia management. Make sure you decide what group each question you encounter falls into as it will impact on your approach to answering it.

Questions Relating to New Guidance or Reports

Questions based on these topics tend to appear within two years of their publication. Search the likely websites (Royal College of Anaesthetists, Difficult Airway Society, Obstetric Anaesthetists' Association, NICE, Association of Anaesthetists of Great Britain and Ireland) and be aware of new national guidelines that are implemented in your place of work. Also, be aware of topical causes of medical error, such as new additions to the list of never events that are relevant to anaesthesia, and statements and alerts from the Safe Anaesthesia Liaison Group. Think about the impact of these guidelines at the organisational level, not just at the point of delivery of anaesthesia.

Questions Relating to Anaesthetic Management of a Specific Operation or Situation

This includes questions about nerve blocks as well. Nerve blocks have peaks of popularity, and the timing of inclusion of questions about them in the SAQ reflects this. Remember to learn the specific complications of such blocks, not just 'bleeding, infection, nerve damage.' It is by listing the specific complications that you demonstrate that you actually know the relevant anatomy.

When considering the anaesthetic management of any operation, think in terms of preoperative, intraoperative and postoperative. Preoperatively, consider history, examination and investigations. However, never state that you would 'take a full history, examine the airway and cardiac and respiratory systems and request ECG, FBC and U&E.' Instead, specify why you are asking this question in this particular patient, what you are seeking in the examination of this particular patient and what investigation anomalies may be found in this particular patient. Intraoperatively, consider mode of anaesthesia, airway management, positioning and its impact, likely duration and its impact, need for warming, thromboprophylaxis, particular needs for monitoring, risk of bleeding and any special issues relating to this type of surgery. This is all as you would in real life. Following the alphabet (see next section) may help you here. Postoperatively, think of where the patient is going to be cared for; ongoing need for oxygen or ventilatory support and why; and how you will manage pain, nausea and thromboprophylaxis. Start to practice this systematic way of thinking in advance of every case you undertake, such that you could write a shopping list and recipe for any case in which you are involved.

Questions Relating to Particular Patient Conditions and Their Impact on Anaesthetic Management

You will all be familiar with using an ABC approach to patient assessment or ABCDE for trauma management. I have just taken that alphabet a little further.

A: airway.
B: respiratory.
C: cardiovascular.
D: neurological, both central and peripheral (disability).
E: endocrine.
F: pharmacology.
G: gastrointestinal.
H: haematology.
I: immunology, infection.
J: cutaneomusculoskeletal (joints).
K: renal (kidneys).
L: hepatic (liver).
M: metabolic.
N: nutrition.
O: obstetric.
P: psychological.

Following this alphabet will help you dredge the depths of your brain for issues that relate to diabetes, rheumatoid arthritis or epidermolysis bullosa. I promise you. Obviously, not all elements of the alphabet are relevant every time, but get into the habit of using it well in advance of the exam. You will see this alphabet used repeatedly in this book.

Finish the Paper

If you miss out a question, you will fail. Do not allow yourself to run out of time. If you run over by 10 minutes on a question you know well and are enjoying answering, you will find it very difficult to make up time elsewhere. You are more likely to gain the majority of the marks overall by writing a few lines down for each section of each question than you are by writing enormous essays for a couple of questions and leaving yourself short for others. Force yourself to move on. Ensure you do some full papers under exam conditions (on lined paper with a nice pen to maximise the clarity of your handwriting) in advance of the big day.

Think About the Timing and Weighting of Questions

The College clearly states how many marks are available for each section of the examination. If there are only 2 marks available for one section of the question, then allocate time accordingly. Two-twentieths of 15 minutes is 1.5 minutes – if you are taking longer than that, then you shouldn't be. Stop. You will not convince the examiner to give you more than the possible 2 marks by writing an essay, so stop wasting your time and move on.

Read the Question

The Chairman's Reports will show you how often candidates run into difficulty for failing to read the question. Sometimes, two questions are asked within one section of a question – make sure you answer both bits. Abbreviations can cause confusion: ASD may mean autistic spectrum disorder or atrioseptal defect, but the College is always careful to specify what any abbreviation means. Another common error is failing to notice the change in the focus of a question. The first part may relate to children with autistic spectrum disorder, the second part may relate to management of any child for dental surgery, not just those with autistic spectrum disorder. Slow down and read carefully; underline key words.

Abbreviations

Beware of using too many abbreviations yourself. Generally, if I have used an abbreviation, I define what I mean by it within that answer. Abbreviations that I have used without defining what they mean are listed in the front of the book and, I think, are commonly accepted.

Lists, Tables and Bullet Points

The Chairman's Reports make it clear that these are welcomed. Imagine the poor examiners having to wade through reams of bad handwriting to try to award marks for key facts scattered here and there. It is much easier for everyone if you get straight to the point.

State the Blindingly Obvious

You will see that some of the Chairman's Reports are very detailed, clearly showing what needs to be written to gain the available points. It has been made clear that there are points available for really obvious things such as stating the need for large bore intravenous access if there is a significant risk of bleeding. Make sure you include such explanations in your answers.

Don't Assume You Don't Know

Don't know the precise definition of cerebral palsy or autistic spectrum disorder? Visualise the people you have met affected by these conditions and describe them. Who: male, female, child, adult. When: lifelong, reversible, terminal. Why: genetic, infection related, trauma related. Keep calm and you will cobble together an answer that will gain you most of the marks available.

Improve Your Clinical Knowledge

The Chairman's Reports have frequently commented on lack of knowledge impacting on answer quality. This is often clinical rather than book-based knowledge. It particularly affects subspecialties such as cardiothoracics and neurosurgery that not all candidates may have rotated through by the time they sit the exam. In the same way that a picture may be worth a thousand words, spending a day in cardiothoracic or neuro theatres will be invaluable. Trainees at my hospital have followed the College's advice and have arranged a couple of days' experience in these subspecialties and have found it very worthwhile. In the same way, you may need to be proactive in getting some experience in vascular surgery, the interventional radiology suite, and magnetic resonance imaging. Failing that, there's nothing you can't find on YouTube.

Remember That You Don't Need to Get Many Marks to Pass

In each paper, two questions are difficult (pass mark 10–11/20), eight are moderately difficult (pass mark 12–13/20), and two are easy (pass mark 14/20 or more). You can therefore miss out great chunks of what is present on the model answer and still pass! This exam is within your grasp.

Practise Past Questions

For a number of reasons, practising past questions is a fantastic way to review. Questions commonly recur: if you encounter a question you have previously practised, you will be able to answer it more quickly and with less brain fatigue, leaving you more time and energy for other questions. Looking at past questions helps you to develop technique, as explained earlier. Also, you will get a feel for the topics that the College considers important by looking at what they have previously included in the exam.

This Book

Thirteen SAQ papers are covered in this book. For each question, the relevant section of the Chairman's Report is reproduced (where available), followed by my answer. I have included diagrams and additional commentary to ensure that this book helps you to learn rather than just providing a list of my suggested model answers. I have no way of knowing how close my answers are to the College's model answers, but they are referenced and have all taken much more time to produce than you will have available to you in the exam. They have also been reviewed by friends (husband) and colleagues with a special interest in each subspecialty. You would not, therefore, need to write this level of detail in order to gain a pass in the exam.

ACKNOWLEDGEMENTS

I am very grateful to those who have read and revised sections of this book:
Drs. Sam Pambakian, Elaine Hipwell, Sharon Pickworth, Irfan Raza, Deepa Jadhav,
Tom Heinink, Mohjir Baloch and Jo Teare, who are colleagues at Frimley Park Hospital;
Dr. Andy Combeer, Epsom and St Helier University Hospitals; Drs. Dom Spray,
Elaine Monahan and Judith Dinsmore of St George's Hospital, London; and Dr. Rik Hawkins,
specialty trainee, St George's School of Anaesthesia. I am indebted to Dr. Kate McCombe,
Mediclinic City Hospital, Dubai, who has read the final proofs from cover to cover, spotting
last-minute errors.

I am very thankful to Paul Hatton, who has kindly produced the excellent diagrams for fun
and because he believes in the NHS and in contributing to education.

My thanks to the Royal College of Anaesthetists for allowing me to reproduce the SAQ
questions and excerpts from the Chairman's Reports.

Finally, thank you to my husband and children for their patience and for allowing me the time
to write this book.

Elizabeth Combeer

1. NEUROSURGERY, NEURORADIOLOGY AND NEUROCRITICAL CARE

a) What characteristic neurological changes occur immediately and in the first three months following transection of the spinal cord at the fourth thoracic vertebra? (25%)

b) What other clinical problems may develop following this type of injury? (40%)

c) List the advantages of a regional anaesthetic technique for a cystoscopy in this patient. (20%)

d) Why and when may suxamethonium be contraindicated in a patient with spinal injury? (15%)

September 2011

Underline the key words in a question; make sure you are always answering the question asked and that you don't miss out a section, as would be easy to do here.

a) What characteristic <u>neurological</u> changes occur <u>immediately</u> and in the <u>first three months</u> following <u>transection</u> of the spinal cord at the fourth thoracic vertebra? (25%)

	Immediate	Changes at three months
Sensory	Complete sensory loss below the level of injury (and, to a variable extent, above the level of transection due to secondary injury; haemorrhage, oedema, ischaemia).	Ongoing anaesthesia. Development of chronic neuropathic and nociceptive pain.
Motor	Spinal shock: flaccid paralysis. Even reflexes are obliterated as these depend on tonic descending facilitation.	Hyper-reflexia with spasticity. Initially, upregulation of receptors facilitates reflexes, then new interneurones develop.
Autonomic	Neurogenic shock: loss of sympathetic function (in injuries at T4 or above, but also at lower levels if significant secondary neurological damage occurs) with unopposed parasympathetic activity. Results in hypotension, bradycardia and sometimes other arrhythmias. Loss of other autonomic reflexes (voiding, bowel emptying, coital).	Autonomic dysreflexia (or sympathetic hyper-reflexia): abnormal synapse development in spinal cord distal to lesion results in non-noxious stimuli causing reflex sympathetic output below level of lesion, resulting in lower body and splanchnic vasoconstriction. The resulting rise in blood pressure activates baroreceptors, thus causing vasodilatation above the level of the lesion and bradycardia, which is insufficient to reduce blood pressure to normal. Onset is variable, may take up to a year to develop. Bowel emptying, voiding and coital reflexes return, but may not be efficient and so many patients require catheterisation.

b) What other clinical problems may develop following this type of injury? (40%)

Follow the alphabet to categorise your answer and ensure you are able to extract as many facts from your brain as possible.

Respiratory:
> Loss of innervation of intercostal muscles results in failure of expansion of ribcage and, therefore, reduced tidal volumes.
> Inefficient seesaw breathing: the diaphragm contracts, pushes abdominal contents down and out due to loss of abdominal wall tone and the chest wall is sucked in.
> Breathing worse in the sitting position. Abdominal contents pull down on the diaphragm, thus expanding expiratory intrathoracic volume, so reducing volume for expansion in inspiration. A high proportion of minute ventilation therefore spent on ventilating dead space, resulting in V/Q mismatch and atelectasis.
> Difficulty clearing secretions: inefficient coughing due to loss of abdominal wall tone.

Cardiovascular:
> Neurogenic shock (may last 24 hours to several weeks): vasodilatation and bradycardia resulting in hypotension. Sensitive to position with postural hypotension. Sensitive to fluid depletion, especially with positive pressure ventilation.
> Later, autonomic dysreflexia predisposes to periods of uncontrolled hypertension, risking headache, flushing, nasal congestion, seizures, retinal haemorrhages, stroke, coma, death.
> Long-term, patients are at risk of ischaemic heart disease due to physical inactivity and development of diabetes.
> Difficulty with intravenous access due to fragile skin, reduced surface blood flow.

Endocrine:
> Initial stress response may result in hyperglycaemia which may exacerbate secondary neurological injury.
> Increased risk of developing diabetes in the longer term.

Gastrointestinal:
> Reduced gastrointestinal motility: delayed gastric emptying (aspiration risk), paralytic ileus, constipation, pseudo-obstruction.
> Increased risk of gall stones and their complications.
> Prone to stress ulceration due to unopposed vagal activity.

Haematological:
> Immobility and thrombogenicity of trauma predispose to thromboembolic disease. Risk falls after three months (possibly due to muscle spasm facilitating the muscle pump of venous return, decreased venous distensibility and femoral artery atrophy).
> Anaemia is common.

Immune, infection:
> Risk of nosocomial colonisation with multi-resistant organisms.

Cutaneomusculoskeletal:
> Contractures resulting from spasticity cause pain and further reduction in function.
> Osteoporosis results from loss of limb use.
> Risk of pressure sores including in unusual places such as occiput.

Renal and genitourinary:
> Nephrogenic bladder. Impaired sensory and motor function may lead to incomplete voiding (predisposing to infection) and uncoordinated voiding (predisposing to vesico-ureteral reflux and, thus, chronic kidney disease). Intermittent or long-term catheterisation is usually required.

Metabolic:
> Poor temperature regulation: vasodilatation may predispose to cooling, whilst lack of ability to sweat below level of injury may cause hyperthermia.

Psychological:
> At risk of depression, suicide, drug addiction.

c) List the advantages of a regional anaesthetic technique for a cystoscopy in this patient. (20%)

> Avoids autonomic dysreflexia.
> Avoids the need for intubation of a patient who may have previously had a tracheostomy with its attendant complications, e.g. tracheal stenosis.
> Avoids deterioration in lung function associated with general anaesthesia, thus reducing the risk of postoperative respiratory complications.
> Avoids opioid use with associated respiratory depression.
> Reduces the risk of aspiration associated with delayed gastric emptying.
> Avoidance of unopposed parasympathetic response to airway instrumentation (bradycardia, cardiac arrest).

d) Why and when may suxamethonium be contraindicated in a patient with spinal injury? (15%)

Upregulation of nicotinic acetylcholine receptors in extrajunctional sites results in massive potassium release with suxamethonium use.

This effect is seen between approximately 72 hours following injury and six months.

References
Bonner S, Smith C. Initial management of acute spinal cord injury. *Contin Educ Anaesth Crit Care Pain*. 2013; 13 (6): 224–231.
Petsas A, Drake J. Perioperative management for patients with a chronic spinal cord injury. *Contin Educ Anaesth Crit Care Pain*. 2015; 15 (3): 123–130.

a) What are the symptoms (10%) and signs (20%) of raised intracranial pressure (ICP) in an adult?

b) Describe the physiological principles underlying the management of raised ICP. (40%)

c) What methods are used to manage or prevent acute rises in ICP? (30%)

September 2012

Chairman's Report

56% pass rate.

Many candidates failed to attempt to answer b) Physiological mechanisms of raised intracranial pressure and instead wrote about areas of clinical management only then to repeat the same points in section c). Key points are never repeated in any question.

A number of candidates advised a 30-degree head-up tilt rather than the 15–20* recommended in this question. Perhaps there was confusion with the head-up tilt to avoid ventilator-associated pneumonia.

Just to confuse you, more recent guidance suggests a 15–30-degree head-up tilt.

a) What are the symptoms (10%) and signs (20%) of raised intracranial pressure (ICP) in an adult?

Symptoms:
> Headache: bursting, throbbing. Exacerbated by sneezing, exertion, recumbency. Worse in morning after a period of recumbency, raised $PaCO_2$ associated with sleep, reduced CSF reabsorption.
> Vomiting.
> Visual disturbance.

Signs:
> Respiratory irregularity, Cheyne-Stokes breathing, neurogenic hyperventilation due to tonsillar herniation.
> Cushing's triad: hypertension with high pulse pressure, bradycardia and associated irregular respirations.
> Eye signs: papilloedema, fundal haemorrhages, pupillary dilatation, ptosis, impaired upward gaze (midbrain compression), abducens palsy.
> Progressive reduction in consciousness due to caudal displacement of midbrain.

b) Describe the physiological principles underlying the management of raised ICP. (40%)

The Chairman's Report said that some candidates wrote the same points for (b) and (c). I am aware that there is some overlap in my answers but am unsure how better to address the question.

The cranium is a closed compartment (Monroe–Kelly doctrine). The sum of its contents (brain, CSF, blood, other) must therefore remain the same. If the amount of one component increases, some compensation can occur by reducing the amount of one of the other components. Once these compensatory mechanisms are exhausted, ICP will rise, ultimately causing pressure on the brain, herniation and thus direct tissue damage. Physiological manipulation of the quantity of each of the components can limit ICP rise.
> Reduce CSF: diuretics, mannitol, hypertonic saline, elevation of head of bed 15–30 degrees, CSF drain.
> Reduce blood:
  • Optimise venous drainage: avoid tight tube ties, head-up tilt 15–30 degrees, paralyse to reduce valsalva, treat seizures with anticonvulsants, avoid excessive PEEP and peak airway pressures.
  • Avoid excessive arterial flow: maintain PaO_2, keep $PaCO_2$ low-normal, anaesthetise to reduce cerebral metabolic rate of oxygen ($CMRO_2$) and avoid pyrexia.

> Reduce brain: mannitol, avoid hyperglycaemia, avoid hypotonic fluid administration.
> Reduce other: evacuate clot, excise tumour.
> Stop the cranium being a closed compartment: decompressive craniectomy.

One of the main issues of a rising ICP is the impact it has on cerebral perfusion pressure (CPP), according to the equation:

$$CPP = MAP - ICP \text{ (or JVP, whichever is higher)}$$

Therefore, in the early stages of rising ICP (before direct pressure brain damage occurs), the effects can be mitigated by maintaining CPP through manipulation of mean arterial pressure (MAP) and jugular venous pressure (JVP).

> Maintain MAP: avoid dehydration and pyrexia, and use vasopressors to target a MAP of 80 mm Hg (this value depends on ICP, which may not be known).
> Reduce JVP: as previously, optimise venous drainage.

c) What methods are used to manage or prevent acute rises in ICP? (30%)

Airway:
> Intubate.

Respiratory:
> Aim PaO_2 >13 kPa and $PaCO_2$ 4.5–5 kPa, keep PEEP <15.
> Hyperventilation to $PaCO_2$ 4–4.5 kPa may be used for short time periods in emergency situations with refractory intracranial hypertension.

Cardiovascular:
> 15–30-degree head-up tilt, tube ties not too tight/tape tube, head in neutral position, increase sedation and paralyse if coughing or straining, ensure that MAP >80 (depends on ICP, if being monitored).

Neurological:
> Adequate sedation to reduce $CMRO_2$, treat seizures, treat pyrexia, monitor for and manage hyperglycaemia (target 6–10 mmol/l).

Pharmacological:
> Mannitol 0.25–1 g/kg.
> Hypertonic saline 5% 2 ml/kg.
> Consideration of CSF drain, under expert guidance.
> Decompressive craniectomy in specialist centre.

References
Dinsmore J. Traumatic brain injury: an evidence-based review of management. *Contin Educ Anaesth Crit Care Pain*. 2013; 13 (6): 189–195.
Tameem A, Krovvidi H. Cerebral physiology. *Contin Educ Anaesth Crit Care Pain*. 2013; 13 (4): 113–118.

A 45-year-old male with acromegaly presents for an elective trans-sphenoidal hypophysectomy.

a) What is the cause of acromegaly in this patient? (10%)

b) List the clinical features of acromegaly of relevance to the anaesthetist. (45%)

c) How do the surgical requirements for this procedure influence the conduct of the anaesthesia? (45%)

March 2013

Chairman's Report

57% pass rate.

It was clear that many candidates had not had experience of managing these patients for this type of surgery. Some candidates quoted the prone position for surgical access!

In section c) perhaps it would be easier to organize your thoughts in the form of a table or list.

Surgical Requirement	Conduct of Anaesthesia
Use of operating microscope	"Hypotensive" anaesthesia
Head-up supine position	Potential for air embolism
Operation on head	Airway under drapes, armoured tube

This approach makes it so much easier for examiner to spot the scoring answers.

This question was the second best discriminator of the paper.

A little bit of revision about the anatomy and function of the pituitary (as I don't want you to be one of the people who think that it is best accessed from the back of the head).

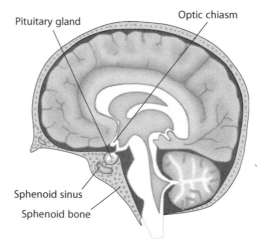

Sagittal section of the pituitary gland

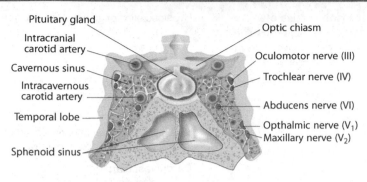

Coronal section of the pituitary gland

Adenohypophysis or anterior pituitary: hypothalamus releases inhibitory or secretory factors, which travel via the portal system to the anterior pituitary, where they control the release of the anterior pituitary hormones.

Neurohypophysis or posterior pituitary: neurosecretory cells in the hypothalamus make oxytocin and vasopressin, which travel down axons to be released from the posterior pituitary.

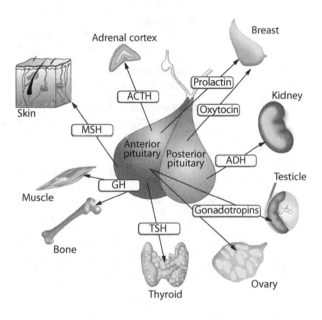

Key:	
ACTH	Adrenocorticotrophic hormone
ADH	Antidiuretic hormone, vasopressin
GH	Growth hormone
MSH	Melanocyte stimulating hormone
TSH	Thyroid stimulating hormone

Pituitary gland hormones

a) What is the cause of acromegaly in <u>this</u> patient? (10%)

b) List the clinical features of acromegaly of relevance to the anaesthetist. (45%)

Hypersecretion of growth hormone from a pituitary adenoma.

Now you are being asked about the features of acromegaly generally...

Airway:
> Large lips, macroglossia, macrognathia, thickening of pharyngeal tissues, laryngeal stenosis. Possibility of difficult airway should be considered.

Respiratory:
> Obstructive sleep apnoea (OSA) with risk of hypoventilation and respiratory failure postoperatively.

Cardiovascular:
> Hypertension, left ventricular hypertrophy, cardiomyopathy with diastolic dysfunction, valvular regurgitation, ECG changes.
> Increased peripheral soft tissue deposition may make cannulation difficult.

Neurological:
> Raised ICP (obstruction of the 3rd ventricle).
> Spinal cord compression. Meticulous care with padding and positioning required.
> Peripheral neuropathies due to impingement by soft tissue or bony overgrowth.

Endocrine:
> Diabetes mellitus. Blood glucose should be monitored and managed with insulin intraoperatively if necessary.

Gastrointestinal:
> Increased risk of colonic polyps and cancer – may necessitate surgery.

Cutaneomusculoskeletal:
> Osteoarthritis, bony overgrowth around joints, limited movement. Care with positioning and padding.

Renal:
> Renal dysfunction may impact on perioperative drug choices.

c) How do the surgical requirements for this procedure influence the conduct of the anaesthesia? (45%)

Even if you have never seen this operation before, experience of ENT surgery will give you some knowledge of the logistics of anaesthesia where the patient's head is distant to the anaesthetist and access to the airway is restricted.

Surgical requirement	Conduct of anaesthesia
Use of operating microscope.	'Hypotensive' anaesthesia, intra-arterial monitoring, immobile patient (muscle relaxant or remifentanil infusion). Preparation of nasal mucosa with e.g. Moffat's solution or phenylephrine.
Periods of intense stimulation and periods of minimal stimulation.	Blood pressure may be very labile, necessitating intra-arterial monitoring. Remifentanil is ideal for management of periods of intense stimulation.
Supine position with head-up tilt.	Potential for air embolism. Ensure adequate intravenous filling.
Operation on head.	Airway under drapes, armoured tube, anaesthetist distant from airway, meticulous securing of tube, protection of eyes, nerve stimulator on leg, circuit extensions for breathing system and for intravenous fluids.
Risk of bleeding from internal carotid or cavernous sinus.	Intubate (anticipate difficult airway), throat pack, two group and save samples preoperatively.
Rapid emergence, need ability to assess neurology as soon as possible postoperatively.	Use of short-acting and rapidly reversible agents.
Suprasellar portion of tumour may need pushing into surgical field.	Lumbar drain with injection of saline or, less commonly, controlled ventilation to ensure high-normal $PaCO_2$.
Avoid postoperative surges in ICP, especially if CSF leak has occurred.	Smooth emergence, adequate reversal, adequate antiemetic, airway and CPAP for known OSA.

Reference

Menon R, Murphy P, Lindley A. Anaesthesia and pituitary disease. *Contin Educ Anaesth Crit Care Pain*. 2011; 11 (4): 133–137.

A 34-year-old man is scheduled for a posterior fossa tumour excision.

a) List patient positions that might be employed for this operation. (10%)

b) What potential intraoperative problems are associated with posterior fossa craniotomy? (25%)

c) What monitoring techniques can specifically detect the presence of venous air embolism during surgery and for each method used, give the features that would indicate the diagnosis? (40%)

d) How would you manage a significant venous air embolism in this patient? (25%)

September 2013

Chairman's Report

48.4% pass rate.

Section (b) was poorly answered. Clearly, inexperience in anaesthesia for this type of surgery was apparent.

The model answer to b) included:
> Problems associated with positioning: including hypotension from pooling of blood, spinal cord injury and peripheral nerve damage.
> Brainstem damage: including the respiratory/cardiovascular centre and cranial nerve nuclei.

Knowledge of the diagnosis and management of an intraoperative air embolism was satisfactory.

a) List patient positions that might be employed for this operation. (10%)

Search for images of the different positions for neurosurgery. It will really help you retain the information about their associated complications. The sitting position is associated with significant risk but is good for access to midline lesions. Gravity assists venous and CSF drainage, thus improving the surgical field, and access to deeper structures is facilitated.
> Sitting.
> Lateral.
> Prone.
> Supine.
> Park bench.

b) What potential intraoperative problems are associated with posterior fossa craniotomy? (25%)

Surgery itself:
> Venous air embolism (VAE), paradoxical air embolism. Air entrainment can happen whenever the venous sinuses are open, but the risk is increased if the open sinuses are elevated, as occurs in e.g. sitting position, thus increasing the pressure differential between them and atmosphere further.
> Cardiovascular instability (hypo- or hypertension, brady- or tachycardia, arrhythmia) due to stimulation of cranial nerve nuclei and other brainstem structures.
> Bleeding, cerebellar haematoma.
> Brainstem damage: respiratory and cardiovascular centres and cranial nerve nuclei.
> Long tract damage.
> CSF leak.
> Meningitis, wound infection.

Positioning:
Sitting:
• Airway: tube displacement, jugular venous obstruction due to flexed neck causing laryngeal and tongue oedema.
• Cardiovascular: VAE, hypotension due to reduced venous return.
• Neurological: cord or brainstem ischaemia due to head flexion and hypotension, sciatic nerve damage, pneumocephalus.
• Cutaneomusculoskeletal: compartment syndrome, lumbosacral pressure sores.

Other positions:

- All other positions that involve moving the patient after induction involve risk of tube dislodgement.
- Each position has its unique pressure points, elbow, knee, ankle for lateral, genitalia and knees for prone. Also, each position has its individual risks for nerve palsies, such as brachial plexus compression in lateral position, brachial plexus stretch and ulnar nerve damage with prone, brachial plexus stretch and common peroneal compression with park bench.
- Prone position has the additional issues of reflux due to raised intragastric pressure, decreased venous return, corneal damage, central retinal artery occlusion, ischaemic optic neuropathy.

c) What monitoring techniques can specifically detect the presence of venous air embolism during surgery, and for each method used, give the features that would indicate the diagnosis? (40%)

Transoesophageal echo:

> Air in right-sided cardiac chambers. In the presence of patent foramen ovale, it can detect air in the left heart also. Not necessarily suitable for long operations where the head is flexed.

Precordial Doppler:

> Sound heard if air present in cardiac chambers.

d) How would you manage a significant venous air embolism in this patient? (25%)

This is a medical emergency, and I would alert the theatre team, call for help and adopt an ABC approach, assessing and managing issues simultaneously. The aims of management are as follows:

> Prevent further air entry: flood site with saline, fluid load, lower patient so that the surgical site is below the right atrium if possible, apply sustained positive airway pressure until this is all achieved.

> Reduce size: stop nitrous oxide if it is being used, administer 100% oxygen, aspirate air from right atrium via central line.

> Overcome mechanical obstruction: left lateral or Trendelenberg positioning may help force bubble above the right ventricular outflow. Inotropic support may be required. If the patient suffers cardiac arrest, chest compressions may assist in dispersing the bubble.

Reference

Jagannathan S, Krovvidi H. Anaesthetic considerations for posterior fossa surgery. *Contin Educ Anaesth Crit Care Pain*. 2014; 14 (5): 202–206.

A 64-year-old man is scheduled for a stereotactic brain biopsy. He is taking dual antiplatelet therapy following the insertion of a drug-eluting coronary artery stent six months earlier.

a) Explain the issues that may arise from antiplatelet therapy in this patient. (30%)

b) Summarise the perioperative strategies to minimise the above issues. (40%)

c) What are the specific contraindications (15%) and complications (15%) of a stereotactic brain biopsy under sedation?

March 2014

Chairman's Report

32.9% pass rate.

There was a low pass rate because candidates misread or misinterpreted the question. Most did not appreciate that the management of antiplatelet therapy requires a balance of risks in a patient for whom intraoperative bleeding could be a critical event. Many candidates mentioned stent thrombosis and intracranial/extracranial haemorrhage but did not explain why these events would be important even though the question specifically asks for these details. In part (b), the question asks for strategies to avoid the risk issues, but many candidates only described administration of neuroanaesthesia. Contraindications and complications were answered marginally better than the other two sections.

a) Explain the issues that may arise from antiplatelet therapy in this patient. (30%)

Contrary to the Chairman's Report, I do not think that the question has specifically asked for the details of why stent thrombosis and intracranial/extracranial haemorrhage would be important. However, the amount of points assigned to this part of the question and the fact that they have asked you to explain, rather than list, should indicate that they want a bit more detail.

If dual antiplatelet therapy (DAPT) continues, the patient is at very high risk of bleeding as a result of the biopsy, into a closed skull, without access for diathermy, with consequent pressure damage on surrounding structures causing brain damage, obstruction of CSF drainage and seizures. Even aspirin alone is associated with a significantly increased mortality risk in neurosurgery. Excessive bleeding from the scalp may occur, but this is unlikely to be a significant issue.

Premature cessation of DAPT renders patient at significant risk of in-stent thrombosis, which carries a mortality of about 50%.

Cessation of ADP receptor antagonist may be associated with a rebound phenomenon, which, in association with the stress response to surgery, may render the patient at even higher risk of thrombosis than usual in the perioperative period.

b) Summarise the perioperative strategies to minimise the above issues. (40%)

Multidisciplinary decision: cardiologist, anaesthetist, surgeon, patient. The decision needs to balance the risks of premature cessation of DAPT against the urgency of the biopsy. DAPT usually continues for one year after insertion of a drug-eluting stent (DES) but factors that may increase the risk of in-stent thrombosis and therefore mandate more prolonged DAPT include impaired renal function, ejection fraction <30%, multiple overlapping stents, stents at bifurcations, diabetes mellitus.

Options:
> Delay biopsy until planned time for DAPT has finished. Although one year is usually the minimum duration for DAPT after DES, the risk of in-stent thrombosis decreases after six months. This is only an option if the indication for biopsy is not unduly urgent.
> Stop ADP receptor antagonist for an appropriate duration prior to surgery but, ideally, continue aspirin if the surgeon and cardiologist are in agreement that the risk of stopping the aspirin outweighs risk of continuing (although the surgeon is unlikely to proceed with biopsy with ongoing aspirin).

> Stop both ADP receptor antagonist and aspirin (a week) prior to surgery if the surgeon and cardiologist are in agreement that the risks of bleeding outweigh the risk of in-stent thrombosis. Restart aspirin as soon as possible after surgery.

> Consideration of bridging with a short-acting GP IIb/IIIa inhibitor, starting within 24 hours of stopping ADP receptor blocker, restarting after surgery and then restarting ADP receptor antagonist the day after surgery if satisfied with haemostasis. This is not, however, a licenced indication for use of this drug.

> If the patient is deemed at high risk of in-stent thrombosis and the ADP receptor antagonist +/– aspirin are to be discontinued, consideration should be given to performing the biopsy in a centre with on-site 24-hour interventional cardiology support to attempt to mitigate the severity of any thrombosis that occurs.

c) What are the specific contraindications (15%) and complications (15%) of a stereotactic brain biopsy under sedation?

Contraindications:

> Lesions too small to safely target.

> Coagulopathic patient.

> Highly vascular tumour or lesions that could possibly be vascular malformations.

> Patient conditions causing inability to comply with procedure (difficulties communicating, confusion, movement disorders).

Complications:

> Haemorrhage (and no direct access to the site for diathermy).

> Airway compromise in awake or asleep patient with poor access to airway due to frame (if being used).

> Air embolism.

> Failure to obtain diagnostic specimen.

> Seizure.

> CNS infection.

References

Barron T et al. Management of antithrombotic therapy in patients undergoing invasive procedures. *N Engl J Med*. 2013; 368: 2113–2124.

DeVile M, Foëx P. Antiplatelet drugs, coronary stents, and non-cardiac surgery. *Contin Educ Anaesth Crit Care Pain*. 2010; 10 (6): 187–191.

Dorairaj I, Hancock S. Anaesthesia for interventional neuroradiology. *Contin Educ Anaesth Crit Care Pain*. 2008; 8 (3): 86–89.

A 54-year-old patient is admitted to the Emergency Department following a traumatic brain injury. A CT scan reveals only cerebral oedema.

a) What is secondary brain injury and when is it likely to occur? (2 marks)

b) Outline the main physiological and cellular changes associated with secondary brain injury. (7 marks)

c) How can secondary brain injury be minimised in this patient? (11 marks)

March 2015

Chairman's Report

Pass Rate 8.3%, 59.2% of candidates received a poor fail.

The pass and poor fail rates for this question are disturbing, and this question had only moderate discriminatory power as the candidate cohort performed so poorly. Management of head injury not requiring neurosurgery is common to most intensive care units. Many candidates were unable to define secondary injury or give an appropriate time frame. Most were unaware of the pathophysiological cellular mechanisms and focused solely on the Monroe–Kelly doctrine. Overall knowledge of NICE guidelines was superficial and most candidates did not define the physiological goals for therapy in enough detail. Treatment options were too narrow in scope although the information given was usually sensible. Examiners were left with the overall impression that many candidates have little theoretical knowledge or practical experience of care of the brain injured patient.

a) What is secondary brain injury, and when is it likely to occur? (2 marks)

Primary brain injury occurs due to the initial insult, depends on the nature, intensity and duration of impact. Macroscopically: fracture, contusion, haematoma, cerebral oedema, diffuse brain injury. Microscopically: cell wall disruption, increased membrane permeability disrupting ionic haemostasis.

Secondary brain injury is the deleterious changes that happen over hours to days in the brain as a consequence of the initial injury, mediated by inflammatory, neurogenic and vasogenic processes.

b) Outline the main physiological and cellular changes associated with secondary brain injury. (7 marks)

> Primary injury (due to e.g. intracerebral bleeding) may exhaust the compensatory capacity of the brain, leading to a raised ICP. Initially, as one component in the closed compartment of the cranium increases in size, it is compensated for by a reduction in another component (intravascular blood or CSF). This is the Monroe–Kelly doctrine. Ultimately, this compensation will reach its limit and ICP will start to rise. This results in cerebral ischaemia and hypoxia.

> Inflammation and local tissue damage cause excessive release of excitatory neurotransmitters (excitotoxicity), resulting in calcium influx to cells, cell oedema and death.

> Dying cells release mediators (platelet activating factor, leukotrienes, oxygen free radicals) that affect blood vessel permeability, resulting in vasogenic fluid accumulation, raising ICP further, contributing to hypoperfusion, cerebral ischaemia, and neurodegeneration.

> Loss of cerebral autoregulation exacerbates cerebral oedema and raised ICP.

> Hypoxia, hypotension, hyper- or hypocapnia and hyper- or hypoglycaemia will exacerbate secondary brain injury, worsen ability to autoregulate, cause direct changes to brain tissue size and therefore impact on ICP and perfusion, thus perpetuating a downward vicious cycle.

> Seizures will cause increased ICP, exacerbating poor cerebral perfusion if untreated. Seizures will also lead to raised $PaCO_2$ and reduced PaO_2, which will further decrease the brain's autoregulatory capacity and increase its metabolic demand.

c) How can secondary brain injury be minimised in this patient? (11 marks)

This is similar to the information required in the question from September 2011. It doesn't say whether the patient is already intubated, so I have included the factors that indicate the necessity to intubate. This answer is based on NICE CG176, which was published in 2014 and then featured in the exam a year later. However, even if you haven't read the guidance, I believe that anyone who has managed a few head injured patients in the emergency department knows this answer.

I would assess and manage this patient simultaneously adopting an ABCDE approach:

Airway:
> Intubate and control ventilation if:
  * Unable to protect own airway.
  * Loss of laryngeal reflexes.
  * GCS less than 8.
  * Hypoxic.
  * Hypercarbic.
  * Seizures.
> Cervical spine control with airway management: immobilise if there is possibility of injury but ensure that collar does not obstruct venous return.

Respiratory:
> Target PaO_2 greater than 13 kPa, $PaCO_2$ 4.5–5.0 kPa.
> PEEP to maintain oxygenation, ideally less than 15 cm H_2O.
> Oxygen saturation and $etCO_2$ monitoring.

Cardiovascular:
> Cannulate.
> Maintain mean arterial pressure (MAP) greater than 80 mm Hg (higher if ICP is raised) using isotonic fluids and vasopressors as necessary. Guide with intra-arterial blood pressure (BP) monitoring.
> Head neutral, tube ties not too tight, 15–30 degree head-up tilt to optimise venous return. Paralyse if coughing/straining on tube.
> Catheterisation to guide fluid balance.

Neurological:
> Target cerebral perfusion pressure >60 mm Hg, ICP less than 20 mm Hg (if have capabilities of monitoring in this hospital).
> Sedate adequately to reduce $CMRO_2$.
> Treat seizures.
> Maintain blood glucose 6–10 mmol/l.
> Treat any raised temperature (which raises $CMRO_2$).
> Manipulation of ICP spikes:
  * Temporising measures: hyperventilation, mannitol 0.25–1 g/kg, 5% hypertonic saline 2 ml/kg (keep Na less than 155 mmol/l, plasma osmolality less than 320 mOsm/l).
  * Definitive: discuss with neurosurgical unit if ongoing coma, ongoing confusion, seizures without recovery, progressive neurological abnormality; consider transfer for decompressive craniectomy or other neurosurgical intervention.

Exposure, environmental control:
> Seek other injuries causing blood loss, which may make maintaining MAP or haemoglobin at adequate levels for brain perfusion a problem.

References

Dinsmore J. Traumatic brain injury: an evidence-based review of management. *Contin Educ Anaesth Crit Care Pain*. 2013; 13 (6): 189–195.

National Institute for Health and Care Excellence. Head injury: assessment and early management CG176. 2014, updated 2017.

A 19-year-old patient has suffered a complete transection of the spinal cord at the first thoracic vertebral level due to a fall, but has no other injuries.

a) Outline the sequence of neurological effects that may develop in the first three months following injury. (6 marks)

b) Which disturbances of the cardiovascular, respiratory and gastrointestinal systems may subsequently occur? (8 marks)

c) When and why may suxamethonium be contraindicated in this patient? (2 marks)

d) Give the advantages of a regional anaesthetic technique for a patient having elective lower limb surgery 2 years after a high thoracic spine transection. (4 marks)

September 2015

Chairman's Report

49.4% pass rate.

This question had the highest correlation with overall performance; i.e. candidates who did well in this question performed well overall in the SAQ. The examiners commented that part (d) about the advantages of regional anaesthesia for elective lower limb surgery, was not well answered. Candidates tended to give general answers such as 'avoids the need for general anaesthesia' or 'maintains cardiovascular stability' rather than specific advantages such as 'reduces the risk of autonomic dysreflexia' or 'avoids postoperative respiratory inadequacy due to general anaesthesia'.

The knowledge required for this question is exactly the same as that required for the question on spinal cord injury in September 2011. If candidates had prepared themselves by addressing the topics covered in past papers, more than half would have passed.

A 54-year-old male with acromegaly presents for a trans-sphenoidal hypophysectomy.

a) What is acromegaly? (2 marks)

b) List the <u>clinical</u> features of acromegaly which are of relevance to the anaesthetist. (8 marks)

c) What other clinical presentations of a pituitary adenoma may be encountered? (2 marks)

d) What <u>specific</u> considerations, including surgical factors, may influence the conduct of anaesthesia in this patient? (8 marks)

March 2016

Chairman's Report

58.8% pass rate.

The examiners felt that this question was answered well despite it having been adjudged to be hard. However, few candidates either knew that acromegaly was a multisystem disease or could list the other possible clinical presentations of a pituitary adenoma, e.g. mass effects. Candidates who performed poorly in part (d) failed to describe the specific issues when anaesthetising a patient for this procedure and focused more on general neuroanaesthetic principles. This is a common mistake that has occurred in many questions across many exams. This question also correlated well with overall performance.

A score of only 10-11/20 is required to pass a 'hard' question. This question is very similar to that from March 2013; only parts (a) and (c) are different.

a) What is acromegaly? (2 marks)

> Acromegaly is the condition that results from excessive growth hormone secretion after the growth plates have fused.
> In this patient and 90% of cases, it results from hypersecretion from a pituitary adenoma.
> Occasionally, it may result from an ectopic pituitary adenoma near, but not in, the sella turcica.
> Rarely, it results from secretion of growth hormone releasing hormone or growth hormone by lung, pancreatic or adrenal tumours.

c) What other clinical presentations of a pituitary adenoma may be encountered? (2 marks)

Non-secretory presentation:
> Local pressure effects causing visual disturbance (bitemporal hemianopia), headache.
> Raised intracranial pressure: cranial nerve palsies, hydrocephalus due to 3rd ventricle outflow blockage.

Hypersecretory presentation:
> Cushing's disease: hypersecretion of adrenocorticotrophic hormone (ACTH) resulting in fatigue, truncal obesity, striae, moon face, buffalo hump, hypertension, glucose intolerance, hirsuitism, depression, anxiety.
> Hyperpituitarism: hypersecretion of any/all anterior pituitary hormones.

Hyposecretory presentation:
> Pituitary apoplexy: internal haemorrhage of the adenoma, or when the adenoma outgrows its blood supply, causing tissue necrosis and swelling. Therefore, there is loss of anterior pituitary hormones. Symptoms include visual loss, sudden-onset headache, cardiovascular instability.
> Central diabetes insipidus: a macroadenoma may cause damage to posterior pituitary blood supply, thus (rarely) causing diabetes insipidus with polyuria and polydipsia.
> Pituitary-related hypothyroidism: generally less severe than hypothyroidism of thyroid origin.
> Adrenocortical insufficiency: again, not as severe as adrenocortical insufficiency of adrenal origin.

a) What is Guillain–Barré syndrome and what are its causes? (3 marks)

b) What are the clinical features of Guillain–Barré syndrome? (6 marks)

c) List the investigations with their findings that may be used to support the diagnosis. (2 marks)

d) What are the specific considerations when anaesthetising a patient recovering from Guillain–Barré syndrome? (9 marks)

September 2016

Chairman's Report

53.3% pass rate.

This was surprisingly poorly answered, with some candidates becoming confused between Guillain–Barré syndrome and myaesthenia gravis. In section (c), some candidates lost marks by not mentioning the findings of investigations. Part (d) was answered with regard to general principles of intraoperative management of a critically ill patient, rather than the measures specific to a patient recovering from GB.

a) What is Guillain–Barré syndrome and what are its causes? (3 marks)

Don't get your neurological disorders all mixed up – there are two great CEACCP articles that succinctly summarise the different disorders and their main issues.

What is Guillain–Barré?
> Acute, immune-mediated, pre-junctional, ascending demyelinating polyneuropathy affecting sensory, motor and autonomic nerves.

What are its causes?
> Associated with respiratory or gastrointestinal infection (especially *Campylobacter*) in preceding weeks.
> Autoimmune in nature – antibodies attack the myelin sheath or, more rarely, the axon itself.

b) What are the clinical features of Guillain–Barré syndrome? (6 marks)

Whenever you are describing a neurological condition, be clear in your mind whether it is upper or lower motor neurone; whether it affects motor, sensory or autonomic nerves; and whether the defect is of the axon, myelin sheath or neuromuscular junction.
> Variable presentation depending on subtype; different forms associated with immune attack on different parts of the neurone. Recovery is variable, ranging from full recovery to relapsing, remitting form.
> Motor: typically ascending symmetrical weakness (flaccid, areflexic paralysis), may ascend to involve respiratory muscles and also to cause facial nerve palsies with bulbar weakness and opthalmoplegia.
> Sensory: ascending sensory impairment associated with pain.
> Autonomic: arrhythmias, labile BP, urinary retention, paralytic ileus, hyperhydrosis, sudden death.
> Miller Fisher syndrome: this is a variant typified by ataxia, areflexia, opthalmoplegia +/– weakness.

c) List the investigations with their findings that may be used to support the diagnosis. (2 marks)

There are only 2 marks available for this part, so I am pretty sure I have overdone it! However, it is difficult to narrow down precisely what tests they are after. No doubt that, as with other questions, you will get your 2 marks if you mention two tests from a whole list included in their model answer. Be systematic when you think about investigations, go through a mental list of the different types, thinking what goes wrong in this particular condition.

Blood tests:
> Variable, not specific or sensitive: low sodium, renal dysfunction, raised ALT and GGT raised CK.
> Elevated ESR +/– CRP.
> Antiganglioside antibodies (antibodies against a component of the axon itself, increased association with *Campylobacter*, worse prognosis) in 25%.

> Serology for *Campylobacter*, CMV, EBV, HSV or *Mycoplasma pneumoniae* may be positive.
> ABG may show development of respiratory failure.

Stool:
> GI infections, especially *Campylobacter*.

CT brain:
> Normal: to exclude other causes.

MRI spine:
> Selective anterior spinal nerve root enhancement with gadolinium.

Lumbar puncture:
> Normal cell count and glucose, elevated protein levels (although even this may be normal early in the disease).

Nerve conduction studies:
> Depends on subtype: majority show demyelinating pattern, some show axonal loss.

Respiratory function tests:
> Reduced vital capacity.

d) What are the specific considerations when anaesthetising a patient recovering from Guillain–Barré syndrome? (9 marks)

Back to the alphabet. Note that this is anaesthesia for a patient RECOVERING from Guillain–Barré, not the initial management of the disease process. However, a future question could ask about the anaesthetic management of a patient at the time of initial diagnosis.

Airway:
> Bulbar weakness, poor cough, increased risk of aspiration. Intubation required – consider need for rapid sequence induction.
> May still have tracheostomy in situ if still requiring ventilatory support or assistance with secretion clearance.

Respiratory:
> Increased risk of pneumonia secondary to aspiration and poor ventilatory function. Make full assessment of this – history, nature of secretions, temperature, chest auscultation. Treat as required, delay non-urgent surgery if necessary.
> Significantly reduced ventilatory capacity, assess likelihood of requiring noninvasive or invasive ventilation postoperatively.

Cardiovascular:
> Autonomic instability, labile BP (with sensitivity to commonly used vasoactive drugs), risk of arrhythmia. Invasive monitoring indicated including cardiac output monitoring to guide fluid administration (ensure full circulation as dehydration will exacerbate lability).
> Prolonged illness, multiple cannulations, access may be tricky.

Neurological:
> Neuropathic pain common – may already be on antineuropathic drugs +/– opioid analgesia. Need to plan postoperative pain relief, involve acute pain team.

Pharmacology:
> Suxamethonium: contraindicated due to risk of hyperkalaemia following the development of extrajunctional nicotinic receptors.
> Non-depolarising neuromuscular blocking agents: increased sensitivity – reduce dose.
> Opioids: increased sensitivity to respiratory depressant effect in the presence of existing respiratory compromise, may already be taking opioids and so dose adjustments may be necessary.

Haematology:

> Risk of deep vein thrombosis due to prolonged immobility – continuation of thromboembolic deterrent stockings and pneumatic compression devices and pharmacological prophylaxis (check timing if planning neuraxial technique).

Cutaneomusculoskeletal:

> Prolonged illness may be associated with weight loss – care with positioning and padding.

Renal:

> Check renal function – may dictate drug choices.

References

Marsh S, Ross N, Pittard A. Neuromuscular disorders and anaesthesia. Part 1: generic anaesthetic management. *Contin Educ Anaesth Crit Care Pain*. 2011; 11 (4): 115–118.

Marsh S, Pittard A. Neuromuscular disorders and anaesthesia. Part 2: specific neuromuscular disorders. *Contin Educ Anaesth Crit Care Pain*. 2011; 11 (4): 119–123.

A 19-year-old patient has suffered a complete transection of the spinal cord at the 6th cervical vertebral level due to a fall, he has no other injuries.

a) Explain the sequence of neurological effects that may develop in the first three months following injury. (6 marks)

b) What disturbances of the cardiovascular (3 marks), respiratory (3 marks) and gastrointestinal systems (2 marks) may occur after three months?

c) List the advantages of choosing a regional anaesthetic technique if this patient is subsequently listed for lower limb surgery. (4 marks)

d) When, and why, may suxamethonium be contraindicated in this patient? (2 marks)

September 2017

49.3% pass rate.

This question had also been used before and was also answered better on this occasion. It was considered to be of moderate difficulty. Most marks were lost in part (a), with some candidates being unable to give a coherent explanation of the sequence of neurological events following a spinal cord injury.

This question is very similar to those from September 2011 and September 2015, except that the level of the injury is now at the 6th cervical vertebra. Be especially careful to read familiar-looking questions carefully. Cord transection at this level may result in secondary neurological injury to a few segments higher and so partial phrenic nerve denervation must be considered, with consequent need for intubation and ventilation.

2. CARDIOTHORACIC SURGERY

a) List the indications for endoscopic thoracic sympathectomy (ETS). (25%)

b) Outline the general (30%) and airway (15%) implications of managing a patient for ETS under general anaesthesia.

c) What are the most likely problems to be encountered in the intraoperative (15%) and postoperative (15%) period?

September 2012

Chairman's Report

26.5% pass rate.

This question was universally answered badly. Clearly, most candidates had never anaesthetized a patient for the procedure nor had any knowledge about the procedure despite being part of the syllabus. Knowledge of the effects of one-lung anaesthesia, effects of a capnothorax and indications for a sympathectomy were relevant in the answer. The pass mark had been adjusted to reflect the level of difficulty ('hard').

These ten key facts would have been sufficient for a pass (there were 23 in the model answer).

a) Indications for transthoracic sympathectomy
   Hyperhidrosis
   Chronic pain/upper limb regional pain syndrome
b) General implications
   Large-bore IV access
   Potential for major haemorrhage
   May need arterial line
   Airway implications
   May need double lumen tube
c) Intraoperative problems
   Hypotension from capnothorax
   Hypoxia
   Postoperative problems
   May have residual pneumothorax
   May be painful

The mean score was 7.7/20. The question was a strong discriminator.

Whilst the question appeared difficult most of the answers required a systematic approach.

You will need a score of 10–11/20 in order to pass a 'hard' question. The level of detail from the Chairman's Report is very useful here: it is reassuring to see that the majority of marks can be gained by writing sensible things like ensuring large-bore intravenous access and that a double lumen tube may be required. The topic was addressed in a CEACCP article from three years previously. Make sure you make use of these articles as they are so often the basis of a question.

a) List the indications for endoscopic thoracic sympathectomy (ETS). (25%)

> Palmar, axillary or craniofacial hyperhidrosis.
> Chronic regional pain syndromes.
> Facial blushing.
> Chronic angina pectoris, unmanageable by pharmacological or cardiac intervention (very unusual indication now).

b) Outline the general (30%) and airway (15%) implications of managing a patient for ETS under general anaesthesia.

General:
> Patients are predominantly young and fit, but may be older with comorbidities especially if the indication is for refractory angina pectoris: consider need for additional assessment and investigation preoperatively.
> Complications are rare but can be catastrophic: ensure the patient has full understanding of risks versus benefits.
> Occasionally, conversion from laparoscopic to open surgery is necessary: prep and drape ready for thoracotomy.
> Risk of major haemorrhage: ensure large-bore intravenous access and two group and save samples for rapid blood issue.
> Periods of hypoxia common: shunt due to one-lung ventilation, atelectasis and failure to fully inflate the first lung before proceeding with surgery on the second side.
> Periods of hypotension due to capnothorax likely: consider invasive blood pressure monitoring or more frequent noninvasive monitoring.
> Consider the complications of positioning:
  • Usually supine, reverse Trendelenberg, arms abducted, with risk of brachial plexus injury.
  • Sometimes prone, with risk of facial or eye damage, dislodgement of airway, difficulty with ventilation, nerve traction and injury.
  • Sometimes lateral positioning with potential difficulty with ventilation, dislodgement of injury, damage to pressure points such as common peroneal nerve.

Airway:

Need to achieve collapse of one lung followed by the other for bilateral surgery. Options include the following:

> One-lung ventilation via double lumen tube.
> One-lung ventilation via endotracheal tube with bronchial blocker.
> Endotracheal tube with intrathoracic carbon dioxide insufflation.
> Laryngeal mask airway with intrathoracic carbon dioxide insufflation.

c) What are the most likely problems to be encountered in the intraoperative (15%) and postoperative (15%) period?

Intraoperative:

Airway:
> Malposition of double lumen tube or bronchial blocker may cause hypoxia.

Respiratory:
> One-lung ventilation causes shunt and, therefore, hypoxia. Efforts to improve this may actually worsen hypoxia (oxygen insufflation or CPAP to the deflated lung may reduce hypoxic pulmonary vasoconstriction; PEEP to the ventilated lung may increase resistance to blood flow to the ventilated side).

> With bilateral surgery, atelectasis of the reinflated lung may cause significant hypoxia when operating on the second side. Consider reinflation under direct vision.

Cardiovascular:
> Hypotension due to capnothorax, rarely cardiac arrest due to rapid insufflation.
> Cardiac arrhythmia induced by intrathoracic diathermy.
> Rarely, bleeding due to inadvertent damage to blood vessels on port insertion. May be catastrophic.

Postoperative:
> Ongoing hypoxia due to atelectasis and residual pneumothorax.
> Risk of acute lung injury in the days following operation if protective one-lung ventilation not used.
> Chest pain during the immediate postoperative period requiring intravenous morphine – may necessitate overnight stay.

References

Martin A, Telford R. Anaesthesia for endoscopic thoracic sympathectomy. *Contin Educ Anaesth Crit Care Pain*. 2009; 9 (2): 52–55.

National Institute for Health and Care Excellence. Endoscopic thoracic sympathectomy for primary facial blushing. [IPG480]. 2014.

National Institute for Health and Care Excellence. Endoscopic thoracic sympathectomy for primary hyperhidrosis of the upper limb. [IPG487]. 2014.

a) What are the theoretical advantages of 'off-pump' coronary artery bypass grafting (OPCAB) compared to 'on bypass' technique? (35%)

b) What causes haemodynamic instability during OPCAB? (20%)

c) Which strategies help to minimise this haemodynamic instability? (25%)

d) Outline the measures that help to minimise perioperative hypothermia during OPCAB. (20%)

September 2012

Chairman's Report

37.3% pass rate

Cardiothoracic anaesthesia is currently a mandatory unit of training, and as such, a question will feature in each SAQ paper. The Royal College recognizes that candidates taking the exam at ST3 level may not have yet had significant experience of this sub-speciality, and for this reason, this question was designated as difficult. Nevertheless, it was felt that this question would be able to be answered by candidates using some basic principles (similar to question 4). Again, this question was poorly answered. Many candidates answered (b) and (c) with on-pump rather than off-pump issues.

A pass would have been achieved by writing these ten key points:

a) Theoretical advantages of OPCAB
- Reduced platelet dysfunction
- Reduced neurological injury

b) Causes of haemodynamic instability
- Mechanical displacement of heart
- Arrhythmias

c) Strategies to minimize haemodynamic instability
- Avoid electrolyte disturbance
- Suspend surgical manipulation

d) Minimising perioperative hypothermia (as with any anaesthetic)
- Increase ambient theatre temperature
- Warm IV fluids
- Use hot-air warmers

The only answers that were specific to OPCAB surgery were to (a), the other answers were generic. There were 24 key facts in the model answer.

Factors contributing to poor performance were lack of knowledge, inexperience and failure to read the question. This question was the best discriminator in the paper.

This is from the same paper as the question on ETS – two cardiothoracic surgery questions in one paper. Once again, it was judged to be difficult; hence a score of 10–11/20 is needed to pass, and once again, a really useful report that shows that calm application of common sense can gain many marks.

a) What are the theoretical advantages of 'off-pump' coronary artery bypass grafting (OPCAB) compared to 'on bypass' technique? (35%)

Don't know anything about 'off-pump' surgery? Basically, it means not using cardiopulmonary bypass (the pump) to facilitate heart surgery, operating on the beating heart instead. An immobilisation device is used to reduce movement of the area of myocardium being operated on at the time. Search for a video of off-pump surgery if you haven't seen it before. Think of all the issues that are associated with 'on-pump' surgery and what might therefore be avoided by staying 'off-pump.'

> Avoidance of complications of CPB:
>   • Platelet dysfunction.
>   • Consumption of clotting factors.
>   • Accelerated fibrinolysis.
>   • Blood transfusion due to coagulation defects.
>   • Renal dysfunction.
>   • SIRS.
>   • Air emboli.
>   • Neurological dysfunction.
>   • Fluid overload/depletion.
>   • Electrolyte disturbance.
> Earlier extubation, shorter/no ICU stay, reduced cost.
> Overall reduced morbidity and mortality.

b) What causes haemodynamic instability during OPCAB? (20%)

Think logically: the operation is being performed directly on a beating heart, which is still responsible for perfusion of the body at the time.

> Ischaemia due to vessel anastomosis (shunts are used to minimise this).
> Manipulation of the heart for access to lateral and posterior aspects: lifting of heart vertically out of pericardial sac, ventricular filling must then happen vertically upwards, mitral and tricuspid annulus deformation resulting in reflux.
> Impaired filling due to immobilisation device.
> Arrhythmias induced by ischaemia, manipulation, reperfusion.
> Bleeding.

c) Which strategies help to minimise this haemodynamic instability? (25%)

> Good communication between the anaesthetist and the surgeon.
> Minimise manipulation, stop if major instability.
> Periods of ischaemia minimised, including through the use of shunts.
> Keep heart rate low/normal: minimises oxygen requirement, reduces effect of periods of ischaemia.
> Monitor and treat electrolyte disturbances: keep potassium over 4.5 mmol/l; give magnesium routinely.
> Ensure that patient is adequately filled, guided by cardiac output monitoring.

d) Outline the measures that help to minimise perioperative hypothermia during OPCAB. (20%)

Comply with NICE guidance on avoidance of perioperative hypothermia:
> Preoperative: check patient temperature, use extra bedding or forced air warming if necessary.
> Intraoperatively: monitor temperature; minimise periods of leaving patient uncovered; use warmed fluids, forced air warming blanket, under-body warming mattress, heat conserving hat and ambient theatre temperature at a minimum of 21°C.
> Postoperatively: continue to monitor temperature; use extra bedding and forced air warming as necessary.

References

Hett D. Anaesthesia for off-pump coronary artery surgery. *Contin Educ Anaesth Crit Care Pain*. 2006; 6 (2): 60–62.

National Institute for Health and Care Excellence. Hypothermia: Prevention and management in adults having surgery [CG65]. 2016.

a) What are the indications for 'one-lung ventilation' (OLV)? (30%)

b) How can the risks associated with lung resection be quantified preoperatively? (30%)

c) How would you manage the development of hypoxaemia during OLV? (40%)

March 2013

Chairman's Report

'Easy'

88.6% pass rate.

This area has been covered in previous SAQ exams (2006 and 2009) and was a very straightforward test of knowledge. Significant numbers of candidates scored 16/20 or more.

a) What are the indications for 'one-lung ventilation' (OLV)? (30%)

> Isolation of lung to prevent cross-contamination, e.g. empyema, massive haemorrhage.
> To control distribution of ventilation, e.g. for bronchopleural fistula.
> To facilitate surgery, e.g. thoracoscopic surgery, oesophagectomy, pneumonectomy, lobectomy, scoliosis surgery.
> Unilateral lung lavage for treatment of alveolar proteinosis.

b) How can the risks associated with lung resection be quantified preoperatively? (30%)

> Measure forced expiratory volume in 1 second (FEV_1) and diffusing capacity for carbon monoxide (DLCO).
> Calculate the predicted postoperative (PPO) FEV_1 and DLCO based on anatomic calculation, ventilation/perfusion scans or CT evaluation.
> If PPO FEV_1 and DLCO are greater than 60%, the patient is low risk.
> If PPO FEV_1 or DLCO is less than 60% but both are greater than 30%, proceed to stair climb or shuttle walk assessment. If good performance, the patient is low risk; if poor performance, proceed to cardiopulmonary exercise testing.
> If PPO FEV_1 or DLCO is less than 30%, poor performance on stair climb or shuttle walk assessment or high risk according to cardiac evaluation (including thoracic revised cardiac risk index score), then proceed to cardiopulmonary exercise testing. If VO_2max is greater than 10 ml/kg/min, the patient is moderate risk; if less than 10, the patient is high risk.

c) How would you manage the development of hypoxaemia during OLV? (40%)

Hypoxaemia during any anaesthetic is an emergency situation. Alert the theatre team, request help, conduct simultaneous assessment and management of the patient following an ABC approach.

A:
> 100% oxygen, take over manual ventilation of patient.
> Check for obvious equipment failure such as disconnection.
> Check for double lumen tube or bronchial blocker dislodgement.
> Check for secretions or blood that may have occluded the tube.
> Use bronchoscope to assess and clear secretions if necessary.

B:
> Assess for compliance, capnography waveform, oxygen saturations.
> Auscultate the chest (if feasible whilst patient is draped) and consider bronchospasm, pneumothorax of ventilated lung, inadequate paralysis.

C:
> Assess for cardiovascular stability; check for sources of bleeding.

If assessment is otherwise normal, the likely cause is the abnormal lung physiology caused by one-lung ventilation. Options to manage hypoxia include the following:

> CPAP or high-frequency oscillatory ventilation to the non-ventilated lung to reduce the shunt effect caused by ongoing perfusion to the non-ventilated lung.

> Intermittent two-lung ventilation.
> High-frequency jet ventilation to both lungs. Not an option if need complete lung collapse or if there are concerns about cross-contamination.
> If the surgery is for pneumonectomy, early clamping of pulmonary artery will resolve shunt issues.
> Increase PEEP to the ventilated, dependent lung to counteract the effect of mediastinal weight on functional residual capacity in the lateral decubitus position.
> Decrease PEEP to reduce possible compression of pulmonary capillaries by excessive intra-alveolar pressure.
> Increased airway pressure to ventilated lung to ensure adequate tidal volume (however, excessive airway pressures risk impairing perfusion).
> Optimise CO and haemoglobin to ensure oxygen delivery. Does not improve hypoxia but mitigates its effects.

References

Brunelli A, Kim A, Berger K, Addrizzo-Harris D. Physiological evaluation of the patient with lung cancer being considered for resectional surgery. Diagnosis and management of lung cancer, 3rd ed: American College of Chest Physicians evidence-based clinical practice guidelines. *Chest*. 2013; 143 (5 suppl): e166S–e190S.

Ng A, Swanevelder J. Hypoxaemia during one-lung anaesthesia. *Contin Educ Anaesth Crit Care Pain*. 2010; 10 (4): 117–122.

You are asked to review a 65-year-old man on the cardiac intensive care unit who underwent coronary artery bypass surgery earlier in the day.

a) Which clinical signs suggest the development of acute cardiac tamponade? (40%)

b) List the investigations and their associated derangements that could confirm the diagnosis of acute cardiac tamponade. (15%)

c) What is the management of acute cardiac tamponade in this patient? (45%)

September 2013

Chairman's Report

57.6% pass rate.

This question was designated an 'easy' question by the exam board and was a good discriminator. The investigations and associated derangements were linked, and 1 mark was awarded for both correct answers. The management of acute pericardial tamponade was generally answered in a generic way (ABC, call for help etc.), but a number of candidates wasted time and effort on managing an anaesthetic in this situation.

Many failed to monitor the clotting and administer blood products or reversing agents if indicated.

a) Which clinical signs suggest the development of acute cardiac tamponade? (40%)

The question asks for _signs_ and asks for those which _suggest acute tamponade_, so I have tried to restrict my answer to precisely that.

> Classically, Beck's triad: hypotension, raised jugular venous pressure, muffled heart sounds.
> Shock (hypotension, tachycardia, clammy, cool peripheries, poor capillary refill, reduced cerebration, cardiac arrest) resistant to fluids and inotropes.
> Pericardial rub.
> Pulsus paradoxus: abnormally large reduction in systolic pressure during inspiration.*
> Kussmaul's sign: rise/lack of fall of JVP with inspiration.**

* During spontaneous inspiration, the full right heart encroaches on the left and blood pools in the pulmonary vasculature, both of which reduce left heart filling, thus causing a decrease in systolic pressure. In tamponade, the effect is exacerbated and the difference in pressure between the right and left heart is lost. Positive pressure ventilation results in a reversal of timings.

**Due to failure of the constricted right heart to accommodate the increase in venous return that occurs with the drop in intrathoracic pressure that accompanies spontaneous inspiration.

b) List the investigations and their associated derangements that could confirm the diagnosis of acute cardiac tamponade. (15%)

I struggled a bit with this. They obviously want more than one investigation as the plural is used, but only echo is confirmatory in the time frame allowed by an acutely developing tamponade.

Transoesophageal or transthoracic echo:
> Pericardial separation of more than 1 cm (however, pericardial collections may be atypical in appearance following cardiac surgery yet still cause significant haemodynamic compromise).
> Sequentially, with worsening tamponade, right atrial free wall collapse in systole, right ventricular free wall collapse in diastole, left atrial free wall collapse in systole.
> Exaggerated respiratory variation in trans-tricuspid and trans-mitral flow.
> Left shift of the interventricular septum.
> Inferior vena cava dilatation without respiratory variation in size.
> 'Swinging heart.'

> Chest radiograph: enlarged cardiac silhouette ('flask shaped').
> ECG: small complexes, electrical alternans.*

* *Varying waveform size due to movement of the heart within the pericardial sac from beat-to-beat.*

Other diagnostic investigations are unlikely to be useful given the time frame of acute tamponade:

> Ultrasound-guided pericardiocentesis: aspiration of free-flowing blood – relatively contraindicated in patients with ongoing anticoagulation.

Neither cardiac catheter studies (equalisation of chamber pressures) nor CT scan (presence of blood or clot in pericardial space) should be considered in an acute, decompensated setting.

c) What is the management of acute cardiac tamponade in this patient? (45%)

> Cardiac tamponade following cardiac surgery is likely to be due to failed haemostasis and, therefore, rapidly progressive with risk of cardiac arrest and high mortality. I would plan for decompressive sternotomy on the intensive care unit as no time permitted for transfer to the operating theatre. Opening the sternum usually reverses the life-threatening haemodynamic compromise. I would follow an ABC approach, assessing and managing the patient simultaneously.
> Fast-bleep team and call for resternotomy trolley:
>   • The surgical team should be ready before induction.
>   • Anaesthetic and ODP support should be requested but may need to proceed without their assistance if the patient is rapidly deteriorating.
>   • Perfusionist to be contacted – may need to go back on bypass.
>   • Major haemorrhage protocol to be activated.
> Patient management:
>   • A: 100% oxygen reduces cardiac workload.
>   • B: Intubate (if not still intubated from earlier surgery). Positive pressure ventilation will have deleterious effect on cardiac filling, and PEEP and high airway pressures should be avoided. Do not induce until surgeons are poised ready to go. Maintain oxygenation with minimal ventilation.
>   • C: Large-bore intravenous access should be secured (if not already present from theatre). Intravenous filling to attempt to maximise effective venous return. Use of vasopressor if necessary.
>   • D: If the patient is sufficiently stable for induction drugs to be used, consider use of opiates, ketamine, benzodiazepines. Avoid causing myocardial depression. If the patient is periarrest, it may be inappropriate to use any induction drugs.
>   • H: Massive haemorrhage protocol should be activated. However, tamponade is not always associated with large blood loss. The patient may already be coagulopathic from recent bypass surgery or may develop coagulopathy with blood loss. Haemoglobin and coagulation should be monitored with near patient testing, with blood administration, reversal of heparin and administration of other clotting products as indicated. Alternatively, management of anticoagulation to go back on bypass may be needed.

Reference
Carmona P et al. Management of cardiac tamponade after cardiac surgery. *J Cardiothorac Vasc Anesth*. 2012; 26 (2): 302–311.

A 71-year-old patient requires a rigid bronchoscopy for biopsy and possible laser resection of an endobronchial tumour.

a) Outline the options available to maintain anaesthesia (20%) and manage gas exchange. (30%)

b) How will use of the laser change the management of anaesthesia? (15%)

c) What are the possible complications of rigid bronchoscopy? (35%)

March 2014

Chairman's Report

60.8% pass rate.

This question proved discriminatory between candidates who gave a mature and thoughtful answer and those who did not understand the implications of 'tubeless' ENT/thoracic surgery. Weaker candidates proposed the use of laser-proof endotracheal tubes, and even double lumen endobronchial tubes and cardiac bypass, to facilitate gas exchange. Part (a) tended to score badly, whilst parts (b) and (c) were better known. Focus in part (c) was dominated by traumatic complications, with candidates forgetting 'anaesthetic' issues such as laryngospasm and bronchospasm, pneumothorax/barotrauma/volutrauma from jet ventilation, cardiovascular disturbances, pulmonary infection, hypoxaemia, hypercarbia and awareness.

a) Outline the options available to maintain anaesthesia (20%) and manage gas exchange. (30%)

Maintenance of anaesthesia: determined primarily by method of management of gas exchange.

> Volatile: use of volatile not possible with jet ventilation, and awareness more likely if volatile used with intermittent ventilation technique.
> Total intravenous anaesthesia: can be used with any option for gas exchange management.
> Immobility should be assured for resection with muscle relaxant or remifentanil infusion, and short-acting opioids are useful due to the highly stimulating nature of rigid bronchoscopy.

Management of gas exchange: depends on the specific bronchoscope used as not all options are compatible with all bronchoscopes.

> Intermittent ventilation with or without oxygen insufflation via side-port. This may be sufficient for the diagnostic aspect of the procedure but does not offer sufficiently reliable ventilation for resection.
> Controlled ventilation via the side port of a ventilating bronchoscope.
> Manual low-frequency jet ventilation, e.g. with Sanders manual jet ventilator.
> Automated high-frequency jet ventilation.

b) How will use of the laser change the management of anaesthesia? (15%)

Use of laser changes the way a case is managed in theatre and, more specifically, how anaesthesia is managed. Due to the difficulty in deciding on a definitive difference between the two, I have included all of the changes.

Patient safety:
> Maintain inspired oxygen concentration as low as possible, certainly less than 0.4 – therefore, use with jet or conventional ventilation.
> Saline-soaked gauze over mouth, teeth.
> Goggles for patient.
> Ensure that all equipment that will be used to instrument the airway is laser-compatible.

General theatre safety:
> Goggles for staff.
> Signage on doors.
> Lock theatre doors.
> Blinds down.

> Presence of laser-trained staff member.
> Assurance of equipment maintenance.

Readiness for airway fire:
> Alertness.
> Syringes of saline ready for flooding airway.
> Airway equipment prepared in case surgery needs to be abandoned and the patient needs to be intubated and ventilated on 100% oxygen.

c) What are the possible complications of rigid bronchoscopy? (35%)

Anaesthetic complications:
> Barotrauma associated with jet ventilation: pneumothorax, pneumomediastinum, pneumopericardium, pneumoperitoneum, subcutaneous emphysema.
> Awareness: secondary to intermittent anaesthesia delivery.
> Inadequate gas exchange: hypercapnia, hypoxia. Patient with existing lung pathology at higher risk.
> Laryngospasm, bronchospasm.
> Impaired venous return: high intrathoracic pressures associated with gas trapping, resulting in cardiovascular instability.
> Dysrhythmia and associated cardiovascular instability associated with jet ventilation.
> Airway contamination: ventilation without airway protection.

Surgical:
> Soft tissue trauma: lips, tongue, vocal cords, trachea, bronchi. Airway oedema may cause airway compromise or obstruction post-procedure.
> Dental damage.
> Haemorrhage: associated with soft tissue damage or resection of lesion.
> Pneumothorax: due to resection or biopsy.
> Cervical spine damage: assess range of movement preoperatively. Consider radiological assessment if the patient has a risk factor such as rheumatoid arthritis.

References

English J, Norris A, Bedforth N. Anaesthesia for airway surgery. *Contin Educ Anaesth Crit Care Pain*. 2006; 6 (1): 28–31.

Evans E, Biro P, Bedforth N. Jet ventilation. *Contin Educ Anaesth Crit Care Pain*. 2007; 7 (1): 2–5.

Pathak V et al. Ventilation and anesthetic approaches for rigid bronchoscopy. *Ann Am Thorac Soc*. 2014; 11 (4): 628–634.

Roberts S, Thornington R. Paediatric bronchoscopy. *Contin Educ Anaesth Crit Care Pain*. 2005; 5 (2): 41–44.

a) What are the purposes (3 marks), typical composition (4 marks) and physiological actions (5 marks) of cardioplegia solutions?

b) By which routes can solutions of cardioplegia be administered? (2 marks)

c) What are the possible complications of cardioplegia solution administration? (6 marks)

September 2014

Chairman's Report

16.5% pass rate.

Cardioplegia is an important basic tool in cardiothoracic anaesthesia, although it is not used invariably in current surgical procedures. It was evident from the answers which candidates had undertaken an attachment in this area of practice or had read an appropriate textbook. The importance of considering the mandatory units of training in preparation for the Final FRCA examination has been emphasised previously.

a) What are the purposes (3 marks), typical composition (4 marks) and physiological actions of cardioplegia solutions? (5 marks)

Stay calm. There aren't many marks for each of these individual sections so I cannot imagine that they want a detailed list of the precise concentrations of the electrolytes in cardioplegia – there is a variety of solutions available, after all. However, they want you to demonstrate that you know what the point of its use is, and some aspects of how it works are closely tied up with its constituents, hence my presentation in tabulated form.

Purposes:
> Myocardial protection:
  • Cardiac arrest in diastole and manipulation of the extracellular environment to minimise ongoing metabolic activity and its deleterious consequences during a period of suboptimal perfusion.
  • Cooling of the heart.
> Facilitation of surgery:
  • Still, relaxed heart.
  • Bloodless field.

Typical composition	Physiological actions
High potassium concentration, approximately 20 mmol/l.	Arrest of heart in diastole – high extracellular potassium levels prevent repolarisation of myocytes, causing inactivation of the fast inward voltage sensitive sodium channels that are important in phase 0 of the action potential.
Calcium at a lower concentration than plasma.	Calcium is required to maintain cell membrane integrity, but keeping the concentration low reduces the amount of calcium available for contraction, thus avoiding myocardial activity.
Magnesium concentration exceeding normal plasma level.	Prevents magnesium loss from the cells, thus maintaining its role as enzymatic cofactor, and competes with calcium, thus reducing calcium-induced contraction.
Sodium and chloride usually at levels near those found in plasma.	(Alternatively, low sodium concentration can be used as the mechanism to induce cardiac arrest.)
Bicarbonate, histidine or other buffer.	To offset tendency to metabolic acidosis associated with ischaemia.
Mannitol.	To raise the osmolarity of the solution, thus reducing tissue oedema.
Other additives: Procaine. Blood.	Reduction of arrhythmia at reperfusion. Oxygen carrying capacity.

b) By which routes can solutions of cardioplegia be administered? (2 marks)

> Anterograde: cannula into ascending aorta or coronary ostia (dependent on adequate root pressure, good coronary perfusion and competent aortic valve to reach all of the myocardium).
> Retrograde: cannula into the coronary sinus.

c) What are the possible complications of cardioplegia solution administration? (6 marks)

Remember to include the issues that may arise from the method of administration as well as from the cardioplegia itself.

> Direct damage associated with the cannulae.
> Failure to attain widespread cardiac perfusion with the cardioplegia, leaving areas of myocardium warm and active whilst ischaemic.
> Fluid overload.
> Myocardial oedema, haemorrhage and injury resulting from high infusing pressures.
> Postoperative electrolyte derangement with consequent risk of arrhythmia.
> Air bubbles in the cardioplegia solution can cause air emboli in the coronary arteries – bubble trap used.

References

Chambers D, Fallouh H. Cardioplegia and cardiac surgery: pharmacological arrest and cardioprotection during global ischemia and reperfusion. *Pharmacol Ther*. 2010; 127: 41–52.

Jameel S, Colah S, Klein A. Recent advances in cardiopulmonary bypass techniques. *Contin Educ Anaesth Crit Care Pain*. 2010; 10 (1): 20–23.

Machin D, Allsager C. Principles of cardiopulmonary bypass. *Contin Educ Anaesth Crit Care Pain*. 2006; 6 (5): 176–181.

A 67-year-old patient is to undergo coronary artery surgery on cardiopulmonary bypass (CPB).

a) What dose of heparin is used to achieve full anticoagulation for CPB and how is it given? (2 marks)

b) Which laboratory and 'point-of-care' tests determine the effectiveness of heparin anticoagulation in CPB patients? Give the advantages and/or disadvantages of each test. (10 marks)

c) What are the causes of inadequate anticoagulation in a patient whom it is believed has already received heparin? (5 marks)

d) Describe the possible adverse reactions to protamine. (3 marks)

March 2015

Chairman's Report

61.5% pass rate; 17.2% of candidates received a poor fail.

This question proved straightforward to candidates who had rotated through a cardiac unit or had read a textbook on cardiothoracic anaesthesia. Many weak candidates neither had knowledge of the intraoperative dosing of heparin for bypass surgery nor aspects of appropriate monitoring. Again, inexperience was the predominating factor in success or failure in this item.

a) What dose of heparin is used to achieve full anticoagulation for CPB and how is it given? (2 marks)

> Check patient's baseline activated clotting time (ACT) via arterial sample.
> Give 300–400 iu/kg via a central venous cannula (CVC) (check line patency first).
> Take another arterial sample after three to five minutes.
> Ensure ACT is 3× baseline or greater than 480 before initiating CPB.
> Recheck every 30 minutes during CPB.

b) Which laboratory and 'point-of-care' tests determine the effectiveness of heparin anticoagulation in CPB patients? Give the advantages and/or disadvantages of each test. (10 marks)

> Activated partial thromboplastin time (APTT), lab test:
   Cheap test.
   Slow turnaround time, which may result in less-well-directed management.
> Anti-Xa Assay, lab test:
   Not widely used for this purpose, poor inter-laboratory correlation.
> ACT, point-of-care (POC):
   Rapid information, cheap, familiar.
   Thrombocytopenia, antiplatelet agents, hypothermia, haemodilution, aprotinin may all prolong ACT.
   ACT has poor correlation with clinical anti-Xa activity.
> Heparin concentration monitoring, POC:
   Measuring of heparin concentration once haemodilution has occurred with CPB may be more appropriate to direct heparin administration than ACT, which is prolonged by commencing CPB. Higher doses of heparin will therefore be required when using heparin concentration measurement.
   Expensive, not widely available.

c) What are the causes of inadequate anticoagulation in a patient whom it is believed has already received heparin? (5 marks)

Error:
> Wrong drug administered.
> Drug not given.
> CVC not patent.
> CVC not flushed after dose given.

Pharmacokinetic factors:

Heparin is highly protein bound, so an increase in the presence of certain proteins reduces free and therefore active amount:

> Acutely ill patients.
> Malignancy.
> Peri- or post-partum.

Lack of antithrombin III:
> Drug induced: recent heparin use.
> Accelerated consumption: DIC, sepsis.
> Dilution: CPB.
> Decreased synthesis: liver cirrhosis.
> Increased excretion: protein-losing states.
> Familial: 1/2,000–20,000.

d) Describe the possible adverse reactions to protamine. (3 marks)

> Arterial hypotension.
> Reduced CO.
> Pulmonary vasoconstriction.
> Anaphylaxis.
> Unbound protamine inhibits platelet reactivity, adhesion and aggregation. An excessive dose therefore promotes bleeding.

References

Machin D, Allsager C. Principles of cardiopulmonary bypass. *Contin Educ Anaesth Crit Care Pain*. 2006; 6 (5): 176–181.
Srivastava A, Kelleher A. Point-of-care coagulation testing. *Contin Educ Anaesth Crit Care Pain*. 2013; 13 (1): 12–16.

a) What are the central and peripheral neurological complications of coronary artery bypass surgery? (7 marks)

b) What are the risk factors for central neurological complications? (6 marks)

c) How can the incidence of central neurological complications be reduced? (7 marks)

September 2015

Chairman's Report

54.6% pass rate.

Candidates who did well in this question tended to do well overall. There was quite a spread of scores, with some candidates having a very clear idea of the answers and others seemingly not very much idea at all. Whether this reflects the fact that some candidates sitting the exam have no experience of cardiac anaesthesia is not clear. However, as stated in previous reports, candidates who have no exposure to the mandatory units of training should endeavour to spend a few sessions gaining firsthand experience prior to sitting the SAQ paper.

a) What are the central and peripheral neurological complications of coronary artery bypass surgery? (7 marks)

It hasn't specified on-pump or off-pump surgery, so you should include the complications of both. Complications of prolonged surgery, surgery in an arteriopath, the issues related to going on-pump and periods of hypotension should all be included, as well as the specific complications caused by the different surgical approaches.

Central:
> Postoperative cognitive dysfunction – short- and long-term.
> Stroke: ischaemic, embolic (from existing patient thrombus/vessel lesions or as a result of CPB) or haemorrhagic.
> Transient ischaemic attack.
> Gas emboli.
> Subtle behavioural or personality changes.
> Ischaemic spinal cord injury.
> Delirium.

Peripheral:
> Brachial plexus injury: central line insertion, positioning, sternal retraction (rotation of first rib, pushes clavicles into retroclavicular space putting traction on plexus) and internal mammary artery (IMA) harvesting (wider retraction necessary).
> Ulnar nerve injury: positioning associated with artery harvesting.
> Phrenic nerve injury (left phrenic nerve passes between lung and mediastinal pleura so at greater risk) with IMA harvesting.
> Recurrent laryngeal nerve injury: intubation (prolonged), surgical dissection, especially of IMA.
> Saphenous nerve injury: damage occurring during saphenous vein harvesting due to close proximity at ankle.
> Intercostal nerve damage: minimally invasive direct coronary artery bypass (MIDCAB), where the incision is between the ribs rather than sternotomy.

b) What are the risk factors for central neurological complications? (6 marks)

Patient factors (these are most significant):
> Age.
> Hypertension.
> Hypercholesterolaemia.
> History of stroke.
> Diabetes mellitus.
> Carotid stenosis.

> Preoperative cognitive dysfunction, including that due to Alzheimer's, Parkinson's and cerebral vascular disease.
> Poor left ventricular function.

Surgical factors:
> Duration of surgery (possibly relating to stress response, disruption of the blood–brain barrier and altered autoregulation).
> Microemboli from diseased aorta when clamped, cannulated or handled.
> Microemboli from cardiopulmonary bypass (CPB) circuit.
> Rapid rewarming after hypothermia can cause loss of autoregulation, resulting in cerebral oedema.
> Failure to maintain adequate brain perfusion pressure during CPB.

Anaesthetic factors (least significant):
> Low mean arterial pressure and so cerebral perfusion pressure.
> Prolonged deep hypnotic time.

c) How can the incidence of central neurological complications be reduced? (7 marks)

Preoperative:
> Patient assessment, identification of high-risk patients and consider whether appropriate to proceed.

Intraoperative:
> Minimally invasive techniques to reduce overall stress response.
> Adequate priming of CPB circuit, if used, and use of bubble traps and embolus filters.
> Surgical care to avoid disrupting aortic plaques on clamping and cannulation.
> Maintenance of haemodynamic stability to ensure adequate cerebral and cord perfusion pressure.
> Careful anticoagulation monitoring and management.
> Careful neck positioning, especially if there are risk factors that may already compromise blood supply to cervical cord.
> Optimal blood glucose management.
> Possibly avoiding excessive periods of excessively deep anaesthesia with the use of depth of anaesthesia monitoring.
> Monitoring and management of acid–base balance to avoid deleterious effects on brain autoregulation.
> If hypothermia induced, avoidance of fast rewarming which predisposes to cerebral oedema.
> Cerebral regional oximetry monitoring with appropriate management in response to decreases.

Postoperative:
> Avoidance of hypoxia.
> Management of modifiable cerebrovascular disease risk factors such as blood glucose, blood pressure, cholesterol.

Reference
Miang Ying Tan A, Amoako D. Postoperative cognitive dysfunction after cardiac surgery. *Contin Educ Anaesth Crit Care Pain*. 2013; 13 (6): 218–223.

A 70-year-old woman with aortic stenosis presents for an open aortic valve replacement (AVR).

a) What is the pathophysiology of worsening aortic stenosis? (8 marks)

b) Which specific cardiac investigations may be used in assessing the severity of this woman's disease? (3 marks)

c) Give values for the peak aortic flow velocity, mean pressure gradient and valve area that would indicate that this woman has severe aortic stenosis. (3 marks)

d) What would be your haemodynamic goals for the perioperative management of this patient? (6 marks)

March 2016

Chairman's Report

41.8% pass rate.

The pass rate for this question was the second lowest overall. Aortic stenosis is a common condition, and its pathophysiology and management should be known to candidates sitting this exam. In part (a), many candidates simply gave the symptoms of aortic stenosis rather than describing the pathophysiology. This could have been due to not reading the question carefully enough but may also reflect lack of knowledge. As mentioned in previous reports, candidates should endeavour to arrange tester sessions in modules such as cardiac anaesthesia if they have not done them prior to sitting the SAQ paper.

a) What is the pathophysiology of worsening aortic stenosis? (8 marks)

Always look at the number of points available for a part of a question: there are 8 points here and so it should have been obvious to candidates that they were after more than just a description of symptoms.

Latent phase:
> Left ventricular outflow obstruction due to abnormal valve (rheumatic fever, congenital bicuspid valve, age-related calcification).

Compensatory phase:
> Left ventricle hypertrophies to overcome outflow obstruction, maintaining ejection fraction.
> Consequent increased oxygen demand but poorer supply and diastolic dysfunction.

Decompensation:
> Subendocardial ischaemia due to poor oxygen delivery to hypertrophied myocardium.
> Increased left ventricular end-diastolic volume and pressure result in increased pulmonary capillary pressure with pulmonary oedema, mitral regurgitation.
> Ejection fraction starts to fall as hypertrophy increases in the face of worsening outflow obstruction.

Symptomatic phase:
> As blood passes through the narrowed valve, it accelerates, gaining kinetic energy. By the law of conservation of energy, it therefore loses pressure, resulting in reduced perfusion pressure of the coronary arteries, thus reducing oxygen delivery to an already embarrassed myocardium. The consequences are angina, breathlessness, syncope, sudden death.

b) Which specific cardiac investigations may be used in assessing the severity of this woman's disease? (3 marks)

Echocardiography (transoesophageal or transthoracic):
> Assess valve: Doppler assessment of peak flow velocity, mean pressure gradient, effective orifice area, presence of regurgitation.
> Assess consequences of its stenosis: left ventricular dimensions and function; mitral valve competence, left atrium, pulmonary artery pressure, right ventricular function, post-stenotic ascending aortic dilatation.

Left heart catheter study:
> Retrograde catheterisation of aortic valve to assess pressure gradient.

MRI:
> To assess the consequences of stenosis.

ECG:
> Will demonstrate the consequences of stenosis: left ventricular hypertrophy, ischaemia, arrhythmias.

c) Give values for the peak aortic flow velocity, mean pressure gradient and valve area that would indicate that this woman has severe aortic stenosis. (3 marks)

Peak aortic flow velocity: greater than 4 m/s.

Mean pressure gradient: greater than 40 mm Hg.

Valve area: less than 1 cm².

d) What would be your haemodynamic goals for the perioperative management of this patient? (6 marks)

Take the opportunity to think through the 'haemodynamic goals' of all sorts of valve or cardiac disorders.

> Maintain myocardial oxygen delivery with adequate systolic and diastolic blood pressure within 20% of normal values (as monitored by invasive BP monitoring).
> Maintain contractility (balanced anaesthetic technique, adequate filling as guided by cardiac output (CO) monitoring, may need inotropic support if left ventricle is poorly functioning).
> Optimise pre-load with filling (guided by CO monitoring).
> Maintain sinus rhythm at a rate of 60–80 bpm (5-lead ECG, avoidance of tachycardia by managing pain, use of beta-blockers, possible need for pacing post-bypass due to surgical interruption of conduction pathway).
> Maintain afterload. Coronary artery filling is dependent on aortic root pressure (avoid excessive doses of intravenous induction agents or inhalational agents, may need alpha agonist, as guided by CO monitoring).

Reference

Chacko M, Weinberg L. Aortic valve stenosis: perioperative anaesthetic implications of surgical replacement and minimally invasive interventions. *Contin Educ Anaesth Crit Care Pain.* 2012; 12 (6): 295–301.

You are asked to review a 65-year-old woman on the cardiac intensive care unit who has undergone coronary artery bypass surgery earlier in the day.

a) What clinical features might suggest the development of cardiac tamponade? (9 marks)

b) Describe specific investigations with their findings that could confirm the diagnosis of cardiac tamponade. (2 marks)

c) Outline the management of acute cardiac tamponade in this patient. (9 marks)

September 2016

Chairman's Report

81.4% pass rate.

This question had the highest pass rate in the paper. It is an important topic and it is good to see that candidates are aware of the signs and symptoms and treatment options for this emergency.

This question is virtually identical to the one that featured in the September 2013 paper except that the patient has changed gender, part (a) asks for 'clinical features' not signs, and part (b) asks for investigations to be 'specific' and now only has 2 marks assigned to it. Perhaps the 2013 cohort had the same difficulties that I did in terms of thinking of enough investigations that would realistically be useful in the likely time frame of acute tamponade.

a) What clinical features might suggest the development of cardiac tamponade? (9 marks)

As it has asked for clinical features, I would start with symptoms before moving on to the signs that were detailed in answer to the 2013 question, and then a quick mention of changes in monitoring that are not signs but not really investigations either, which are covered in part (b).

Symptoms:
> Shortness of breath.
> Sharp chest pain radiating to the shoulder, neck, back, abdomen; may be pleuritic.
> Anxiety, restlessness, dizziness, drowsiness.

Monitoring:
> Increasing CVP.
> Progressive hypotension or increasing dose of vasopressor required to maintain blood pressure.
> Reduction or sudden loss of chest drain output.
> Equalisation of atrial and LVEDP if in pulmonary artery catheter in situ.
> Oliguria – although rapid timeframe may mean that this is not observed before the patient is periarrest.

a) What are the theoretical advantages of 'off-pump' coronary artery bypass grafting (OPCAB) compared to an 'on-bypass' technique? (7 marks)

b) What are the potential causes of haemodynamic instability during OPCAB? (5 marks)

c) Which strategies help to minimise this haemodynamic instability? (8 marks)

March 2017

Chairman's Report

60.4% pass rate.

It is encouraging that the pass rate for this question was high. Hopefully, this reflects the fact that candidates are ensuring they get exposure to the subspecialty of cardiac anaesthesia prior to sitting the exam. Some candidates did not give enough detail in parts (b) and (c), concerning the causes and mitigation of haemodynamic instability during off-pump cardiac surgery, and so failed to score well. This question correlated well with overall performance; i.e. those candidates who scored well in this question did well in the exam overall.

Apart from some tiny tweaks to the wording, the only difference between this question and the one from September 2012 is that this question does not ask about temperature maintenance. Anyone who had bothered to look at past papers must have been delighted when this question came up again.

a) What is meant by counter pulsation in the context of an intra-aortic balloon pump (IABP)? (1 mark)

b) Briefly explain the effect of counter pulsation from an IABP on coronary blood flow and the left ventricle. (4 marks)

c) What are the indications for (6 marks) and contraindications to (3 marks) the use of an IABP in an adult?

d) List possible complications of an IABP. (6 marks)

September 2017

Chairman's Report

58.7% pass rate.

This question correlated well with overall performance and was generally well answered in the clinical sections (parts c and d). However, part (b), which required an explanation of the physiological effects of counter-pulsation, was answered poorly.

a) What is meant by counter pulsation in the context of an intra-aortic balloon pump (IABP)? (1 mark)

Inflation of the balloon in diastole and deflation in early systole.

b) Briefly explain the effect of counter pulsation from an IABP on coronary blood flow and the left ventricle. (4 marks)

Inflation:
> Forces blood proximally, increasing the pressure within the proximal aorta compared to the left ventricle, thus improving perfusion of coronary arteries, increasing oxygen delivery.
> Forces blood distally, thus augmenting the apparent output from the left ventricle.
> Augments Windkessel effect.

Deflation:
> Decrease in afterload reduces myocardial wall stress during systole, thus reducing myocardial oxygen demand.

c) What are the indications for (6 marks) and contraindications to (3 marks) the use of an IABP in an adult?

These indications are under scrutiny as a result of recent evidence showing failure to confer benefit in some groups and so may change in the future.

Indications:
> Cardiogenic shock due to myocardial infarction if revascularisation planned.
> Acute mitral regurgitation or ventricular septal defect due to acute myocardial infarction.
> Refractory ventricular arrhythmias whilst awaiting definitive treatment.
> Refractory unstable angina if treatment option available.
> Refractory left ventricular failure if destination treatment planned.
> Perioperative support for high-risk coronary artery bypass surgery.
> Perioperative support for high-risk non-cardiac surgery.

Contraindications:
Absolute
> Aortic regurgitation, dissection or stent.
> Chronic end-stage heart disease with no further possible intervention.

Relative
> Uncontrolled sepsis.
> Abdominal aortic aneurysm, severe peripheral vascular disease or arterial reconstruction surgery.
> Uncontrolled bleeding disorder.
> Tachyarrhythmias.

d) List the possible complications of an IABP. (6 marks)

> Haemodynamic compromise due to poor timing of counterpulsation or malposition.
> Limb, spinal cord or visceral (especially renal) ischaemia.
> Compartment syndrome.
> Aortic dissection.
> Vascular injury causing bleeding, haematoma, false aneurysm, arteriovenous fistula.
> Cardiac tamponade.
> Thromboembolism.
> Thrombocytopaenia and haemolysis.
> Infection.
> Balloon rupture resulting in gas embolus.

References

Krishna M, Zacharowski K. Principles of intra-aortic balloon pump counterpulsation. *Contin Educ Anaesth Crit Care Pain*. 2009; 9 (1): 24–28.

MacKay E et al. Contemporary clinical niche for intra-aortic balloon counterpulsation in perioperative cardiovascular practice: an evidence-based review for the cardiovascular anesthesiologist. *J Cardiothorac Vasc Anesth*. 2017; 31: 309–320.

3. AIRWAY MANAGEMENT

a) Which nerves supply sensation to i) the nasal air passages (10%), ii) the oropharynx (10%) iii) the larynx? (10%)

b) Outline the techniques for achieving local anaesthesia of these areas? (15%)

c) What are the indications (15%) and contraindications (15%) for awake fibreoptic intubation?

d) List the complications of awake fibreoptic intubation. (25%)

September 2011

a) Which nerves supply sensation to: i) the nasal air passages (10%), ii) the oropharynx (10%) iii) the larynx? (10%)

Nasal air passages = ophthalmic and maxillary divisions of trigeminal nerve:

> Anterior septum and nares: anterior ethmoidal nerve (V1).
> Elsewhere: greater and lesser palatine nerves (V2).

Oropharynx = glossopharyngeal nerve.

Larynx = vagus:

> Above vocal folds: internal laryngeal branch of superior laryngeal nerve.
> Below vocal folds: recurrent laryngeal nerve.

b) Outline the techniques for achieving local anaesthesia of these areas? (15%)

Outline. More than a list, less than a full explanation….and only 15% of the marks.

> Spray as you go. Co-phenylcaine mucosal atomisation device to nostrils, 1% lignocaine spray to tongue and oropharynx, 2% lignocaine via epidural catheter to larynx above and below the cords.
> Topicalisation with local anaesthetic soaked pledgets in nasal passages (disadvantages: does not reduce sensation of any other area).
> Nebulised local anaesthetic (disadvantages: easy to exceed maximum local anaesthetic doses, does not work for larynx, requires the patient to take good breaths, which is often not possible in patients requiring awake intubation).
> Individual nerve blocks: glossopharyngeal nerve, superior laryngeal nerve block, recurrent laryngeal nerve block etc. (disadvantages: patient discomfort, especially in a patient who already has airway compromise; multiple blocks needed; and expertise in unusually performed blocks required).
> Cricothyroid puncture for translaryngeal block (disadvantages: anaesthetises larynx only, patient discomfort).

c) What are the indications (15%) and contraindications (15%) for awake fibreoptic intubation?

Indications:
> Previous difficult airway for intubation or face mask ventilation.
> Predicted difficult airway:
>   • Dentition.
>   • Limited mouth opening (facial fractures, rheumatoid arthritis, dental abscess, scleroderma).
>   • Limited neck movement (rheumatoid arthritis, ankylosing spondylitis, previous cervical spine surgery or trauma).

- Airway anatomy abnormality (thyroid, tongue, tonsillar or laryngeal tumours, epiglottitis, Ludwig's angina, airway oedema or burns, obesity, retrognathia, previous neck radiotherapy).
- Syndromes associated with difficult airway (Pierre-Robin, Treacher-Collins).

> Need for intubation but requirement to stay awake, e.g. need for neurological examination following intubation.

Contraindications:
> Patient refusal.
> Patient not able to comply (confusion, young age etc.).
> Local anaesthetic allergy.
> Operator inexperience.
> Subglottic airway issue (i.e. if the predicted difficulty in the airway is below the glottis, it won't be overcome by fibreoptic intubation).
> Significant laryngeal stenosis.
> Threat of airway obstruction.
> Airway bleeding or risk of airway bleeding due to e.g. vascular tumour.

d) List the complications of awake fibreoptic intubation. (25%)

Drugs related:
> Failure to achieve adequate anaesthesia of airway resulting in patient discomfort.
> Local anaesthetic toxicity.
> Nerve damage secondary to nerve blocks if used.
> Apnoea, loss of consciousness and loss of airway due to sedation, if used.

Airway related:
> Trauma to any of the structures en route.
> Airway obstruction due to fibreoptic scope and tube, airway oedema, bleeding, laryngospasm.
> Failure to achieve secure airway due to operator inexperience, patient noncompliance, airway more problematic than anticipated.
> Aspiration of blood from trauma of procedure or pre-existing bleeding, or secondary to full stomach. Consequent risk of lower respiratory tract infection etc.
> Bronchospasm.

Reference
Leslie D, Stacey M. Awake intubation. *Contin Educ Anaesth Crit Care Pain*. 2015; 15 (2): 64–67.

a) What airway, respiratory and cardiovascular problems may follow the removal of a tracheal tube? (50%)

b) List the patient and surgical factors that may contribute to a high-risk extubation. (30%)

c) Outline the strategies used to prevent airway complications if a difficult extubation is anticipated in the operating theatre. (20%)

September 2011

Of all the airway issues reported to NAP4, 1-in-6 complications occurred at emergence and 1-in-6 in recovery. NAP4-based topics have come up repeatedly in the exam, in pure airway questions and also under other headings such as intensive care medicine. The Difficult Airway Society produced guidelines to help structure the management of extubation. In the lead-up to the exam, it is really important to stay up to date with publications and guidelines that are of relevance to anaesthesia.

a) What airway, respiratory and cardiovascular problems may follow the removal of a tracheal tube? (50%)

A simple list is required here, and the examiners have already helped you with headings for classification. Leave space at the end of each of the three lists so that you can add to them when things pop into your head later on.

Airway:
> Sore throat, hoarseness.
> Foreign body causing obstruction: teeth, throat pack, blood clot.
> External compression of airway due to surgical site swelling/bleeding.
> Laryngospasm: triggered by blood, secretions and airway manipulation during light anaesthesia.
> Laryngeal oedema.
> Laryngeal trauma caused during intubation (e.g. bougie use), causing bleeding, swelling, tears.
> Vocal cord paralysis: direct trauma/pressure.
> Vocal cord dysfunction.
> Tracheomalacia: erosion/softening of tracheal rings due to prolonged intubation, retrosternal thyroid, large thymus or tumour.
> Tracheal stenosis after prolonged intubation.

Respiratory:
> Coughing.
> Mucociliary dysfunction.
> Diffusion hypoxia.
> Basal atelectasis causing ventilation/perfusion mismatch.
> Inadequate minute ventilation due to ongoing sedation.
> Post-obstructive pulmonary oedema.
> Bronchospasm.
> Pulmonary aspiration.
> Respiratory failure due to any respiratory or airway complications.

Cardiovascular:
> Catecholamine release causing tachycardia and hypertension.
> This may result in reduced ejection fraction in patients with coronary artery disease.
> Risk of silent or overt myocardial infarction due to increased myocardial oxygen demand (effect exacerbated if there is hypoxaemia due to other complications of extubation).

b) List the patient and surgical factors that may contribute to a high-risk extubation. (30%)

Patient factors:
> Airway: dysmorphia, musculoskeletal disease contributing to airway difficulties (rheumatoid arthritis, ankylosis), airway pathology (tumour), obesity. These issues may have been detected at preoperative assessment or at intubation: difficult airway assessment, difficult face mask ventilation, difficult intubation, complications at intubation.

> Breathing: respiratory disease including asthma, obstructive sleep apnoea, chronic obstructive pulmonary disease, recent upper respiratory tract infection (especially in children), smoking.
> Cardiovascular: ischaemic heart disease, unstable arrhythmias.
> Neurological: posterior fossa tumour, head injury, Guillain–Barré, myasthenia gravis, multiple sclerosis.
> Gastrointestinal: full stomach, reflux, hiatus hernia.
> Muscular: muscular dystrophy, dystrophia myotonica.

Surgical factors:
> Site: airway, head, neck, thorax, posterior fossa, cervical spine. Any surgery requiring use of double-lumen tube.
> Complications of surgery or double-lumen tube use: bleeding, swelling, infection.
> Duration: prolonged intubation predictive of problems with extubation.
> Position: Trendelenberg exacerbates development of laryngeal oedema.
> Intraoperative issues not directly related to airway: difficulty achieving adequate ventilation, hypothermia, significant blood loss, electrolyte imbalance, fluid shifts.

c) Outline the strategies used to prevent airway complications if a difficult extubation is anticipated in the operating theatre. (20%)

There are three options here: extubate now but take steps to make it safer, extubate later or don't extubate at all.

The decision depends on the likely issues anticipated.

Extubate in theatre:
> Pre-medicate with proton pump inhibitor if appropriate.
> Plan A, plan B, plan C.
> Involve colleagues with specific airway skills +/– ENT.
> Ensure full difficult airway kit to hand.
> Ensure cardiovascular, respiratory and metabolic stability.
> Optimise oxygenation prior to starting, ongoing full monitoring.
> Ensure full reversal of neuromuscular blockade.
> Position: left lateral head down or sitting up.
> Extubation wide awake: good grip, tongue protrusion, adequate minute ventilation.

Consideration of additional techniques:
> Exchange of tube for SAD when deep +/– still paralysed.
> Use of airway exchange catheter.
> Use of nasopharyngeal or oropharyngeal airway.
> Flexible bronchoscope through the LMA to visualise the larynx and vocal cords to check for cord paralysis and tracheomalacia (if indicated due to type of surgery).
> Extubation onto noninvasive ventilation or high-flow humidified oxygen.
> Use of remifentanil to manage awake extubation.

Delayed extubation if reversible contributing factors:
> Transfer to ICU with a plan for delayed extubation.
> Avoid positive fluid balance.
> Ensure normothermia.
> Normalise electrolytes.
> Allow any airway swelling to settle; consider need for steroid therapy.

Surgical tracheostomy if contributing factors are not readily reversible:
> Nature of surgery: flaps, spinal fixation, complications from airway tumour.

References

Batuwitage B, Charters P. Postoperative management of the difficult airway. *BJA Educ*. 2017; 17 (7): 235–241.

Cook T, Woodall N, Frerk C (eds.). *4th National Audit Project of the Royal College of Anaesthetists and the Difficult Airway Society. Major Complications of Airway Management in the United Kingdom*. London: The Royal College of Anaesthetists and Association of Anaesthetists of Great Britain and Ireland; 2011.

Popat M et al. Difficult Airway Society Guidelines for the management of tracheal extubation. *Anaesthesia*. 2012; 67: 318–340.

4. CRITICAL INCIDENTS

a) List the implications for the patient of an inadvertent wrong-sided peripheral nerve block. (25%)

b) Summarise the recommendations of the 'Stop Before You Block' campaign and list factors that have been identified as contributing to the performance of a wrong-sided block. (45%)

c) Define the term 'never event' as described by the National Patient Safety Agency and list three never events of relevance to anaesthetic or intensive care practice. (30%)

September 2012

Chairman's Report

40.5% pass rate.

It is disappointing that many candidates displayed a relative unfamiliarity with the Stop Before You Block Campaign. This is an important national patient safety initiative that was introduced recently to reduce the incidence of inadvertent wrong-sided nerve blocks. Many examinees left some sections unanswered. Some candidates could not adequately define the term 'never event' despite its topicality.

A virtually identical question came up in March 2017 – this again highlights the importance of looking at past questions. I have written the question in full here so you can see the wording but will answer it in the March 2017 question. The National Patient Safety Agency ceased to exist in 2012, the current home of Never Event publications being NHS Improvement.

The 4th National Audit Project (NAP4) was published in 2011.

a) Which factors are most likely to lead to an adverse airway event when using a supraglottic airway device (SAD)? (30%)

b) How would you recognise that a patient has regurgitated and aspirated gastric contents during an anaesthetic administered via a SAD? (30%)

c) How would you manage this patient? (40%)

September 2012

Chairman's Report

78.4% pass rate.

Generally well answered. There was significant variation in the knowledge detailed in the NAP4 relating to the safe use of supraglottic airways. The diagnosis and management of aspiration was of appropriate standard.

a) Which factors are most likely to lead to an adverse airway event when using a supraglottic airway device (SAD)? (30%)

This answer is easy if you've read the vignettes in the NAP4 SAD chapter. However, it should also be straightforward to anyone who regularly makes the decision of whether to use an SAD or to intubate.

Patient factors:
> Obesity.
> Known/predicted difficult airway.
> Irritable airway: asthma, recent chest infection.
> Obstructive sleep apnoea.
> Aspiration risk: obesity, reflux, hiatus hernia, raised abdominal pressure, pregnancy, drugs or conditions (recent trauma, recent pancreatitis, pain, ileus, bowel obstruction, diabetes mellitus, chronic kidney disease) affecting gastric emptying.

Surgical factors:
> Urgent surgery, inadequate fasting time.
> Lithotomy, prone, semi-prone or Trendelenberg positioning.
> Prolonged surgery.
> Abdominal surgery.
> Laparoscopic surgery.
> Shared airway surgery.

Anaesthetic factors:
> Junior anaesthetists, inadequate training, poor supervision, poor attention to detail, poor patient selection, poor judgment.
> Use of SAD to avoid intubating patients with known/predicted difficult airway.
> Difficulty siting SAD, resulting in problems during maintenance or emergence.
> Light anaesthesia.
> First-generation SAD use.

b) How would you recognise that a patient has regurgitated and aspirated gastric contents during an anaesthetic administered via a SAD? (30%)

A:
> Gastric contents visible in the oropharynx/tube of SAD.

B:
> Desaturation.
> Cyanosis.
> Bronchospasm.
> Increased airway pressures/reduced tidal volumes in ventilated patient.
> Abnormal auscultation.

C:
> Tachycardia.

c) How would you manage this patient? (40%)

This is an anaesthetic emergency. I would alert the theatre team, call for help and adopt an ABC approach, assessing and managing the patient simultaneously.

A:
> Head down tilt +/– lateral tilt.
> Remove SAD.
> Oropharyngeal suction.

B:
> 100% oxygen.
> RSI (with cricoid pressure and avoidance of stomach inflation).
> Ideally, tracheal suction prior to ventilation but oxygenation is paramount.
> Positive pressure ventilation with PEEP.
> Symptomatic treatment with bronchodilators if necessary.

C:
> Ensure cardiovascular stability; manage as appropriate.

Once the patient is stable:
> Early bronchoscopy if particulate matter has been aspirated.
> Decision to continue with surgery depends on circumstances.
> Extubation or ventilation on ICU: dependent on clinical condition.
> If extubated, extended recovery stay for observation of respiratory rate, oxygen saturations, other signs of respiratory distress.
> CXR.
> Maintain a high index of suspicion for aspiration pneumonia and treat early (antibiotics not routinely advocated).
> Discussion with patient and/or family followed up by written information of what symptoms should prompt the patient to seek medical help.

References

Cook T, Woodall N, Frerk C (eds.). *4th National Audit Project of the Royal College of Anaesthetists and the Difficult Airway Society. Major Complications of Airway Management in the United Kingdom*. London: The Royal College of Anaesthetists and Association of Anaesthetists of Great Britain and Ireland; 2011.

Robinson M, Davidson A. Aspiration under anaesthesia: risk assessment and decision-making. *Contin Educ Anaesth Crit Care Pain*. 2014; 14 (4): 171–175.

a) Define the types of unintentional awareness that may occur during general anaesthesia. (20%)

b) What factors may increase the likelihood of intraoperative awareness? (55%)

c) What monitoring techniques can be employed to reduce the risk of awareness during general anaesthesia? (25%)

March 2013

Chairman's Report

Easy

79.8% pass rate.

A straightforward and topical question (National Audit Project 5) that had been widely predicted by candidates and trainers! A question on awareness has featured in 1996, 1998, 2000 and 2006 papers.

An easy question requires you to score 14/20 in order to pass, or 70% back when questions were weighted by percentage instead of points.

a) Define the types of unintentional awareness that may occur during general anaesthesia. (20%)

Explicit awareness:
> May have spontaneous recall, or recall prompted by questioning.
> May occur with or without pain.
> May result in psychological harm, sleep disturbance, nightmares, anxiety or even post-traumatic stress disorder (PTSD).

Implicit awareness:
> No conscious recall but may affect behaviour and performance in the future.

b) What factors may increase the likelihood of intraoperative awareness? (55%)

See the question about awareness from March 2016 – this section of the question was asked again in an almost identical manner, but by that date, the outcomes from NAP5 were available to help answer the question.

c) What monitoring techniques can be employed to reduce the risk of awareness during general anaesthesia? (25%)

Think systematically and incrementally again. Firstly, there is the presence of you and the things that you can monitor without monitors, then there are the monitors you use as standard during anaesthesia and then there are the monitors that have been developed specifically for the purpose of measuring depth of anaesthesia.

Clinical monitoring:
> Presence of the anaesthetist throughout the case.
> Eye position.
> Pupillary dilatation and reactivity to light.
> Sweating.
> Lacrimation.
> Tachypnoea.
> Movement.
> Retching on tube/LMA.

General monitoring:
> Full equipment checks and ongoing monitoring during anaesthesia (pumps, anaesthetic machine, vaporisers).
> Heart rate, respiratory rate and tidal volume (if not paralysed), blood pressure.
> End tidal anaesthetic gas (ETAG) monitoring.
> TIVA pump effect-site or plasma-site concentration.
> Train-of-four monitoring to ensure that neuromuscular blockade is reversible before ending anaesthesia.

Specific depth of anaesthesia monitoring:

> Processed EEG monitors convert the frontal signal into a dimensionless number, 1–100 (100 = fully awake). BIS (target 40–60 for absence of postoperative recall), M-Entropy and Narcotrend.
> Other specific monitors use auditory evoked potentials as a measure of depth of anaesthesia.

Reference

Pandit J, Cook T, the NAP5 Steering Panel. *NAP5. Accidental Awareness During General Anaesthesia*. London: The Royal College of Anaesthetists and Association of Anaesthetists of Great Britain and Ireland; 2014.

a) What factors predispose to inadvertent intra-arterial (IA) drug injection that could lead to severe extremity injury? (35%)

b) Outline the possible intravascular mechanisms of injury. (15%)

c) What are the acute clinical features of inadvertent IA injection? (20%)

d) What is the early management of an acute IA injection injury? (30%)

September 2013

Chairman's Report

71.9% pass rate.

This question was answered well and proved to be a good discriminator. The factors that predispose to intra-arterial injection were broken down to patient factors, anatomical anomalies and the appreciation that some drugs are particularly harmful when injected intra-arterially. One candidate sadly misread the question and wrote about local anaesthetic toxicity, confusing the abbreviation (IA) with (LA). All abbreviations are explained before using them later in the question. This resulted in a 'poor fail' for that particular question but an overall pass for the paper. It should be pointed out that a poor fail in four or more questions is likely to result in an overall fail for the paper.

a) What factors predispose to inadvertent intra-arterial (IA) drug injection that could lead to severe extremity injury? (35%)

Take care to read the question – it doesn't just ask what factors are likely to lead to inadvertent intra-arterial injection, but what factors then increase the likelihood of this error causing harm.

Patient factors:
> Unconscious so unable to indicate pain on cannulation/injection.
> Hypotension or hypoxia, causing failure to recognise cannula as arterial.
> Anatomically anomalous artery accidentally cannulated, thoracic outlet syndrome with loss of radial pulse on abduction or rotation of arm.

Staff factors:
> Poor training resulting in failure to differentiate between artery and vein.
> Failure to check which line is being accessed.
> Failure to label line as arterial.

Drug factors:
> Some drugs have greater potential for harm than others, e.g. vasoactive drugs, hyperosmolar drugs.

b) Outline the possible intravascular mechanisms of injury. (15%)

> Arterial spasm resulting in distal ischaemia: secondary to the drug itself or due to mediators released in response to drug.
> Chemical arteritis: direct tissue damage causing endothelial damage.
> Initiation of release of harmful endogenous substances, e.g. thromboxane, which cause endothelial damage and activation of platelets resulting in thrombosis.
> Drug precipitation and crystal formation in distal microcirculation causing ischaemia and thrombosis.

c) What are the acute clinical features of inadvertent IA injection? (20%)

> Failure of drug to have intended effect.
> Pain at and distal to the injection site.
> Pallor, cyanosis and coolness of limb, or redness and warmth.
> Paraesthesia.

d) What is the early management of an acute IA injection injury? (30%)

> Stop injection.
> ABC assessment of patient, to include intravenous access and administration of drug by intended route if urgent.
> Keep cannula in situ for consideration of IA sympatholysis (with, for example, iloprost or local anaesthetic) but ensure no other use.

> Elevation of extremity to improve venous and lymphatic drainage.
> Pain control.
> Consideration of anticoagulation with heparin.
> Documentation.
> Explanation and apology to patient/patient's family, followed up in writing.
> Incident report.
> Plastics referral.
> Consideration of stellate ganglion/lower limb sympathetic blocks.

Reference

Lake C, Christina Beecroft L. Extravasation injuries and accidental intra-arterial injection. *Contin Educ Anaesth Crit Care Pain*. 2010; 10 (4): 109–113.

a) Which human factors contribute to intravenous drug administration errors in theatre-based anaesthetic practice? (30%)

b) Outline the organisational strategies that might minimise intravenous drug administration errors. (70%)

March 2014

Chairman's Report

39.2% pass rate.

Relatively few candidates had good insight into the factors associated with drug errors and were able to suggest strategies to reduce the incidence. The Safe Anaesthesia Liaison Group (SALG) has generated a number of publications specifically aimed at this subject matter and strong candidates had taken advantage of these.

Even if you hadn't read the reports from SALG, you should still have attended enough M&M meetings to have insight into what causes these sorts of errors. When you see a question in the exam that you know that you have done no formal revision for, don't panic. Many questions can be answered with the knowledge you absorb in your day-to-day work and a logical approach. The subheadings here are much less important than the actual factors.

a) Which human factors contribute to intravenous drug administration errors in theatre-based anaesthetic practice? (30%)

Lack of knowledge:
> Unfamiliarity with a particular drug, its route of administration etc.

Human cognition:
> Human memory – cannot be relied upon to remember all infusion mixtures, dose variations etc.
> Difficulty with complex calculations, e.g. paediatrics, infusions.
> Lack of knowledge of certain unfamiliar drugs.

Distraction:
> Needing to address other tasks whilst also drawing up drugs, prescribing drugs, calculating doses, giving drugs.
> High noise levels.

Stress and fatigue:
> Tiredness, e.g. due to night work.
> Non-work emotional issues causing reduced work performance.

Lack of teamwork:
> Lack of double checking of drugs.
> Failure to feel able to voice lack of knowledge about a particular drug and its administration.
> Failure to implement a 'no blame culture,' lack of encouragement of reporting and learning from errors.
> Poor communication, poor handover: failure of one member of a team to give explicit instructions to another about the administration of a particular drug or whether a drug has already been given.

Excessive physical demands:
> Excessive workload, e.g. high turnover list.

Physical environment:
> Cluttered workspace, low light levels.
> Drugs with similar packaging, changes in packaging without notice, unclear or too small labelling and lettering size.

b) Outline the organisational strategies that might minimise intravenous drug administration errors. (70%)

Processes:
> Standardisation of cross-checking, handover etc.
> Standardisation of infusion doses, diluents etc.
> Availability of reference databases for doses, calculations, diluents.
> Regulations regarding what is drawn up and by whom and at what stage in the care of a patient.
> Avoidance of distraction during drug preparation.
> Checklist to ensure prescription chart checked before administration of drugs by anaesthetist to avoid double-dosing or omitted doses.
> Investigation of possibility of pre-mixed infusions.
> Flushing all lines as standard before leaving theatre and recovery.

Physical environment:
> Standardisation of lay-out and contents of anaesthetic carts.
> Ensure intrathecal/epidural drugs kept separate from intravenous drugs.
> Removal of non-essential, rarely used drugs from cart which have high injury risk if inadvertently given.
> Ensuring label availability at all times.
> Process for dealing with unused ampoules to prevent them from being returned to incorrect box (e.g. second-person check or discard altogether).
> Ensure adequate lighting levels.
> Sourcing of products with clear labelling, sufficiently large lettering etc., where possible.

Team working:
> Simulation sessions to highlight risks to all team members.
> Unusual drugs to be dealt with in the team briefing.
> Encouragement of working environment where any team member feels able to voice concern.
> Inclusion of pharmacist in team: notification of team members about changes in product appearance, education about new drugs for inclusion in anaesthetic carts etc.

Management of error:
> Open incident reporting with no-blame culture, lead clinician who will analyse factors contributing to error and be responsible for national reporting. Morbidity and mortality meetings for education of all team members about pitfalls that may lead to error.
> Communication of e.g. Safe Anaesthesia Liaison Group reports to all team members to help everyone learn from errors that have occurred nationally.

References

Glavin R. Drug errors: Consequences, mechanisms, and avoidance. *Br J Anaesth*. 2010; 105 (1): 76–82.

Safe Anaesthesia Liaison Group. *Patient Safety Update Including the Summary of Reported Incidents Relating to Anaesthesia, 1 March 2012 to 30 March 2012*. National Patient Safety Agency; 2012.

Toff N. Human factors in anaesthesia: Lessons from aviation. *Br J Anaesth*. 2010; 105 (1): 21–25.

a) List the factors that may have contributed to an increase in the prevalence of asthma in developed countries in the last 20 years. (5 marks)

b) What are the possible causes of acute bronchospasm during general anaesthesia in a patient with mild asthma? (5 marks)

c) Outline the immediate management of acute severe bronchospasm in an intubated patient during general anaesthesia. (10 marks)

March 2015

Chairman's Report

47.0% pass rate; 8.5% of candidates received a poor fail.

The poor pass rate for this question is of concern as patients with asthma are regularly encountered in daily practice. The treatment of common co-existing medical disorders is specified in the syllabus for the CCT. In general, the management of acute bronchospasm was more thoroughly answered than the aetiology and causation sections. This was reflected in a lower poor fail rate compared to other questions, which is reassuring for patient safety under general anaesthesia.

a) <u>List</u> the factors that <u>may</u> have contributed to an increase in the prevalence of asthma in <u>developed</u> countries in the last 20 years. (5 marks)

Make sure you underline key words in the question, as I have done, before starting your answer; it will help you focus your thoughts. There are a number of suggested theories that have not been proven.

> Better identification of cases, influenced by targets for asthma management in primary care.
> Hygiene hypothesis: cleaner environment associated with increased rates of allergy-associated asthma.
> Obesity: increases an individual's risk due to altered airway mechanics and chronic inflammatory state.
> Urbanisation.
> Asthma development following survival from premature birth.
> Increased use of drugs such as beta-blockers, NSAIDs, aspirin.

b) What are the possible causes of acute bronchospasm during general anaesthesia in a patient with mild asthma? (5 marks)

> Pre-existing upper respiratory tract infection, poor asthma control, smoking.
> Airway irritation: cold inspired gases, airway secretions, airway suctioning, laryngoscopy, intubation, extubation, aspiration, carinal stimulation or endobronchial intubation.
> Drugs causing histamine release, muscarinic block or allergy.
> Vagal stimulation: peritoneal or visceral stretch etc.

c) Outline the immediate management of acute severe bronchospasm in an intubated patient during general anaesthesia. (10 marks)

This is an emergency situation and I would alert the theatre team, call for help and assess and manage the patient simultaneously following an ABC approach.

> Stop surgical/drug triggers where possible.
> A: Ensure ETT patent, ensure position is correct (carinal or endobronchial placement may have triggered bronchospasm), suction if required (avoiding stimulation of trachea), 100% inspired oxygen.
> B: Auscultate chest, confirm wheeze or even absence of breath sounds; check SpO_2, manually ventilate to assess compliance and apply higher, sustained pressure for ventilation and longer expiratory flow time; and increase inspired anaesthetic gas concentration.
> C: Check heart rate and blood pressure, increase intravenous filling as increasing intrathoracic pressure reduces venous return, reducing cardiac output and causing a tamponade-type effect.
> Drugs:
>   • Salbutamol MDI via airway adaptor on breathing circuit, 10 puffs.
>   • Salbutamol IV 100–300 mcg bolus in extremis/5–20 mcg/min ivi.
>   • Magnesium 1.2–2 g/20 min IV bolus.

- Adrenaline IV 0.2–1 mg bolus in extremis/1–20 mcg/min ivi.
- Hydrocortisone 200 mg IV.

> Once acute situation has resolved, monitor response with arterial blood gas, assess whether safe to proceed with case or whether to abandon, to keep intubated and take to ICU or whether safe to wake the patient up.
> Incident reporting.
> Consideration of need for referral for optimisation of asthma control.
> Full explanation to patient and/or family, including a written explanation of what has occurred.

Reference

Stanley D, Tunnicliffe W. Management of life-threatening asthma in adults. *Contin Educ Anaesth Crit Care Pain*. 2008; 8 (3): 95–99.

a) What are the factors associated with an increased risk of accidental awareness under general anaesthesia (AAGA)? (14 marks)

b) What monitoring devices can be used to help reduce the incidence of AAGA? (2 marks)

c) What are the possible consequences to the patient of an episode of AAGA? (4 marks)

March 2016

Chairman's Report

57.1% pass rate.

This question had the highest correlation with overall performance. Most candidates obviously had good knowledge of the recent NAP5 publication and this resulted in a relatively high pass rate. Candidates who presented their answers in an organized way tended to score more highly than those who did not, probably reflecting their greater knowledge. Again, some candidates disadvantaged themselves by not reading the question carefully.

NAP5 is a recent publication that is of real importance to the world of anaesthesia, and the question has come up a number of times before. Despite this, only 57.1% of candidates passed the question.

Some key statistics from NAP5:

> *Incidence of AAGA: approximately 1/19,000.*
> *Incidence of AAGA if NMBD used: 1/8,000.*
> *Incidence of AAGA if no NMBD used: 1/36,000.*
> *Incidence of AAGA in obstetrics: 1/670.*
> *Incidence of AAGA in cardiothoracics: 1/8,600.*

a) What are the factors associated with an increased risk of accidental awareness under general anaesthesia (AAGA)? (14 marks)

The following is lifted straight from the executive summary of the NAP5 report:

Drug factors: NMBD, thiopentone, TIVA.

Patient factors: female gender, young adults, obesity, previous AAGA, possibly difficult airway.

Surgical factors: obstetric, cardiac, thoracic, neurosurgical.

Organisational: emergencies, junior anaesthetists, out of hours operating.

More detail can be added in after reading through the individual chapters, but the majority of the marks could have been obtained by reading the executive summary only.

Drug factors:
> TIVA results in a full range of human and equipment error issues: tissued cannula, pump failure, failure to switch the pump on, pump wrongly programmed.
> Neuromuscular blocking drug (NMBD): 97% of the episodes of awareness reported to NAP5 included use of NMBD. Failure to reverse, failure to monitor depth of block, human error causing syringe switches, failure to label syringes properly, mixed up ampoules.
> Increased incidence of awareness associated with thiopentone use.
> RSI.

Patient factors:
> Female gender.
> Young adults.
> Difficult airway.

> Obesity: difficulties with drug dosing and increased risk of difficult airway.
> Previous awareness: possible genetic component.
> Sick, cardiovascularly compromised patients in whom lower doses of anaesthetic agents were given.

Surgical factors:
> Obstetrics, especially emergency LSCS: anxiety, no pre-medication, physiological changes of pregnancy mask awareness, NMBD used, thiopentone commonly used, may underdose due to failure to take account of body weight, rapid sequence induction, emergency (increased risk of error), junior anaesthetist, out of hours, short period between intubation and commencement of surgery, not giving adequate time for drugs to work. Failed regional is a risk factor according to the reports submitted.
> Cardiac: not many cases in NAP5, but previously high level of awareness reported at start of cardiopulmonary bypass. May also relate to cardiac anaesthesia technique (low hypnotic dose, high opioid dose). May be less likely to report as patients are warned of waking in cardiac ICU with tube still in situ, and older patients may possibly be more tolerant.
> Thoracics: NMBD usually used. Switching tubes (single lumen to double lumen) and failing to maintain anaesthesia by volatile technique. Rigid bronchoscopy – episodes of intense stimulation, intermittent interruption to anaesthesia administration if volatile used, NMBD needed.
> Neurosurgical.

Organisational:
> Out of hours.
> Junior anaesthetist.
> Emergency surgery.

b) What monitoring devices can be used to help reduce the incidence of AAGA? (2 marks)

On this occasion, the College has asked specifically about monitoring devices, so it is not relevant to include information about the presence of an anaesthetist and observance of clinical signs.

General monitoring:
> Full equipment checks and ongoing monitoring during anaesthesia (pumps, anaesthetic machine, vaporisers).
> Heart rate, respiratory rate and tidal volume (if not paralysed), blood pressure.
> ETAG monitoring.
> TIVA pump effect-site or plasma-site concentration.
> Train-of-four monitoring to ensure patient is reversible before ending anaesthesia.

Specific depth of anaesthesia monitoring:
> Processed EEG monitors convert the frontal signal into a dimensionless number, 1–100 (100 = fully awake). BIS (target 40–60), M-Entropy and Narcotrend.
> Other specific monitors use auditory evoked potentials as a measure of depth of anaesthesia.

c) What are the possible consequences to the patient of an episode of AAGA? (4 marks)

Only 4 marks here, a brief explanation only required.

> There may be immediate, delayed or no recall.
> Experiences may be auditory or tactile; may include pain and awareness of paralysis.
> Response very varied: neutral feelings about experience to extreme distress at the time and also subsequently in the form of post-traumatic stress disorder with flashbacks, anxiety and depression, with impact on personal, social and work life.

> May cause avoidance of all medical settings or specifically anaesthesia and loss of trust of healthcare professionals.
> No recall may still cause long-term problems with e.g. unexplained anxiety due to implicit memory.
> Patients tend to benefit from explanation and cognitive behavioural therapy.

Reference

Pandit J, Cook T, the NAP5 Steering Panel. *NAP5. Accidental Awareness During General Anaesthesia*. London: The Royal College of Anaesthetists and Association of Anaesthetists of Great Britain and Ireland; 2014.

A 60-year-old man is having an elective knee arthroscopy and has just aspirated a significant amount of gastric fluid during anaesthesia. He has a supraglottic airway device in place and is breathing spontaneously. His inspired oxygen fraction is 1.0 and the pulse oximeter shows an oxygen saturation of 91%.

a) Describe your immediate management of this patient. (4 marks)

b) List the respiratory complications he could develop in the next 48 hours. (2 marks)

c) What are the possible preoperative risk factors for regurgitation and aspiration of gastric contents in this case? (6 marks)

d) Describe the strategies available to reduce the risk and impact of aspiration of gastric contents in any patient. (8 marks)

September 2016

Chairman's Report

77.5% pass rate.

This was adjudged to be an easy question and most candidates answered it well, demonstrating good knowledge of how to manage such an emergency and of the recommendations of NAP4. The few candidates who did less well wasted time describing general intraoperative safety measures that were not relevant to the scenario outlined.

Parts of this question are very similar to the one concerning aspiration in September 2012.

a) Describe your immediate management of this patient. (4 marks)

There are only 4 points available for this answer and it asks for 'immediate' management only.

This is an anaesthetic emergency. I would alert the theatre team, call for help and adopt an ABC approach, assessing and managing the patient simultaneously.

A:
> Head down tilt +/– lateral tilt.
> Remove SAD.
> Oropharyngeal suction.

B:
> 100% oxygen.
> RSI (with cricoid pressure and avoidance of stomach inflation).
> Ideally, tracheal suction prior to ventilation but oxygenation is paramount.
> Positive pressure ventilation with PEEP.
> Symptomatic treatment with bronchodilators if necessary.

C:
> Ensure cardiovascular stability; manage as appropriate.

b) List the respiratory complications he could develop in the next 48 hours. (2 marks)

> Sustained hypoxia.
> Bronchospasm.
> Pneumonitis.
> Complications of barotrauma, including pneumothorax due to ongoing high airway pressures.
> Lobar collapse.
> Pulmonary infection.
> ARDS.

c) What are the possible preoperative risk factors for regurgitation and aspiration of gastric contents in this case? (6 marks)

From the long list of risk factors for aspiration with an SAD, I have extracted the ones that may relate to a 60-year-old man having an elective knee arthroscopy.

> Obesity.
> Failure of the lower oesophageal sphincter: reflux, heartburn, hiatus hernia, previous upper gastrointestinal surgery, gastro-oesophageal disease.

> Drugs or conditions (recent opioid-based analgesia, recent pancreatitis, diabetes mellitus, chronic kidney disease) affecting gastric emptying.
> Failure to follow starvation advice preoperatively.

d) Describe the strategies available to reduce the risk and impact of aspiration of gastric contents in any patient. (8 marks)

> Avoidance of general anaesthesia by use of regional anaesthesia/local anaesthesia/no surgery.
> Routine preoperative starvation.
> Naso- or orogastric tube insertion and stomach drainage before or during anaesthesia.
> Premedication with prokinetic drugs, antacids, H_2 receptor blockers and proton pump inhibitors.
> Tracheal intubation instead of SAD use.
> Second-generation supraglottic airway device use instead of first generation.

Reference

Cook T, Woodall N, Frerk C (ed.). *4th National Audit Project of the Royal College of Anaesthetists and the Difficult Airway Society. Major Complications of Airway Management in the United Kingdom*. London: The Royal College of Anaesthetists and Association of Anaesthetists of Great Britain and Ireland; 2011.

a) List the implications for the patient of an inadvertent wrong-sided peripheral nerve block. (5 marks)

b) Summarise the recommendations of the 'Stop Before You Block' campaign (4 marks), and list factors that have been identified as contributing to the performance of a wrong-side block. (5 marks)

c) Define the term 'never event' (2 marks) and list four drug-related never events. (4 marks)

March 2017

Chairman's Report

39.0% pass rate.

This question related to an important safety initiative. Candidates did not have adequate knowledge of the factors contributing to the performance of a wrong-side block such as distraction, the patient being lateral or prone, or a site mark being covered by blankets.

This question is almost identical to that from September 2012 and yet only 39% of candidates passed it. There was also a recent CEACCP article on never events that should have offered a clue that the question remained topical and therefore likely for a repeat appearance in the exam.

a) List the implications for the patient of an inadvertent wrong-sided peripheral nerve block. (5 marks)

> Potential adverse effects of unnecessary nerve block (including infection, bleeding, nerve damage, visceral damage).
> Bilateral block may be contraindicated (e.g. interscalene), resulting in cancellation of surgery, suboptimal pain relief or experience of side effects of the alternative pain relief.
> Safe doses of local anaesthesia may be exceeded if correct side subsequently blocked.
> May result in wrong-sided surgery.
> Delayed discharge due to immobility if nerve blocks therefore undertaken on both legs.
> Loss of trust.

b) Summarise the recommendations of the 'Stop Before You Block' campaign (4 marks), and list factors that have been identified as contributing to the performance of a wrong-side block. (5 marks)

Beware, two things are being asked in one section here. It's very easy in the stress of an exam to only answer one part.

Recommendations of the Stop Before You Block Campaign:
> Educate staff, ensure cooperation of all staff, especially anaesthetists and ODPs.
> After WHO checklist, STOP just before needle insertion.
> ODP and anaesthetist to:
  • Visualise arrow indicating the laterality of surgery.
  • Check laterality with patient if conscious, consent form if not.
  • Confirm site and side of block.

Factors identified as contributing to a wrong-side block:

There are all sorts of things that may contribute to a wrong-sided block. These are the factors that have been documented, but if you hadn't read the Stop Before You Block campaign supporting information, you should still be able to have a good attempt at listing some issues that may increase the likelihood of error.

> Long duration since WHO sign-in.
> Patient being turned prone or lateral.
> Busy anaesthetic room; anaesthetist distracted.
> Lower limb blocks: arrow may not be immediately visible if patient covered for warmth or dignity.
> Anaesthetist not regularly performing blocks.

c) Define the term 'never event' (2 marks) and list four drug-related never events. (4 marks)

I've listed more than four...

Never events are serious incidents that are entirely preventable because guidance or safety recommendations providing strong systemic protective barriers are available at a national level and should have been implemented by all healthcare providers.

> Mis-selection of a strong potassium-containing solution.
> Wrong route administration of medication.
> Overdose of insulin due to abbreviations or incorrect device.
> Overdose of methotrexate for non-cancer treatment.
> Mis-selection of high-strength midazolam during conscious sedation.
> Unintentional connection of patient requiring oxygen to an air flowmeter.

Below is the complete list of never events, as defined by NHS Improvement. A large proportion involve anaesthesia and drug administration. Some of them could be the basis of a future question.

> *Wrong site surgery (includes wrong site block).*
> *Wrong implant/prosthesis.*
> *Retained foreign object post-operation.*
> *Mis-selection of a strong potassium-containing solution.*
> *Wrong route administration of medication.*
> *Overdose of insulin due to abbreviations or incorrect device.*
> *Overdose of methotrexate for non-cancer treatment.*
> *Mis-selection of high-strength midazolam during conscious sedation.*
> *Failure to install functional collapsible shower or curtain rails.*
> *Falls from poorly restricted windows.*
> *Chest or neck entrapment in bedrails.*
> *Transfusion or transplantation of ABO-incompatible blood components or organs.*
> *Misplaced naso- or orogastric tube.*
> *Scalding of patients.*
> *Unintentional connection of patient requiring oxygen to an air flowmeter.*
> *Undetected oesophageal intubation.*

References

Adyanthaya S, Patil V. Never events: an anaesthetic perspective. *Contin Educ Anaesth Crit Care Pain*. 2014; 14 (5): 197–201.

French J, Bedforth N, Townsley P. Stop Before You Block Supporting Information. http://salg.ac.uk/sites/default/files/SBYB-Supporting-Info.pdf [Accessed 27th June 2017].

NHS Improvement. Never Events List 2018. https://improvement.nhs.uk /uploads/documents/Never_Events_list_2018_FINAL_v2.pdf [Accessed 25th January 2018].

a) List the anaesthetic factors that predispose to perioperative dental damage. (6 marks)

b) List the dental factors that predispose to perioperative dental damage. (4 marks)

c) You have anaesthetised a 22-year-old man and you notice a missing front tooth after intubation. What is your initial management of this situation? (6 marks)

d) How would you follow this patient up? (4 marks)

September 2017

Chairman's Report

68.3% pass rate.

This question was thought to be easy and the pass rate was correspondingly high. Part (d) concerned the need to be open with patients when things go wrong (duty of candour) and was not as well answered as the parts relating to purely clinical matters. It is important to be aware of how to manage such situations as misunderstandings can lead to great distress for all parties. As mentioned above, some candidates failed to read the question properly and lost marks in part (a) because they listed patient rather than anaesthetic factors that could predispose to dental damage.

a) List the anaesthetic factors that predispose to perioperative dental damage. (6 marks)

> Limited mouth opening.*
> LMA use.
> Laryngoscopy.
> Tracheal intubation.
> Difficult intubation.

I would not have considered limited mouth opening under anaesthetic factors unless I had actually read the Safe Anaesthesia Liaison Group guidance on management of dental trauma during anaesthesia, the document that I assume is the basis of this question.

b) List the dental factors that predispose to perioperative dental damage. (4 marks)

> Primary teeth.
> Poor dental health.
> Crowns, fillings and bridges.
> Patient age over 50 years.
> Prominent upper incisors.
> Isolated teeth.
> Previously traumatised teeth.

c) You have anaesthetised a 22-year-old man and you notice a missing front tooth after intubation. What is your initial management of this situation? (6 marks)

Assess for possibility of airway compromise as a result:
> Alert team, call for senior assistance. Assess airway and ventilation. Check for obvious presence of tooth in airway, check oxygen saturations, auscultate chest, ensure airway pressures and volumes appropriate.

Manage loss of tooth:
> Look for tooth in mouth, on laryngoscope etc. If tooth intact and patient not immunocompromised, insert tooth into the gum, taking care to avoid touching the root. Hold in place for several minutes. Decision as to whether to proceed with surgery depends on urgency and possibility of further trauma to the mouth and teeth. If tooth cannot be reimplanted, it should be stored in saline or milk.

Locate missing tooth:
> If tooth not found on examination of mouth and airway, a chest radiograph should be performed. If tooth has been aspirated, discussion with ENT surgeon regarding retrieval should take place.

d) How would you follow this patient up? (4 marks)

> Written referral to dentist (or onsite dental service if available). Information to be included:
>   - Patient's full details.
>   - Details of damage.
>   - Action taken at the time.
>   - Analgesia given and further recommendations for analgesia if required.
>   - Instructions for self-care.
>   - Details of referrer with contact numbers of anaesthetic department/named person to contact.
> In line with Duty of Candour, speak with the patient postoperatively to explain what has happened, give apologies and explain follow-up.
> Letter to be sent to patient documenting all of the above.
> Complete critical incident form.

References

Milne A, Lockie J. Dental damage in anaesthesia. *Anaesth Int Care Med*. 2014; 15 (8): 370–372.

Paolinelis G, Renton T, Djemal S, McDonnell N. *Dental Trauma During Anaesthesia*. London: King's Dental Unit with Safe Anaesthesia Liaison Group; 2012.

5. DAY SURGERY

A 52-year-old man has been admitted for a tympanoplasty on the morning of surgery. He is a longstanding insulin-dependent diabetic who has failed to attend the preoperative assessment clinic.

a) What specific issues does this patient's diabetes present? (30%)

b) How should his diabetes be managed whilst in hospital? (35%)

c) What are the anaesthetic considerations for tympanoplasty? (35%)

September 2011

This question appeared in the year that 'NHS Diabetes Guideline for the Peri-operative Management of the Adult Patient with Diabetes' was issued. In 2015, the AAGBI issued a guideline that aimed to tailor that advice to anaesthetists and to address some updates in recommendations. This may be an opportunity for the College to include a new question on the perioperative management of diabetes in the exam.

a) What specific issues does this patient's diabetes present? (30%)

The question asks for specific issues. The words to underline to help you focus your thoughts are as follows:

> *52-year-old.*
> *Longstanding.*
> *Failed to attend.*
> *Admitted....on the morning of surgery.*

> Longstanding diabetes, now 52 years old:
> • High probability of micro- (retinopathy, neuropathy, nephropathy) and macrovascular (ischaemic heart disease, cerebrovascular disease) complications.
> Failure to attend preoperative assessment:
> • This may be indicative of generalised poor compliance with medical management, which is associated with a greater burden of complications of diabetes.
> • Need to assess recent control by checking glycosylated haemoglobin (HbA1c). HbA1c greater than 69 mmol/mol is associated with increased postoperative complications risk. Non-urgent surgery should be cancelled and diabetes management optimised.
> • Patient has not had instructions on alteration of insulin regimen and may now be at greater risk of perioperative hypo- or hyperglycaemia.
> • Patient may not have starved appropriately preoperatively.

> Admitted on morning of surgery:
  * Limited time to now undertake thorough assessment and investigation. Still need to make a thorough assessment of symptoms and signs suggestive of serious vascular or renal comorbidity. If further investigation and assessment are indicated, non-urgent surgery should be postponed.

b) How should his diabetes be managed whilst in hospital? (35%)

Exogenous insulin is always required for patients who do not produce insulin in order to prevent catabolism, hyperglycaemia and ketosis. During times of stress such as surgery, the release of pro-catabolic hormones exacerbates this situation further. Insulin may be given as an infusion, or, for short periods of starvation and minor surgery, the normal long-acting insulin dose may be relied upon. Regional anaesthesia and opioids both reduce catabolic hormone secretion helping to improve metabolic management perioperatively. It is important to minimise starvation periods in diabetics, both pre- and postoperatively.

> The patient should be first on morning or afternoon list. Should not be on elective evening list as this is likely to lead to excessive starvation time.
> Monitor capillary blood glucose (CBG) hourly if 'basal-bolus' insulin regimen and starvation time is short (one missed meal). Basal insulin provides continuous insulin release. Bolus is omitted with missed meal and then given when eating restarts. Glucose-containing fluids are to be avoided.
> If period of starvation is likely to be prolonged (more than one meal) or if the patient does not use a long-acting inulin, a variable rate intravenous insulin infusion (VRIII) must be commenced on admission, in combination with glucose and potassium containing fluid (0.45% saline with 5% glucose and 0.15% or 0.3% potassium chloride at 25–50 ml/kg/h). When the patient is ready to eat postoperatively and is not suffering from nausea or vomiting, a pre-meal bolus should be given at 30–60 minutes prior to discontinuation of the VRIII to avoid iatrogenic ketoacidosis.
> CBG target 6–10 mmol/l (up to 12 acceptable) for both regimens.
> Hourly CBG monitoring for both and if otherwise indicated.
> Aim to return to eating and mobilising as soon as possible.

c) What are the anaesthetic considerations for tympanoplasty? (35%)

> Local or general anaesthetic: local anaesthetic avoids loss of consciousness, which may make monitoring for hypoglycaemia easier in a diabetic patient.
> Facial nerve monitoring: if intubated, need to allow paralysis to wear off to facilitate this. Supraglottic airway device use depends on the patient's characteristics. Gastroparesis associated with long-standing diabetes may make this choice inappropriate.
> Day case surgery: need to ensure good analgesia and antiemesis in order to facilitate same day discharge. Tympanoplasty tends to be emetogenic. In a diabetic patient, avoidance of nausea and vomiting is even more important in order to facilitate return to normal insulin regimen. Dexamethasone worsens diabetic control and should be avoided. Total intravenous anaesthesia may be considered. Oral analgesia usually sufficient for tympanoplasty, but NSAIDs may not be appropriate in a diabetic patient with renal complications.
> Hypotensive anaesthesia: optimises surgical field but may be inappropriate in the presence of micro- and macrovascular comorbidities.
> Nitrous oxide: avoid due to emetogenesis and gas diffusion into middle ear cavity with the potential for disruption of tympanoplasty grafts (either at the time that the nitrous is being administered or postoperatively as it washes out causing negative pressure in the cavity).
> Optimisation of ventilatory control: low–normal $etCO_2$ required to avoid vasodilatation, which is associated with blood loss and impaired surgical field.

References

Association of Anaesthetists of Great Britain and Ireland. Peri-operative management of the surgical patient with diabetes 2015. *Anaesthesia*. 2015; 70: 1427–1440.

Dhatariya K, Levy N, Kilvert A et al. NHS Diabetes guideline for the perioperative management of the adult patient with diabetes. *Diabetic Med.* 2012; 29: 420–433.

6. GENERAL, UROLOGICAL AND GYNAECOLOGICAL SURGERY

A 52-year-old woman is to undergo laparotomy for ovarian malignancy having completed 3 cycles of primary chemotherapy. She has a BMI of 23 but massive ascites.

What specific features of this case will affect the anaesthetist's approach to the

a) preoperative (50%),

b) intraoperative (25%) and

c) postoperative management (25%) of this patient?

March 2012

Chairman's Report

46.4% pass rate.

This question was generally not answered well. Again, many candidates wrote a generic answer and therefore missed out on valuable marks. The specific features of the case related to the effects of malignancy, chemotherapy, ascites and how the extent of surgery would affect anaesthesia.

Ovarian malignancy risks: familial (including BRCA 1 and 2 genes), obesity, nulliparity. May be secondary from elsewhere such as bowel or breast. Malignant cells slough off and spread to any intra-abdominal surface or organ (hence surgery may result in removal of large numbers of abdominal and pelvic organs, pelvic exenteration, resulting in ureteric diversion and colostomy formation). Lymphatic spread above the diaphragm may occur. Haematogenous spread occurs to lung parenchyma, pleura, skin, central nervous system, bone. Chemotherapy for debulking prior to surgery followed by postoperative chemotherapy is common: paclitaxel and cisplatin are commonly used agents.

In each part of this question, I have tried to make the answers SPECIFIC to this patient. The College has already classified your answer for you into pre-, intra- and postoperative, but this is a clear case where following the alphabet will really help you pull facts from your brain.

a) Preoperative (50%)

Airway:
> Massive ascites will increase risk of reflux – may require draining preoperatively.

Respiratory:

> Pleural effusion. Assess for likelihood: assess exercise tolerance, auscultate and percuss chest. However, the patient is likely to have recent imaging that will show effusions. Significant effusions can be drained preoperatively to improve lung function.

> Massively reduced functional residual capacity due to ascites. Affects V/Q matching and causes basal atelectasis. Consider need to drain preoperatively.

Cardiac:

> Assess for cardiotoxic effects of paclitaxel and cisplatin. Assess exercise tolerance, echo.

> Pericardial effusions. May be indicated by small complexes on ECG and detected on echo.

> Indwelling venous access may already be in situ for chemotherapy. Need to consider when deciding where to place lines for operation. Veins may be difficult to cannulate due to previous treatment and use.

Pharmacology:

> Paclitaxel and cisplatin cause bone marrow suppression (check full blood count), renal damage (check urea and electrolytes), liver dysfunction (check liver function tests and coagulation), and cardiotoxicity (request echo). Discuss with oncologist regarding any other effects of any chemotherapeutic agents that have been received.

> Diuretics may have been used to attempt to alleviate effusions and ascites; therefore, check for electrolyte imbalance that may need correcting.

> Antiemetics: may already be being used to manage nausea and vomiting associated with chemotherapy. Ensure uninterrupted treatment perioperatively.

> Opioids: may already have opioid requirement, which will have to be considered when planning postoperative analgesia.

Haematological:

> Risk of deep vein thrombosis (procoagulant factors released in cancer state, venous obstruction due to intra-abdominal mass and ascites). Some patients may have already been receiving prophylaxis. Perioperative prophylaxis plan needs addressing.

> Liver dysfunction may cause coagulopathy: check clotting, manage appropriately.

> Risk of significant bleeding with removal of many intra-abdominal and pelvic organs. Cross-match preoperatively.

Immune, infection:

> Bone marrow suppression: renders patient at greater risk of infection. Assess for possible infections preoperatively.

Renal:

> Risk of renal toxicity from chemotherapy. If there is renal impairment, consider impact on drugs to be used intraoperatively.

Liver:

> Risk of liver dysfunction from chemotherapy, from cholestasis secondary to massive ascites and from malignant deposit. Check liver function tests. Consider impact on choice of drugs to be used.

Nutrition:

> Malnutrition and dehydration risk due to anorexia, chemotherapy, ascites. May need intravenous fluid preoperatively and dietician involvement from the outset.

b) Intraoperative (25%)

Airway:
> Intubate: major, prolonged, abdominal surgery, sometimes head down position, risk of reflux from raised intra-abdominal pressure.

Respiratory:
> Reduced functional residual capacity due to ascites. Ensure thorough pre-oxygenation in head up position.
> Capnography and arterial blood gas monitoring to target adequate ventilatory parameters, care with high airway pressures due to ascites (until abdomen opened).

Cardiac:
> Two large cannulae – risk of significant bleeding.
> Arterial line: beat-to-beat blood pressure monitoring and electrolyte monitoring useful in face of large fluid shifts.
> Cardiac output monitoring: massive fluid shifts due to further loss of ascites (this must be done slowly) and large amounts of tissue removal.

Neurological:
> Pain management: NSAIDs and paracetamol may be contraindicated if there is renal and liver dysfunction. May already be on opioids; therefore, higher doses may be required. Avoid renally excreted opioids in the presence of significant renal dysfunction. Consideration of epidural if clotting permits. Consideration of rectus sheath catheters for opioid-sparing effect.

Haematological:
> Significant blood loss may occur due to ooze from many tissue surfaces. Monitor with near patient testing for haemoglobin and coagulation.
> Risk of DVT: automated intermittent leg compression devices intraoperatively.

Immune, infection:
> Bone marrow suppression renders patient at greater risk of infection. Scrupulous asepsis required.

Cutaneomusculoskeletal:
> Prolonged surgery, care with positioning and padding. Care if known bony metastases.

Renal:
> Catheterise to monitor urine output to assist with managing fluid balance in the presence of significant fluid shifts.
> Use of drugs whose metabolism is independent of renal function if patient has renal impairment, e.g. remifentanil infusion, atracurium.
> Risk of liver dysfunction; consider drug suitability before giving.

Metabolic:
> Prolonged surgery: monitor temperature, use under body warming mattress, warmed fluids, insulating hat.
> Arterial blood gas analysis to monitor lactate and base excess in the presence of large fluid shifts.

c) Postoperative management (25%)

Consideration of location of postoperative care: level 1 or 2 if, for example, there has been significant blood loss or if there is significant preoperative or intraoperative organ dysfunction. May possibly need level 3 care.

Respiratory:
> Postoperative oxygen especially if opioid PCA. May need additional respiratory support such as noninvasive ventilation.

Cardiac:
> Postoperative heart rate, blood pressure and cardiac output monitoring to guide ongoing fluids (reaccumulation of ascites may result in intravascular depletion).

Neurological:

> Pain management to be optimised by involving the acute pain management team. Oxycodone or fentanyl may be indicated if there is renal impairment.

Haematological:

> Risk of DVT: use of thromboembolic deterrent stockings, low-molecular-weight heparin if no contraindications, early mobilisation.

Renal:

> Urine output monitoring to help guide ongoing fluid management.

Nutrition:

> Re-establish enteral nutrition as soon as possible or consideration of parenteral nutrition if this is likely to be delayed.

Reference

Morosan M, Popham P. Anaesthesia for gynaecological oncological surgery. *Contin Educ Anaesth Crit Care Pain*. 2014; 14 (2): 63–68.

A 45-year-old man is scheduled for a laparoscopic Nissen fundoplication under general anaesthesia. He is graded ASA 1.

a) Describe how <u>laparoscopy</u> can cause adverse effects in this patient. (70%)

b) How may these effects be minimised? (30%)

September 2013

Chairman's Report

72.5% pass rate.

This was a modification of a question on the adverse effects of abdominal laparoscopy previously used in the May 2006 paper. The effect of steep head-up position and not Trendelenberg tilt was not appreciated by a number of candidates. A significant number of answers incorrectly referred to the effects of a Trendelenberg position raising intracranial and intraocular pressure. The question was otherwise answered with a good systematic approach to the physiological effects of a pneumoperitoneum and the adverse effects of performing a laparoscopy.

This question is virtually identical to one from 2006, and then recurs in 2016. I am slightly unclear as to why the College underlined the word laparoscopy when they clearly wanted you to discuss issues related to the position of the patient. Generally, though, if they mention the type of operation a patient is having, it is for a reason. Cancer surgery? Minimal opportunity for delaying for optimisation, consider impact of radio- and chemotherapy. Pelvic or lower abdominal laparoscopic surgery? Often Trendelenberg position, with its attendant issues. Ear surgery? Consider nausea and vomiting. Day case surgery? Think about optimising analgesia and antiemesis in order to get the patient out within 24 hours. However, note that the College was approving of those who had used a 'good systematic approach'.

a) Describe how <u>laparoscopy</u> can cause adverse effects in this patient. (70%)

Trocars:
> Unintended visceral or vascular injury.
> Risk of intravascular carbon dioxide embolus.
> Surgical emphysema.

Steep head-up position:
> Airway: accidental extubation.
> Cardiovascular: venous pooling, decreased venous return, decreased cardiac output, hypotension, myocardial ischaemia.
> Neurological: reduced intracerebral perfusion pressure.
> Cutaneomusculoskeletal: pressure points, security on table.

Pneumoperitoneum:

> **Respiratory:**
  • Reduced functional residual capacity (already reduced due to anaesthesia), atelectasis, V/Q mismatch, reduced compliance.
  • Carbon dioxide absorption increasing $PaCO_2$.
  • Risk of barotrauma due to elevated airway pressures used to maintain tidal volume and $etCO_2$ against raised intraperitoneal pressure.

> **Cardiac:**
  • On inflation, autotransfusion from splanchnic vessels.
  • Then, compression of inferior vena cava causing reduced venous return in the face of increased intrathoracic pressure. Stroke volume falls resulting in reflex tachycardia.
  • Compression of aorta and release of neurohumoral factors (renin–angiotensin–aldosterone system, catecholamines) cause an increase in systemic vascular resistance and so cardiac output is maintained overall. Myocardial workload is therefore increased, risking ischaemia in susceptible individuals.

> **Neurological:**
>   - Raised $PaCO_2$ (if uncorrected) causes cerebral vasodilatation.
>   - If cardiac output is significantly reduced in the head-up position, may compromise cerebral perfusion pressure.

> **Gastrointestinal:**
>   - Patient already at risk of reflux as evidenced by the need for this surgery – further risk due to raised intra-abdominal pressure.
>   - Compromised splanchnic blood flow.

> **Haematological:**
>   - Venous stasis, risk of deep vein thrombosis.

> **Renal:**
>   - Raised intra-abdominal pressure causes increased renal vascular resistance, with raised renal venous pressure causing reduced glomerular flow rate, reduced urine output.
>   - Risk of acute kidney injury in susceptible individuals or with prolonged surgery.

> **Hepatic:**
>   - Reduced liver perfusion.

b) How may these effects be minimised? (30%)

In the exam, you could present your answer in two columns: the adverse effects alongside methods by which the risks can be minimised.

Patient selection (ensure that the patient has sufficient cardiac and respiratory reserve to cope with the process), good surgical technique (thus minimising risk of trocar damage and limiting duration and pressure of pneumoperitoneum).

A: Check tube position after movement, inflation of abdomen.

B: Intubate, positive pressure ventilation to control PaO_2 and $PaCO_2$, use PEEP.

C: Ensure adequate circulating volume, management of hypotension with inotropic rather than vasopressor drugs, ensure that airway pressures do not further compromise cardiac output. Consider intra-arterial blood pressure monitoring and cardiac output monitoring for long procedures or in patients with cardiac comorbidities. Avoid excessive intraperitoneal pressure and limit duration.

D: Adequate filling and blood pressure.

G: Minimise face mask ventilation pre-intubation to reduce gastric distension and obscuration of surgical field, thus reducing risk of stomach injury. Deflate stomach with oro- or nasogastric tube if this has occurred. Intubation reduces risk of reflux due to raised intra-abdominal pressure. Rapid sequence or modified rapid sequence induction may be indicated for pre-existing reflux.

H: Thromboembolic deterrent stockings, pneumatic compression devices, postoperative low-molecular-weight heparin.

J: Padding, ensure secure positioning on the table.

K: Adequate filling and blood pressure.

L: Adequate filling and blood pressure.

Reference

Hayden P, Cowman S. Anaesthesia for laparoscopic surgery. *Contin Educ Anaesth Crit Care Pain*. 2011; 11 (5): 177–180.

A 45-year-old patient is reviewed in the preoperative assessment clinic prior to surgery for excision of a phaeochromocytoma.

a) What are the characteristic symptoms (15%) and signs (30%) of a phaeochromocytoma?

b) Which specific biochemical (10%) and radiological (5%) investigations might confirm the diagnosis of a phaeochromocytoma?

c) What therapeutic options are available to optimise the cardiovascular system prior to surgery? (40%)

March 2014

Chairman's Report

44.7% pass rate.

Most candidates knew the radiological/diagnostic tests for this condition. Some candidates confused the signs and symptoms of phaeochromocytoma with carcinoid syndrome and thereby lost marks. Most candidates knew that alpha blockade had to be started before beta blockade but did not mention optimizing circulating volume, nor drugs such as calcium channel blockers and magnesium.

Phaeochromocytomas are catecholamine-secreting neuroendocrine tumours usually arising from the adrenal medulla. Some are malignant (risk of spread to liver), some are inherited in an autosomal dominant manner, some are bilateral. When hereditary, they may be part of a multiple endocrine neoplastic (MEN) syndrome or in association with neuroectodermal dysplasia, e.g. Von Hippel-Lindau or Von-Recklinghausen's. They predominantly secrete noradrenaline, followed by adrenaline and then, to a much lesser extent, dopamine. However, familial ones predominantly secrete adrenaline. They affect both genders and present mainly in the third to fifth decade of life.

a) What are the characteristic symptoms (15%) and signs (30%) of a phaeochromocytoma?

	Symptoms	Signs
Respiratory	Shortness of breath, orthopnoea, reduced exercise tolerance.	Crackles on auscultation (pulmonary oedema due to heart failure due to cardiomyopathy).
Cardiovascular	Palpitations, ischaemic chest pain.	Hypertension, tachycardia, tachyarrhythmias.
Neurological	Severe headache, anxiety, visual disturbance due to malignant hypertension.	Tremor. Hypertensive encephalopathy: altered mental state, focal neurological signs, seizures.
Gastrointestinal	Nausea, vomiting, abdominal pain (splanchnic vasoconstriction).	
Metabolic	Sweating.	Weight loss.

b) Which specific biochemical (10%) and radiological (5%) investigations might confirm the diagnosis of a phaeochromocytoma?

Biochemical:
> Plasma and urinary metanephrine, normetanephrine, dopamine and homovanillic acid.

Radiological:
> MRI or CT will confirm diagnosis in patient with positive biochemical diagnosis.
> MIBG (meta-iodobenzylguanidine) scanning important for assessing extra-adrenal tumours or adrenal tumours with risk of spread. MIBG is a radiopharmaceutical agent, similar in structure to noradrenaline, so is taken up by adrenergic neurones and concentrated in phaeochromocytomas or paragangliomas.

c) What therapeutic options are available to optimise the cardiovascular system prior to surgery? (40%)

Overall aims: reduce blood pressure and systemic vascular resistance, fill the circulation, control tachycardia, aim to see a consequent improvement in cardiac function.

Alpha blockers:
> Start one to two weeks preoperatively.
> Lowers blood pressure.
> Increases intravascular capacity – adequate filling of patient must then take place, monitor with serial haematocrits.
> Reduced afterload reduces myocardial strain and dysfunction.
> Reduces chance of hypertensive surges with tumour manipulation.
> Non-selective α blocker; phenoxybenzamine. Irreversible. Protects against blood pressure surges with tumour manipulation. BUT α_2 blockade prevents presynaptic noradrenaline reuptake, resulting in uninhibited noradrenaline release and consequent tachycardia via β_1 receptors, and can cause resistant hypotension postoperatively. Must be stopped a couple of days before surgery.
> Selective α_1 blocker; doxazosin, prazosin. Does not block α_2 receptors so avoids tachycardia. However, they are competitive inhibitors and so may be overwhelmed by catecholamine release with tumour manipulation.

Calcium channel blockers:
> May be used in addition to α blocker if resistant hypertension, or instead of α blocker if hypertension is mild.
> Blocks noradrenaline-induced influx of calcium.

Beta blockers:
> To control tachycardia caused by either non-selective α blockade or adrenaline/dopamine secreting tumour.
> Started AFTER α blocker, or blockade of vasodilatory β_2 receptors will cause worsening of hypertension in presence of ongoing action of noradrenaline on α receptors, and heart will lose β_1-mediated inotropy whilst afterload still high, which may precipitate myocardial dysfunction and heart failure.
> Selective β_1 receptor antagonists such as metoprolol or atenolol are used.

Reference
Connor D, Boumphrey S. Perioperative care of phaeochromocytoma. *BJA Educ.* 2016; 16 (5): 153–158.

A patient is to receive a cadaveric renal transplant.

a) Detail the aspects of your preoperative assessment specific to chronic kidney disease (CKD). (11 marks)

b) How can the function of the transplanted kidney be optimised intraoperatively? (3 marks)

c) How may this patient's postoperative pain be optimally managed? (3 marks)

d) Explain why some common postoperative analgesic drugs should be avoided. (3 marks)

September 2014

Chairman's Report

59.1% pass rate.

Overall, this question was answered well and was a very strong discriminator between candidates. Weaker candidates tended to ignore the anaesthetic implications of 1) diseases which lead to chronic renal failure, 2) the importance of preserving dialysis catheters/fistulae sites, 3) the implications of a prior failed renal transplantation and any associated immunosuppressive therapy, and most surprisingly 4) the need for preoperative investigations. Inexperience is the most likely cause of these omissions.

a) Detail the aspects of your preoperative assessment specific to chronic kidney disease (CKD). (11 marks)

Issues relate to:
> CKD itself.
> Underlying cause of the CKD.
> Management of CKD.
> Implications of possible previous transplant *(and I will freely admit I would never have thought of this issue if it hadn't been in the Chairman's Report!).*

Airway:
> Some causes of CKD may contribute to a difficult airway, e.g. scleroderma.

Respiratory:
> Assess for fluid overload.
> Patient may be immunosuppressed due to drugs or disease – assess for possibility of respiratory infection.
> Continuous ambulatory peritoneal dialysis (CAPD) fluid should be drained preoperatively as it may cause diaphragmatic splinting, basal atelectasis, shunt.

Cardiovascular:
> Patients with CKD at risk of accelerated coronary artery disease. Assess symptoms, check recent ECG.
> Hypertension may be underlying cause or result from CKD. Check for end-organ damage in the form of left ventricular hypertrophy on ECG and echo.
> Fistulae/vascaths must be preserved. Do not cannulate or take blood pressure on fistula arm, avoid pressure on it intraoperatively.
> At risk of calcified valvular lesions resulting in stenosis – assess symptoms, auscultate heart sounds, echo if indicated.
> Up-to-date ECG, echo and exercise testing should be done in work-up for transplant list.

Neurological:
> Autonomic neuropathy related to uraemia and diabetes mellitus. Risk of delayed gastric emptying and possible need for proton pump inhibitor premedication and rapid sequence induction.

Endocrine:
> If patient has diabetes mellitus, use variable rate insulin infusion.
> In the absence of diabetes, the patient may still have impaired glucose tolerance due to steroid treatment.
> If having steroid treatment, may need perioperative supplementation.
> Patient may have secondary hyperparathyroidism: check calcium and phosphate levels.

Pharmacology:
> Suxamethonium for rapid sequence induction may be contraindicated in the presence of elevated serum potassium.
> Variable rate insulin infusion if diabetic, or management of oral hypoglycaemic agents according to AAGBI guidelines.
> Omit angiotensin converting enzyme inhibitor or angiotensin II receptor antagonist prior to surgery to avoid hypotension. All other antihypertensives to be continued.
> If patient has previous transplant, may be taking steroids and other immunosuppressive drugs (e.g. tacrolimus, cyclosporin). Even if transplant has failed, these drugs need to remain therapeutic to avoid rejection, so seek advice from renal physicians regarding dosing perioperatively, whilst nil by mouth.

Gastrointestinal:
> Consider autonomic neuropathy due to chronic kidney disease (or diabetes mellitus). Premedication with proton pump inhibitor and rapid sequence induction should be considered.

Haematological:
> May have anaemia due to a variety of underlying reasons: chronic disease, impaired erythropoiesis, blood loss from dialysis, gastrointestinal loss.
> Check full blood count, ensure up-to-date group and save.
> Thrombocytopathy associated with renal failure may contraindicate regional anaesthesia, but this is improved by dialysis and therefore unlikely to be an issue.

Immune, infection:
> Susceptible to infection due to immunosuppression of disease state and/or drugs. Check white cell count; consider urinary tract, respiratory system, and vascular or peritoneal access as possible sources of infection.

Renal:
> Assess fluid status. Some patients with CKD are anuric, some still pass urine. Ensure patient is not hypovolaemic if recent haemodialysis as this increases risk of perioperative hypotension.
> Check electrolytes – may require haemodialysis preoperatively. Abnormalities predispose to arrhythmia.

b) How can the function of the transplanted kidney be optimised intraoperatively? (3 marks)

Airway, respiratory:
> Optimise gas exchange to support oxygen delivery, minimise risk of respiratory acidosis.

Cardiovascular:
> Optimise filling with cardiac output monitoring, central venous pressure monitoring (12–14 cm H_2O).
> Aim for normotension (MAP 90 mm Hg or more in hypertensives).
> Adequate patient warming to avoid vasoconstriction.

Endocrine:
> Glucose control if indicated.

Pharmacology:
> Do not give nephrotoxins including starch solutions.

Immune, infection:

> Early commencement of immunosuppression.

c) How may this patient's postoperative pain be optimally managed? (3 marks)

> Regular pain assessment and management of anxiety through explanation and reassurance.
> Regular paracetamol.
> NSAIDs contraindicated due to effect on renal perfusion.
> Wound catheters.
> PCA: fentanyl and oxycodone do not accumulate in renal failure (graft may not function immediately).
> Epidural: used in some centres, may be contraindicated by recent heparin administration for dialysis. Need to ensure that hypotension does not result.

d) Explain why some common postoperative analgesic drugs should be avoided. (3 marks)

> NSAIDs: reduce renal perfusion, poor perfusion results in reduced function, and can be directly nephrotoxic.
> Morphine: metabolised primarily in the liver to active metabolites that are excreted by the kidney. Postoperative renal impairment (i.e. a graft that is not immediately fully functional) might result in accumulation of these metabolites and cause drowsiness, hypotension and respiratory depression. Smaller doses with longer dosing intervals for short time periods are acceptable.
> Codeine and dihydrocodeine: active metabolites renally excreted so increased risk of sedation, respiratory depression and hypotension in renal failure.

Reference

Mayhew D, Ridgway D, Hunter J. Update on the intraoperative management of adult cadaveric renal transplantation. *BJA Educ*. 2016; 16 (2): 53–57.

A 75-year-old man is having a transurethral resection of the prostate (TURP) under spinal anaesthesia.

a) Which clinical features would make you suspect the patient has TURP syndrome? (6 marks)

b) List the intraoperative factors that may increase the risk of developing TURP syndrome. (7 marks)

c) How would you manage suspected TURP syndrome? (7 marks)

March 2015

Chairman's Report

84.5% pass rate; 4.3% of candidates received a poor fail.

Overall this question was answered very well and was only a moderate discriminator between candidates. However weaker candidates did not mention CNS features and many had not read the question thoroughly and ignored the information that the patient had received neuraxial anaesthesia. Very few candidates mentioned repeated measurements of sodium and osmolality. This clinical problem is an old chestnut which all trainees should be able to manage safely and effectively.

TURP syndrome:

> *Excessive irrigation fluid (glycine 1.5%, 220 mosmol/kg) absorbed into circulation.*
> *Occurs between 15 minutes and 24 hours after start of surgery.*
> *Volume changes cause cardiovascular complications.*
> *Hyponatraemia and hyposmolality cause neurological complications. Free water absorption into brain parenchyma causes raised intracranial pressure, water intoxication, cerebral oedema. Results in burning sensation in the face and hands, headache, visual disturbance, confusion, restlessness, convulsions, coma.*
> *Glycine (an inhibitory neurotransmitter) toxicity causes nausea, headache, transient blindness, myocardial depression. Potentiates NMDA receptor activity causing encephalopathy and seizures. Magnesium stabilises NMDA receptors so useful in managing seizures.*

a) Which clinical features would make you suspect the patient has TURP syndrome? (6 marks)

Respiratory:
> Tachypnoea, hypoxia, respiratory distress, pulmonary oedema.

Cardiovascular:
> Hypertension (due to volume overload) with reflex bradycardia, then acute congestive cardiac failure, hypotension, cardiovascular collapse.
> Broadening QRS complexes, T wave inversion due to hyponatraemia.

Neurological:
> Burning sensation in the face and hands, headache, visual disturbance, confusion, restlessness, convulsions, coma.
> Absence of signs of high block (as this is a differential diagnosis, although both may happen at the same time).

Gastrointestinal:
> Nausea and vomiting.

b) List the intraoperative factors that may increase the risk of developing TURP syndrome. (7 marks)

> Pressure of irrigation fluid: bag height to remain less than 70 cm above the patient.
> Large quantities of irrigation fluid used.
> Low venous pressure (hypotensive or hypovolaemic patient).
> Prolonged surgery (more than an hour).
> Large blood loss (large numbers of open veins increases rate of absorption).
> Capsular or bladder perforation, allowing fluid into the peritoneum, from where it is rapidly absorbed.
> Large prostate.

c) How would you manage suspected TURP syndrome? (7 marks)

This is an emergency situation and I would call for help and manage and treat the patient simultaneously adopting an ABC approach.

Alert the theatre team, stop surgery as soon as possible, stop further irrigation fluid.

A, B:
> 100% oxygen.
> Auscultate chest, check saturations.
> Intubate if necessary.
> Consider intravenous furosemide for pulmonary oedema (but may exacerbate hyponatraemia) or mannitol (100 ml 20%).

C:
> Atropine, inotropes and vasopressors may be required.
> Stop intravenous fluids.
> Take blood for sodium, osmolality and haemoglobin.
> Site arterial line and check blood gas.

D:
> Manage seizures with lorazepam or magnesium.
> If serum sodium less than 120 mmol/l or severe symptoms of hyponatraemia, give 3% sodium chloride to raise sodium by 1 mmol/h (do not raise too rapidly or may cause central pontine myelinolysis).

Level 2 or 3 admission for supportive treatment, ongoing monitoring of osmolality, haemoglobin and sodium.

Reference

O'Donnell A, Foo I. Anaesthesia for transurethral resection of the prostate. *Contin Educ Anaesth Crit Care Pain*. 2009; 9 (3): 92–96.

A 26-year-old patient with stage 4B Hodgkin's disease (spread to lymph nodes and other organs) requires an open splenectomy.

a) List the specific factors that are of importance when planning your anaesthetic management. (10 marks)

b) Outline the options for providing postoperative analgesia for this patient and give a possible disadvantage of each. (6 marks)

c) Which vaccinations should this patient receive and what is the optimal timing of these? (4 marks)

September 2015

Chairman's Report

38.8% pass rate.

Many examiners marking this question felt that either the candidates had not read the question as carefully as they should have done, or they lacked knowledge of the implications of Hodgkin's lymphoma and its treatment for anaesthesia. Rather than focusing on specific factors of importance many candidates wrote about general problems when anaesthetising for a splenectomy. This was reflected in the pass rate.

Hodgkin's Lymphoma:

> *Cancer of the lymphatic system therefore presenting with lymphadenopathy, splenomegaly, hepatomegaly.*
> *B symptoms: fever, night sweats, weight loss, itch, fatigue.*
> *Stages:*
>   • *I: single lymph node involvement (or Ie, single extralymphatic site).*
>   • *II: two or more lymph nodes, same side of the diaphragm (or one lymph node plus contiguous extralymphatic site IIE).*
>   • *III: lymph nodes on both sides of diaphragm, which may include the spleen (IIIS) and/or contiguous extralymphatic site (IIIE, IIIES).*
>   • *IV: disseminated involvement of one or more extralymphatic organs, e.g. liver.*
>   • *If B symptoms absent, add A to the stage; if present, B. S denotes splenic involvement; X, bulky disease.*
>   • *Treatment is with chemo- and radiotherapy.*
>   • *Splenectomy may be indicated due to its sheer size or hypersplenism, i.e. excessive destruction of blood cells and platelets.*

a) List the specific factors that are of importance when planning your anaesthetic management. (10 marks)

As with the question concerning ovarian malignancy, think about the disease process, the treatment so far and the operation.

Airway:

> Upper airway may be compromised by lymph nodes in neck/oropharynx. Meticulous airway assessment.
> Potential for airway compromise by mediastinal mass (cough, dyspnoea, hoarse voice, orthopnoea, syncope with positional change or no symptoms at all). Compression may be at the tracheal or bronchial level. Establish what position the patient is least symptomatic in. Assess with CT thorax. Plan A may include keeping the patient spontaneously ventilating until airway secured, plan B rigid bronchoscopy.
> May have mucositis from chemotherapy. Care with airway instrumentation.

Respiratory:

> Risk of atelectasis and pneumonia due to airway collapse caused by lymph nodes and immunocompromised state. CXR, CT thorax.
> Bleomycin confers lifelong susceptibility to pulmonary toxicity with exposure to high oxygen concentrations. Oxygen saturations to be maintained at 88%–92%, minimising supplemental oxygen where feasible.

Cardiovascular:

> Compression of major vessels or even heart due to mediastinal lymph nodes: risk of cardiovascular collapse under anaesthesia. Check CT thorax.
> Risk of cardiac dysfunction due to chemotherapy.
> Mediastinal radiotherapy may cause damage to valves, vessels, pericardium. Echo to check for myocardial compression, ventricular dysfunction and pericardial effusion.
> May have central venous access/port for chemotherapy.

Neurological:

> Risk of compression of nerves and even spinal cord by lymphoma mass.
> Risk of peripheral or autonomic neuropathies (effect on gastric emptying, may necessitate antacid premedication and RSI) due to chemotherapeutic agents.

Pharmacology:

> Consider the side effects of chemotherapy.

Gastrointestinal:

> May be malnourished due to anorexia associated with treatment, painful mouth due to mucositis, fullness of abdomen from splenomegaly.

Haematological:

> May be pancytopenic, with low platelets and low haemaglobin. This may need to be corrected prior to surgery. Regional anaesthesia may be contraindicated.
> Significant blood loss may be encountered intraoperatively. Plan for adequate intravenous access and cross-match.

Immune, infection:

> Immunocompromised due to disease and chemotherapy; assess for intercurrent infection. Meticulous infection control essential.

Cutaneomusculoskeletal:

> Thrombocytopaenia associated with easy bruising, bleeding from minor cuts etc. Care with positioning and padding.
> Patient may be oedematous from hypoalbuminaemia associated with liver impairment or nephrotic syndrome. Thin, fragile overlying skin, difficulty with venous access.

Renal:

> Risk of renal dysfunction due to chemotherapy.
> Risk of nephrotic syndrome, obstruction of renal vessels or ureters, lymphogranulomatous infiltration of parenchyma, amyloid and consequent renal dysfunction.
> Renal dysfunction impacts on perioperative drug choices and increases the importance of avoiding dehydration and hypotension as these compound the nephrotoxic process.

Liver:

> Risk of liver dysfunction due to chemotherapy or disease: may result in disordered coagulation, may contraindicate regional anaesthesia, may impact on anaesthetic drug handling.

b) Outline the options for providing postoperative analgesia for this patient and give a possible disadvantage of each. (6 marks)

> Oral analgesics: insufficient on their own. NSAIDs may be contraindicated in the presence of renal dysfunction; paracetamol dose may need adjusting in the presence of liver dysfunction. Oral morphine may accumulate in the presence of renal dysfunction.
> Epidural analgesia: may be contraindicated due to thrombocytopaenia and even coagulation disturbance if there is liver involvement. Cardiovascular instability may occur as high block would be required. High block may compromise respiratory function if the patient already has compromise due to mediastinal disease.

> Paravertebral block: avoids the cardiovascular instability that may result from epidural but may still be contraindicated due to thrombocytopenia or disordered clotting.
> Patient-controlled analgesia (PCA): may need high doses to achieve adequate pain relief. Long-acting opioid such as morphine may accumulate in the presence of renal dysfunction, causing respiratory compromise, narcosis. Fentanyl or oxycodone PCA may be an alternative.
> Rectus sheath and transverse abdominis plane blocks: do not manage visceral pain but have a role in reducing analgesic requirements. Might not achieve cover of proximal end of wound. May be feasible at platelet levels where neuraxial blocks would be contraindicated.

c) Which vaccinations should this patient receive and what is the optimal timing of these? (4 marks)

Initial vaccinations at least two (ideally four to six) weeks preoperatively, or two weeks afterwards, and three months after completion of chemo- or radiotherapy:

> Haemophilus influenza b.
> Pneumococcus (booster dose every five years).
> Meningitis B and C.

Annually:
> Influenza.

References

Allan N, Siller C, Breen A. Anaesthetic implications of chemotherapy. *Contin Educ Anaesth Crit Care Pain*. 2012; 12 (2): 52–56.

Davies J et al (British Committee for Standards in Haematology). Review of guidelines for the prevention and treatment of infections in patients with an absent or dysfunctional spleen. *Br J Haematol*. 2011; 155 (3): 308–317.

a) <u>List</u> and <u>briefly state the reasons</u> for the cardiovascular (7 marks) and respiratory (4 marks) effects of laparoscopy in the head-up position for a Nissen fundoplication (anti-reflux procedure).

b) How may these effects be minimised? (9 marks)

March 2016

Chairman's Report

54.5% pass rate.

This question was judged to be of moderate difficulty. It would appear from their answers that many candidates had not seen a Nissen fundoplication and were unable to go back to first principles and talk about the effects of laparoscopy in the head-up position. Also, candidates failed to read part (a) of the question and so did not give the cardiovascular and respiratory effects <u>and</u> their causes.

This is virtually identical to the question from March 2013, and so well-prepared candidates should have been ready for it. This time, the College has been kind enough to tell people that a Nissen's is performed in a head-up position and has changed part (a) so that they are only asking about cardiovascular and respiratory effects. As a moderately difficult question, a score of 12–13/20 would have been required to pass.

A 52-year-old woman, who has completed 3 cycles of primary chemotherapy for ovarian malignancy, is to undergo an open laparotomy for surgical treatment of her disease. She has massive ascites. How do the <u>specific features</u> of this case affect your approach to the patient with regard to:

a) Preoperative assessment? (12 marks)

b) Intraoperative management? (8 marks)

September 2016

Chairman's Report

39.1% pass rate.

This question was not well answered. Candidates tended to talk about general principles of perioperative management rather than those issues that are specific to a patient having surgery as part of treatment for cancer such as possible bone marrow suppression or other organ damage due to chemo- or radiotherapy, cachexia, pleural or abdominal effusions and difficult venous access, to name but a few.

This question is very similar to one from March 2012, the only difference being that it doesn't ask about postoperative management this time. As with cadaveric renal transplant and splenectomy for lymphoma, consider the issues relating to the disease process itself, the treatment of that disease and finally the operation the patient is to have.

A patient is to receive a cadaveric renal transplant.

a) Detail the aspects of your preoperative assessment specific to chronic kidney disease (CKD). (11 marks)

b) How can the function of the transplanted kidney be optimised intraoperatively? (3 marks)

c) How may this patient's postoperative pain be optimally managed? (3 marks)

d) Explain why some common postoperative analgesic drugs should be avoided or used with caution. (3 marks)

March 2017

Chairman's Report

42.1% pass rate.

Renal transplantation is the most frequently undertaken form of transplant surgery, but it seemed that many candidates had not had any practical experience of it. This was particularly noticeable in the answers to part (b), improving the function of the transplanted kidney intraoperatively, and part (c), management of postoperative pain. However, even candidates who have never seen a renal transplant operation should know the principles of analgesic use in renal failure.

This question is identical to that from September 2014 and very similar to the one about anaesthetising a patient with stage 4 CKD from March 2012 (see Perioperative Medicine chapter). Only 42.1% of candidates passed. Have I convinced you yet of the importance of looking at topics and questions that have previously featured in the exam? The question from 2012 asked about the 'organ system effects' of CKD that must be considered – you therefore wouldn't include details about the medications the patient is currently taking. However, in 2014 and 2017, the wording changes to 'detail the aspects of your preoperative assessment specific to CKD', at which point you do need to include F in your alphabet.

A 35-year-old woman presents for splenectomy for idiopathic/immune thrombocytopenic purpura, which is not controlled with medical management.

a) Which vaccinations should this patient receive (3 marks) and when should they be given? (2 marks)

b) List three immunological functions of the spleen in the adult. (3 marks)

c) What are the preoperative considerations related to this patient's condition? (8 marks)

d) Describe the rationale for (1 mark) and principles of (3 marks) conservative management for traumatic splenic rupture.

September 2017

Chairman's Report

34.4% pass rate.

The examiners considered this to be a difficult question, and this would seem to be confirmed by the pass rate. Most marks were available in section (c), which asked for preoperative considerations specifically related to the patient's condition. This would include such things as steroid dependence, anaemia, or antibodies due to previous blood product transfusions. Many candidates answered in too generic a fashion, including only non-specific considerations for anaesthesia for major surgery.

a) Which vaccinations should this patient receive (3 marks) and when should they be given? (2 marks)

Initial vaccinations at least two (ideally four to six) weeks preoperatively, or two weeks afterwards:

> Haemophilus influenza b.
> Pneumococcus (booster dose every five years).
> Meningitis B and C.

Annually:
> Influenza.

b) List three immunological functions of the spleen in the adult. (3 marks)

> Synthesis of antibodies and immune proteins that facilitate phagocytosis.
> Removal from circulation of antibody-coated blood cells and bacteria.
> Reservoir of monocytes that can specialise into dendritic cells and macrophages.

c) What are the preoperative considerations related to this patient's condition? (8 marks)

Splenectomy is undertaken to stop the splenic destruction of platelets. It is indicated if there is insufficient or non-sustained improvement with steroid treatment. The patient may therefore have a very low platelet count preoperatively, and immunoglobulin infusions may be utilised to give a temporary boost. If the platelet count is critically low, there is a risk of spontaneous and catastrophic bleeding, and platelet transfusions may be required.

Airway:
> Risk of swollen soft tissues and tongue due to multiple haematomas with critically low platelet count.
> Difficult airway must be anticipated – plan for airway management involving minimal trauma.

Cardiovascular:
> Aim for minimal surges in blood pressure as bleeding may be precipitated – optimise pain relief, consider use of remifentanil infusion and obtund response to laryngoscopy.

Neurological:
> Pain control plan: neuraxial techniques contraindicated in the presence of low platelet count. Nonsteroidal anti-inflammatory drugs should be avoided.
> Avoidance of surges in blood pressure and straining on tube (use of muscle relaxant or remifentanil) – critically low platelet count renders patient at risk of catastrophic intracerebral bleeding.

Endocrine:

> Consider need for perioperative steroid supplementation if the patient has had recent high-dose treatment.

Gastrointestinal:

> Assess for possibility of gastrointestinal haemorrhage. Consideration of need for rapid sequence induction if stomach is therefore 'full'.

Haematological:

> Platelet transfusion may be required if platelet count very low – liaise with haematologist.
> Cross-matched blood must be available due to possibility of major haemorrhage: atypical antibodies may be present due to past blood transfusions.

Immunological, infective:

> Discuss with the haematologist the need for postoperative antibiotic prophylaxis.

Cutaneomusculoskeletal:

> Consider need for padding and care with handling due to risk of bruising and bleeding secondary to low platelet count.

d) Describe the rationale for (1 mark) and principles of (3 marks) conservative management for traumatic splenic rupture.

Rationale:

> Avoidance of major surgery with its attendant risks.
> Retention of splenic immunological function.

Principles – patient selection based on:

> Haemodynamic stability.
> Grading of splenic injury on CT scanning, lower grades being more amenable to conservative management.
> Local availability of radiological interventions for angioembolisation if necessary.
> Absence of need for laparotomy for any other indication.

References

Hildebrand D et al. Modern management of splenic trauma. *BMJ*. 2014; 348: 27–31.
Trimmings A, Walmsley A. Anaesthesia for urgent splenectomy in acute idiopathic thrombocytopenic purpura. *Anaesthesia*. 2009; 64 (2): 226–227.

7. HEAD, NECK, MAXILLO-FACIAL AND DENTAL SURGERY

A 23-year-old man is brought to the emergency department following an assault in a nightclub. He appears to have suffered significant mid-face fractures and is uncooperative with staff. You are asked to accompany him to the CT scanner.

a) Outline the immediate management plan for this patient. (25%)

b) List the options for securing the airway in this case and any advantage or disadvantage of the methods. (25%)

c) What problems should be anticipated before securing the airway? (50%)

September 2012

Chairman's Report

51.3% pass rate.

Answers to this question were generally appropriate. It should be noted that 'securing the airway' using a laryngeal mask airway as a primary technique was not part of the model answer. Perhaps a rapid sequence induction would be 'plan A' rather than an inhalational induction to achieve the definitive airway.

a) Outline the immediate management plan for this patient. (25%)

This is an emergency trauma situation and so I would assess and manage the patient simultaneously following an ABCDE approach.

Call for help (senior anaesthetic and ODP support, maxillofacial or ENT colleague) and a difficult airway trolley.

Airway:
> Allow the patient to adopt a position that is comfortable for breathing.
> Oxygen 15 l/min via non-rebreathe bag.
> Check for airway obstruction by blood, teeth, displaced bone. If posteriorly displaced midface fracture causes loss of airway, then pull midface forward.
> Assess for indications for immediate intubation: dyspnoea, stridor, drooling, voice change.

C-spine control: if the patient is uncooperative, it is not safe to force them into collar and blocks, but bear in mind the possibility of associated injury.

Breathing:
> Assess for associated injuries: auscultate and palpate chest, assess for bilateral chest movement with respiration, palpate trachea.
> Monitor oxygen saturations and respiratory rate.

Cardiovascular:
> Large-bore intravenous access, take blood for cross-match, full blood count, urea and electrolytes, blood glucose.
> Major midface fractures rarely cause significant hypovolaemia, but the patient may have other injuries causing blood loss.

Disability:
> Patient is uncooperative. Possible causes: alcohol; illicit drug use; brain injury; hypoxia due to airway compromise.
> Check GCS and pupils and assess for any obvious lateralising signs that may indicate an associated brain injury.

Exposure:
> Check for signs of other major and immediately life-threatening injuries and manage appropriately.

b) List the options for securing the airway in this case and any advantage or disadvantage of the methods. (25%)

Rapid sequence induction:
> Preferred option due to low likelihood of cooperation and full stomach.
> Requires videolaryngoscope and full difficult airway trolley availability, skilled assistance, presence of maxillo-facial/ENT colleague if considered necessary.
> Plan B supraglottic airway device, plan C surgical cricothyroidotomy/ emergency tracheostomy.

Advantages:
> Rapidly secures the airway.
> Minimal patient cooperation required.
> Maximum protection of airway from contamination by blood or full stomach.

Disadvantages:
> Potential for difficulty intubating once the patient is rendered apnoeic. Depending on gas exchange and level of consciousness, it may not be possible to wake the patient up again, hence the need for full range of airway adjuncts (remembering that nasopharyngeal airway contraindicated due to risk of base of skull fracture).

Other options:
  Awake fibreoptic:
  • Advantages: maintenance of spontaneous ventilation, useful in the presence of distorted anatomy.
  • Disadvantages: specific skills required, does not protect airway from contamination, requires patient cooperation, requires transfer to theatre of potentially unstable patient, view would be obscured if there is airway bleeding.
  Awake tracheostomy:
  • Advantages: avoids a potentially difficult airway.
  • Disadvantages: requires skilled surgeon, patient cooperation, skilled anaesthetist.

c) What problems should be anticipated before securing the airway? (50%)

> Preoxygenation: uncooperative patient, mask may not fit well/cause pain due to fracture. May be done sitting for patient comfort. Consider high-flow nasal oxygen.
> Difficult laryngoscopy: distorted anatomy, obscured view due to blood, neck immobilisation, hence the need for difficult airway trolley, senior anaesthetic assistance and, possibly, ENT or maxillofacial assistance.
> Airway contamination: blood, teeth, full stomach.
> Tube: smaller diameter tube should be available and leave uncut – potential for significant swelling.
> Cardiovascular stability: may be compromised by other injuries. Resuscitation drugs, fluid boluses, full monitoring should all be ready.

> Drugs: consideration of potential interactions of anaesthetic agents with alcohol and illicit drugs.
> Comorbidities: awareness that history may be limited due to patient's lack of ability to cooperate.

Reference

Morosan M, Parbhoo A, Curry N. Anaesthesia and common oral and maxillo-facial emergencies. *Contin Educ Anaesth Crit Care Pain*. 2012; 12 (5): 257–262.

A 54-year-old patient with base of tongue cancer presents for a hemiglossectomy and radial forearm free flap reconstruction.

a) Which specific factors must the anaesthetist consider when assessing this patient prior to surgery? (10 marks)

b) List the benefits of a free flap reconstruction. (2 marks)

c) What are the causes of flap failure and how may they be prevented in the perioperative period? (8 marks)

September 2014

Chairman's Report

31.5% pass rate.

Inexperience probably accounts for the poor pass rate for this question. Weak candidates suggested assessment of a potentially difficult airway as the important preoperative feature but ignored the comorbidities associated with causative factors such as smoking and alcohol consumption. The impacts of major physiological changes that are caused by such prolonged and invasive surgery were ignored. The role of the anaesthetist in influencing free-flap survival was particularly poorly answered.

a) Which specific factors must the anaesthetist consider when assessing this patient prior to surgery? (10 marks)

The question asks for specific factors – think about the patient, the condition that they have, and the operation that is going to be performed. I followed my usual alphabet approach. The stereotypical patient is a smoker, has high alcohol intake, is malnourished due to high alcohol intake and presence of oral cancer, and may have had radiotherapy and chemotherapy already, which will have contributed to the malnourishment and difficult airway.

Airway:
> May be a difficult airway due to tumour and any preceding radiotherapy.
> Consideration needs to be given to airway plan – may include awake fibreoptic intubation or awake tracheostomy depending on assessment.

Respiratory:
> Likely to be smoker: assess for evidence of smoking-related lung disease.
> Smoking increases risk of flap failure.

Cardiovascular:
> Likely to be a smoker: assess for evidence of ischaemic heart disease.
> Smoking-related peripheral vascular disease may increase risk of flap failure.
> Likely to have a history of high alcohol intake: risk of arrhythmia, dilated cardiomyopathy.
> Consider the cardiovascular effects of preceding chemotherapy.
> Vascular access site will be determined by the donor site – ensure confirmation of planned donor site with surgeon before any cannulations.

Neurological:
> If ongoing high alcohol intake, consider the possibility of withdrawal whilst inpatient and treat appropriately.

Gastrointestinal:
> Risk of poor nutrition associated with high alcohol intake, oral cancer, chemotherapy. Increases risk of poor wound healing and flap failure.
> Consideration of preoperative PEG placement to optimise perioperative nutrition.

Haematological:

> Risk of anaemia: associated with high alcohol intake, malnourishment or chronic disease. Impairs wound healing and flap survival.
> Prolonged surgery: mechanical deep vein thrombosis prophylaxis.

Infection, immune:

> Comorbidities increase propensity to infection: assess for possibility of e.g. respiratory infection preoperatively.

Cutaneomusculoskeletal:

> Often very prolonged surgery and possibly malnourished, underweight patient. Meticulous attention to positioning and protection.

Metabolic:

> Prolonged surgery – warming mattress, warmed fluids and core and surface temperature monitoring required.

Psychological:

> Patient anxiety due to potentially life-changing surgery may need pharmacological management.

b) List the benefits of a free flap reconstruction. (2 marks)

What are the benefits of a free flap reconstruction? Consider what the alternatives are, and it helps to organise your thoughts. Without going into too much plastic-surgical detail, an area of body that has had cancer removed could be covered by a graft (skin and subcutaneous tissues that are taken from elsewhere in the body and rely on development of vascular supply from the recipient site to survive) or a flap. The flap can be local (moving a chunk of tissue to cover a defect locally, taking its blood supply with it), pedicled (excising an area of tissue and moving it to some distant part of the body whilst retaining a pedicle through which the original blood supply still flows, for example a transverse rectus abdominis muscle, or TRAM, flap) and finally a free flap (where tissue is completely removed from the donor site and its blood vessels are anastomosed at the recipient site). You can visualise that a graft of skin and subcutaneous tissues alone will not give the functional or cosmetic result of a flap in this case, nor will it necessarily develop sufficient blood supply to survive when covering such a large area. There are no suitable nearby donor sites that could provide a local or pedicled flap, especially as the use of bone in the reconstruction that this patient will have is so critical to the functional and cosmetic outcome.

Better cosmetic outcome than a graft.

> Better functional outcome than graft: bone used to reconstruct a functioning jaw into which dental implants can ultimately be inserted.
> Lack of suitable local donor sites for local or pedicled flap.
> Better coverage than a graft for large and deep defects.
> Better healing and vascularisation than a graft.
> Possibility of retaining innervation as the whole neurovascular bundle can be reanastomosed.
> Better coverage of delicate underlying structures than a graft.

c) What are the causes of flap failure and how may they be prevented in the perioperative period? (8 marks)

Inadequate perfusion	Blood flow $= \dfrac{\Delta P \pi r4}{8\eta l}$ R, radius of vessels: • Maintain normothermia with active warming, and maintain core:peripheral temperature gradient less than 1°C. Avoid postoperative shivering. • Adequate analgesia: transplanted arteries still respond to catecholamines. Consideration of regional anaesthesia. • Use flow-directed therapy to optimise fluid management and to avoid inappropriate use of vasoconstrictors. • Arterial thrombosis: may be triggered by inflammatory reaction due to reperfusion after prolonged ischaemic time. Avoid excessive ischaemic time. May need anticoagulation to avoid arterial thrombosis. ΔP, pressure gradient along vessels: • Maintain blood pressure. Intra-arterial blood pressure monitoring, cardiac output monitoring, keep cardiac output high. • Avoid extramural pressure on arteries: ensure dressings not tight, drains utilised to avoid haematoma. • Avoid poor venous drainage due to thrombosis. Anticoagulation may be required. Maintain normothermia. • Avoid inadequate venous drainage due to external compression. η, viscosity of blood: • Aim for haematocrit of 0.3 as this offers optimum balance between oxygen delivery and blood flow.
Flap oedema	• Minimise flap handling. • Minimise flap ischaemic time. • Avoid excessive fluid therapy with cardiac output monitoring.
Poor wound healing	• Ensure optimum glucose control if diabetic. • Smoking cessation preoperatively. • Management of any pre-existing malnutrition.
Poor oxygen delivery	• Monitor haemoglobin and haematocrit, transfuse if necessary but ensure balance between haemoglobin level and viscosity is maintained. • Supplemental oxygen therapy.
Anastomosis failure	• Maximise surgical technique. • Avoid surges in blood pressure caused by coughing, retching (consider remifentanil or neuromuscular blocker infusion use, optimise nausea and vomiting prophylaxis).

References

Adams J, Charlton P. Anaesthesia for microvascular free tissue transfer. *BJA CEPD Rev*. 2003; 3 (2): 33–37.

Nimalan N, Branford O, Stocks G. Anaesthesia for free flap breast reconstruction. *BJA Educ*. 2016; 16 (5): 162–166.

a) Which investigations are specifically indicated in the preoperative assessment of a patient presenting for thyroidectomy for treated thyrotoxicosis? (5 marks)

b) What particular issues must the anaesthetist consider during the induction, maintenance and extubation phases of anaesthesia for a euthyroid patient having a total thyroidectomy? (11 marks)

c) Describe the specific postoperative problems that may be associated with this operation. (4 marks)

September 2015

Chairman's Report

31.9% pass rate.

The first and last parts of this question on preoperative tests and postoperative considerations were well answered. The majority of the marks were lost in the middle section on issues to be aware of during anaesthesia for elective thyroidectomy. Many of candidates [sic] concentrated on management of thyroid storm or difficult airway, both of which are relatively rare during such surgery. It is likely that some candidates failed to read the question correctly because it was clearly stated that the patient was euthyroid, making thyroid storm very unlikely.

a) Which investigations are specifically indicated in the preoperative assessment of a patient presenting for thyroidectomy for treated thyrotoxicosis? (5 marks)

Blood tests:
> Thyroid function tests: confirm that the patient is euthyroid.
> Full blood count: carbimazole and propylthiouracil can cause agranulocytosis. Check haemoglobin is adequate.
> Two group and save samples: potential for blood loss.
> Calcium: check preoperatively as level may drop postoperatively due to loss of parathyroid glands.

ECG:
> Should show normal rate if euthyroid. May be bradycardic if ongoing beta blocker use.

Fibreoptic nasendoscopy:
> If concerns about likely ease of visualisation of larynx at laryngoscopy.

CXR or lateral thoracic inlet film:
> May indicate tracheal deviation or narrowing.

CT:
> Assess for retrosternal extension of goitre, tracheal compression.

b) What particular issues must the anaesthetist consider during the induction, maintenance and extubation phases of anaesthesia for a euthyroid patient having a total thyroidectomy? (11 marks)

The College has given you the headings under which you need to categorise your answer – make sure you address each one in turn.

Induction:
> Possibility of deterioration in tracheal compression on lying flat if large goitre (although this should have been elicited by preoperative questioning and investigations). Head-up tilt for induction. Consider need for smaller-diameter endotracheal tube.
> Possibility of slower than usual intubation, if difficult, and, therefore, hypoxia. Pre-oxygenation required; consider use of high-flow nasal oxygen.
> Choice of airway management is determined by preoperative investigations and discussion with the surgeon: straightforward intubation, asleep or awake fibreoptic intubation, awake tracheostomy. Full difficult airway kit should be ready.
> Shared airway: armoured tube.
> If 'can't intubate, can't ventilate' (CICO) situation is encountered due to goitre size, obstruction is likely below the level of a cricothyroidotomy: ENT surgeon ready for rigid bronchoscopy.

Maintenance:

> Shared airway surgery, patient's head distant to anaesthetist:
>   • Padding of eyes (extra care if exophthalmos).
>   • Secure taping of tube.
>   • Be alert to airway dislodgement or tube compression.
>   • Head-up tilt to improve venous drainage but not so as to impair arterial supply.
>   • Extensions on fluid administration set.
>   • Long breathing circuit for anaesthetic machine.
> Drugs:
>   • Maintenance via intravenous or inhalational route.
>   • Remifentanil useful to minimise need for further muscle relaxant and to achieve a degree of hypotension that will improve surgical field.
>   • Vasopressor, e.g. phenylephrine, may be useful to achieve normotension towards the end of surgery to test haemostasis.
>   • High risk of nausea and vomiting: give antiemetics. Dexamethasone has added effect of reducing airway oedema.
>   • Plan for postoperative analgesia: important for blood pressure control postoperatively. Intravenous morphine towards end of surgery, regular paracetamol, NSAIDs if not contraindicated, oral morphine for breakthrough pain usually sufficient in addition to local anaesthetic plus adrenaline infiltration by surgeon. Superficial cervical plexus blocks may also be used.
> Thromboembolic prophylaxis: leg compression devices indicated due to surgery duration.
> Warming mattress/forced air warmer and warmed fluids indicated due to surgery duration.

Extubation:

> Assessment by surgeon for tracheomalacia (fibreoptic scope through tube, tube can be retracted to allow visualisation) or recurrent laryngeal nerve palsy (visualisation of vocal cords with laryngoscopy) if concerns. Extubation can be deferred if such complications have occurred.
> Risk of failure of haemostasis: aim for smooth extubation, can continue remifentanil infusion if used, ensure analgesia sufficient, sitting up.
> Risk of laryngeal oedema increases the risk of problems at extubation: dexamethasone given intraoperatively, then manage extubation in standard manner, ensuring patient sitting up, fully awake, fully reversed (assess train-of-four, appropriate dosing of neostigmine with glycopyrrolate, consideration of sugammadex use if high risk).

c) Describe the specific postoperative problems that may be associated with this operation. (4 marks)

> Failure of haemostasis: causing airway compression, necessitating removal of clips on ward or urgent return to theatre.
> Tracheomalacia: not detected prior to end of surgery, causing airway obstruction necessitating immediate reintubation. Rare.
> Recurrent laryngeal nerve palsy: can be difficult to detect on direct visualisation prior to extubation. Uni/bilateral may cause stridor, difficulty breathing. Unilateral may cause hoarse voice, difficulty phonating.
> Laryngeal oedema: increased likelihood after complex surgery or difficult airway management.
> Hypocalcaemia: due to trauma to or removal of parathyroid glands.
> Pneumothorax: if retrosternal dissection has been necessary due to goitre size.

Reference

Malhotr S, Sodhi V. Anaesthesia for thyroid and parathyroid surgery. *Contin Educ Anaesth Crit Care Pain*. 2007; 7 (2): 55–58.

a) List all of the elements of the STOP-BANG assessment for a patient with suspected obstructive sleep apnoea (OSA) (4 marks) and explain how it is used to quantify their risk. (3 marks)

b) What are the cardiovascular consequences of OSA? (3 marks)

c) How can perioperative risks be minimised in a patient with known severe OSA, but no other cardiovascular or respiratory comorbidities, who is having peripheral surgery involving at least one night in hospital? (10 marks)

September 2017

Chairman's Report

43.3% pass rate.

The pass rate for this question was surprisingly low. Most candidates knew the elements of the STOP-BANG assessment but few knew how to use the score to quantify risk. Most marks were available in part (c), and those who remembered the importance of such things as the use of perioperative CPAP, short acting anaesthetic agents, neuromuscular monitoring and of ensuring full reversal of muscle relaxation scored well here, and tended to do well overall.

a) List all of the elements of the STOP-BANG assessment for a patient with suspected obstructive sleep apnoea (OSA) (4 marks) and explain how it is used to quantify their risk. (3 marks)

Beware of question sections with more than one part – make sure you read the question carefully and answer the whole section.

Elements of STOP-BANG assessment:
S – loud snoring.

T – daytime tiredness.

O – observed cessation in breathing.

P – high blood pressure, treated or untreated.

B – BMI greater than 35 kg/m^2.

A – age greater than 50 years.

N – neck circumference greater than 40 cm.

G – male gender.

Risk quantification:
> Score less than 3 virtually excludes sleep apnoea.
> Score of 3–4 indicates intermediate risk of sleep apnoea.
> Score of 5–8 indicates high risk of sleep apnoea.

b) What are the cardiovascular consequences of OSA? (3 marks)

> Overall increased risk of cardiovascular morbidity and mortality.
> Arrhythmias.
> Hypertension.
> Biventricular dysfunction.
> Pulmonary hypertension.
> Congestive heart failure.
> Myocardial infarction (risk increased by the increased presence of dyslipidaemia, enhanced platelet activation, inflammatory pathway activation and endothelial dysfunction seen in OSA).

Preoperative:
c) How can perioperative risks be minimised in a patient with known severe OSA, but no other cardiovascular or respiratory comorbidities, who is having peripheral surgery involving at least one night in hospital? (10 marks)

> Ensure patient is established on and compliant with CPAP for three months prior to surgery, if clinical condition permits, and continue use in the perioperative period.
> Encourage preoperative weight loss if overweight. Dietician referral if necessary.
> If a smoker, encourage to stop and refer for cessation therapies if necessary.
> Assess for the possibility of associated difficult airway and plan accordingly.

> Consider the possibility of using regional technique only, or regional technique as a method of reducing overall use of systemic drugs that will impact on respiratory drive and alertness.
> Avoid sedative premedication.

Intraoperative:
> If general anaesthesia is used, target normal oxygen saturations and end tidal carbon dioxide.
> Use short-acting agents such as desflurane, propofol and remifentanil.
> Monitor neuromuscular blockade and ensure adequate reversal before extubation. Consider need for sugammadex.
> Extubate awake.
> Use multimodal analgesia to reduce/avoid need for long-acting opioid.

Postoperative:
> Ensure CPAP available for use in PACU.
> Consider prolonged PACU stay.
> Ensure ward is suitable for the level of monitoring, and assistance with CPAP, that the patient requires – dependent on mode of anaesthesia, individual patient and complexity of surgery. Consideration of level 2 care.
> Supplemental oxygen.
> Continuous oxygen saturation monitoring including overnight.

References

Martinez G, Faber P. Obstructive sleep apnoea. *Contin Educ Anaesth Crit Care Pain*. 2011; 11 (1): 5–8.

Chung F, Subramanyam R, Liao P, Sasaki E, Shapiro C, Sun Y. High STOP-BANG score indicates a high probability of obstructive sleep apnoea. *BJA*. 2012; 108 (5): 768–775.

8. MANAGEMENT OF RESPIRATORY AND CARDIAC ARREST

a) What are the cerebral physiological benefits of induced hypothermia following successful resuscitation from cardiac arrest? (25%)

b) How can a patient be cooled in these circumstances? (20%)

c) What adverse effects may occur due to the use of induced hypothermia? (35%)

d) In what other nonsurgical clinical scenarios may the use of induced hypothermia be beneficial? (20%)

September 2011

The NICE guidance from 2011, referenced below, advised cooling to 32–34°C for patients who had suffered cardiac arrest followed by return of spontaneous rhythm. Later that year, this question featured in the final exam. However, subsequent research has found no improvement in outcome when targeting 33°C compared with targeting 36°C, yet hypothermia is associated with significant complications. Therefore, temperature control following cardiac arrest is now called targeted temperature management and aims for 36°C in the hope of gaining the benefits of temperature control and avoidance of pyrexia (common following resuscitation from cardiac arrest) with a lower burden of complications.

a) What are the cerebral physiological benefits of ~~induced hypothermia~~ targeted temperature management following successful resuscitation from cardiac arrest? (25%)

Targeted temperature management avoids the deleterious effects of pyrexia, which occurs commonly after resuscitation from cardiac arrest. Reduction of temperature to 36°C has the following effects:

> Reduced cerebral metabolic rate for oxygen ($CMRO_2$), resulting in reduced oxygen and glucose consumption.
> Suppression of release of oxygen free radicals during reperfusion after cardiac arrest.
> Suppression of destructive neuroexcitotoxic cascade (glutamate release, receptor activation, leading to intracellular calcium overload and cell death).
> Reduction of expression of pro-apoptotic signals.
> Reduction of cerebral oedema associated with reperfusion.

b) How can a patient be cooled in these circumstances? (20%)

Surface cooling:
> Ice packs.
> Surface heat-exchange devices.
> Surface cooling helmet.

Internal cooling:
> Endovascular cooling devices.
> Infusion of cold fluids.

c) What adverse effects may occur due to the use of induced hypothermia? (35%)

This is no longer relevant to this situation now that patients are cooled to only 36°C. However, the knowledge of the systemic risks of hypothermia in the perioperative period was tested in a paper in 2010 and so I list them here for you to learn:

Respiratory:
> Increased risk of pneumonia.

Cardiovascular:
> Initially catecholamine release, increased oxygen demand, increased cardiac output.
> Arrhythmias.
> Shivering increases oxygen demand.

Endocrine:
> Reduced insulin release with increased insulin resistance resulting in elevated blood glucose.

Gastrointestinal:
> Reduced motility compromising enteral nutrition.
> Rarely, pancreatitis.

Haematological:
> Reduced platelet number (sequestered in spleen and liver) and function results in prolonged bleeding time.
> Decreased clotting factor function.

Immune, infection:
> Impaired immune function, overall increased risk of sepsis.

Renal:
> Diuresis and loss of electrolytes resulting in risk of hypovolaemia and effects of electrolyte imbalance such as arrhythmia.

Metabolic:
> Lactic acidosis.
> Hypoxic perinatal brain injury.

d) In what other nonsurgical clinical scenarios may the use of induced hypothermia be beneficial? (20%)

References

National Institute for Health and Care Excellence. Therapeutic hypothermia following cardiac arrest. Interventional procedures guidance [IPG386]. March 2011.

The TTM Trial Investigators. Targeted temperature management at 33°C versus 36°C after cardiac arrest. *N Engl J Med*. 2013; 369: 2197–2206.

Vaity C, Al-Subaie N, Cecconi M. Cooling techniques for targeted temperature management post-cardiac arrest. *Crit Care*. 2015; 19: 103.

9. NON-THEATRE

You are asked to anaesthetise a 75-year-old man for an urgent DC cardioversion on the coronary care unit (CCU). He has a broad complex tachycardia of 150 beats/minute, but is maintaining a systolic blood pressure of 70 mm Hg and has a Glasgow Coma Score of 13/15.

a) List the advantages and disadvantages of providing anaesthesia in the CCU. (30%)

b) What factors must be taken into consideration when choosing an anaesthetic technique for this patient? (30%)

c) What complications may occur as a consequence of the procedure? (40%)

September 2013

Chairman's Report

45.7% pass rate.

This question proved difficult for many candidates.

a) The advantages of providing anaesthesia in a coronary care unit for a maximum of three marks included:

Avoiding the transfer of an unstable patient to theatre

Cardiology department skills readily available

Specialist equipment and drugs are immediately accessible

Allows earlier treatment

The most important disadvantage was anaesthetizing a patient in a remote and unfamiliar environment. This statement needed to be expanded to include the potential lack of monitoring (capnography), anaesthetic drugs, recovery and skilled assistance. Few candidates mentioned the difficulty in complying with the filling in of a WHO checklist.

b) Some of the factors that should have been considered before commencing anaesthesia included valid consent, recent investigations, starvation status and a potential need for intra- or inter-hospital transfer.

c) Required both anaesthetic and cardiological complications; the latter included arterial embolism, myocardial ischaemia, pulmonary oedema, burns to the patient and electrical injury to staff.

a) List the advantages and disadvantages of providing anaesthesia in the CCU (30%).

Advantages	Disadvantages
• Don't need to transfer unstable patient. • Minimises delays to treatment. • Close availability of cardiology specialist equipment/drugs/staff.	• Remote, unfamiliar environment. • Possible lack of availability of monitoring, especially capnography. • Availability of anaesthetic drugs and equipment. • Availability of skilled assistant. • Feasibility of team briefing/WHO checklist/venous thromboembolism assessment. • Availability of adequate recovery care and facilities. • Adequacy of trainee competencies. • Availability of named consultant supervision. • Availability of timely anaesthetic support if problems encountered.

My list of disadvantages of providing anaesthesia on CCU is an abridged version of the issues discussed in the RCoA document 'Anaesthetic Services in Remote Sites.' It is important to keep this list in your mind as it features in other questions concerning non-theatre duties and also in questions in other topics, for example vascular, where anaesthesia may be undertaken in the radiology suite.

b) What factors must be taken into consideration when choosing an anaesthetic technique for this patient? (30%)

> Period of starvation.
> Reflux.
> Anticipated difficult airway.
> Any other investigation results.
> Other medical history. May have limited history as patient has a GCS of 13.
> Likelihood of whether this is an isolated broad complex tachycardia or the presenting feature of an ischaemic myocardial event.
> Post-cardioversion plans, need for transfer elsewhere for further management, e.g. cardiac catheter laboratory.
> Consent.

c) What complications may occur as a consequence of the procedure? (40%)

Anaesthetic:

There are risks associated with all anaesthetics. However, the issues specific to this situation are as follows:

> Aspiration secondary to full stomach.
> Deterioration in cardiovascular stability.
> Failure to gain important anaesthetic history information from patient due to reduced GCS and urgency of situation.
> Risk of awareness.

Cardioversion:
> Arterial embolism causing stroke, cardiac ischaemia.
> Asystole, pulseless ventricular tachycardia, ventricular fibrillation.
> Burns.
> Electrical injury to staff.
> Pulmonary oedema.

References

Knowles P, Press C. Anaesthesia for cardioversion. *BJA Educ*. 2017; 17 (5): 166–171.

Royal College of Anaesthetists. Anaesthetic Services in Remote Sites. 2014. http://www.rcoa.ac.uk/document-store/anaesthetic-services-remote-sites. [Accessed 29th June 2017].

A 55-year-old patient is due to have electro-convulsive therapy (ECT) for severe depression.

a) What are the specific preoperative considerations for ECT? (5 marks)

b) What are the physiological effects of ECT (7 marks) and which physical injuries may occur during treatment? (3 marks)

c) The patient is taking lithium and fluoxetine. What are the anaesthetic implications of these agents during ECT? (5 marks)

March 2015

Chairman's Report

13.3% pass rate; 54.4% of candidates received a poor fail.

Performance on this question was highly variable as reflected by the pass and poor fail rates, and the item was strongly discriminatory. Examiners felt that trainees did not have adequate experience of supervised working in non-theatre locations. Few seem to be attending ECT sessions; for example many candidates did not realise suxamethonium would be given and did not appreciate that myalgia is a common side effect. Many thought that ECT could not be conducted safely in an isolated environment. Consent and mental health issues, problems with patient communication and the likelihood of comorbidity did not feature in many scripts. Of concern was failure to understand the significance of lithium or fluoxetine therapy, as patients appearing on routine theatre lists may be taking these drugs; few candidates made mention of the potentiation of relaxants or volatile anaesthetic agents by lithium.

ECT:
> *Used for severe, medication-resistant depression, mania, catatonia.*
> *Tonic–clonic seizure of specific duration (15–120 seconds) is induced.*
> *Both electrodes on the non-dominant hemisphere minimises cognitive side effects.*
> *Electrode each side if speed of recovery is the most important factor.*
> *Repeat twice a week for up to four weeks or until no further improvement.*

a) What are the specific preoperative considerations for ECT? (5 marks)

> Capacity for consent; patient may be under section.
> Psychiatric illness may make it difficult to obtain full medical history from the patient, may affect compliance with treatment for comorbidities, may affect recent oral intake (consider dehydration and electrolyte disturbance).
> Anaesthetic assessment: check for significant reflux (usually do not use airway adjuncts in ECT), dentition (bite block will be used).
> Assess for comorbidities that specifically affect suitability for ECT: significant ischaemic heart disease, cardiac failure (ventricular dysfunction noted in normal hearts for up to six hours afterwards), significant valvular disease, raised intracranial or intraocular pressure, untreated cerebral aneurysm, recent cerebrovascular accident, unstable fracture or cervical spine (patient is 55 years old, increasing the likelihood of some of these issues being present).
> Check for implantable cardioverter defibrillator (ICD) (which should be deactivated) or permanent pacemaker (which may be set into a fixed mode, depending on underlying pathology). Liaise with cardiac physiologist.
> ECT tends to happen in site remote from main theatres: ensure full staffing, monitoring, equipment, recovery facilities – if patient has significant comorbidities, consider need for relocation to more central, supported site.

b) What are the physiological effects of ECT (7 marks) and which physical injuries may occur during treatment? (3 marks)

Two questions in one – make sure you notice and answer them both.

Physiological effects of ECT:

Airway: risk of laryngospasm, increased salivation secondary to parasympathetic phase.

Respiratory: risk of aspiration.

Cardiovascular: brief (15 seconds) parasympathetic response with bradycardia (risk of asystole), followed by prominent sympathetic response; increased heart rate and blood pressure, therefore increased myocardial oxygen consumption.

Neurological: increased cerebral oxygen consumption and intracranial pressure. Risk of intracranial haemorrhage, transient ischaemic defects, status epilepticus. More commonly, disorientation and memory loss.

Gastrointestinal: increased gastric pressure risking reflux.

Cutaneomusculoskeletal: seizure increases peripheral oxygen consumption and results in raised lactate, raised temperature and myalgia.

Physical injuries that may occur during ECT:

> Dental damage due to seizure plus bite block.
> Intraoral damage due to biting.
> Musculoskeletal damage and fractures rare since use of muscle relaxant.
> Myalgia due to seizure and use of suxamethonium.

c) The patient is taking lithium and fluoxetine. What are the anaesthetic implications of these agents during ECT? (5 marks)

Lithium:

> Potentiation of effect of neuromuscular blocking drugs and volatile agents.
> Nephrogenic diabetes insipidus – consider patient fluid status.
> Narrow therapeutic index – ensure recent level check.
> Renally excreted. NSAIDs reduce lithium excretion and can result in toxic levels.
> Cardiac arrhythmias are a side effect, worse if toxic.
> Omit for 24 hours prior to anaesthesia.

Fluoxetine:

> Tramadol and meperidine contraindicated – risk of serotonin syndrome.
> Inhibits CYP2D6, thus preventing metabolism from codeine to morphine so no analgesic effect would be obtained.

Reference

Uppal V, Dourish J, Macfarlane A. Anaesthesia for electroconvulsive therapy. *Contin Educ Anaesth Crit Care Pain*. 2010; 10 (6): 192–196.

You are asked to transfer an intubated intensive care patient for a magnetic resonance imaging (MRI) scan.

a) What is meant by the terms magnetic resonance (MR) safe, and MR conditional, in relation to equipment used in the MRI scanner room? (2 marks)

b) What precautions can be taken to prevent burns caused by monitoring equipment used in an MRI scanner? (6 marks)

c) List other precautions you would take to minimise the risks associated with MRI. (7 marks)

d) What are the contraindications to an MRI scan? (5 marks)

September 2016

Chairman's Report

45.8% pass rate.

Despite the fact that many candidates will have accompanied patients to the MRI scanner, knowledge of the specific precautions needed to prevent harm during such a procedure was poor. Points were lost by concentrating on the difficulties of anaesthesia in a remote location, which, whilst important, were not what was asked for.

a) What is meant by the terms magnetic resonance (MR) safe, and MR conditional, in relation to equipment used in the MRI scanner room? (2 marks)

MR Safe: these devices pose no MR-related hazards to patients or staff when used according to instructions and can therefore be used in any MR setting.

MR Conditional: this equipment poses no MR-related hazard in a specified MR environment under specific conditions of use, e.g. static field strength, rate of change of magnetic field.

b) What precautions can be taken to prevent burns caused by monitoring equipment used in an MRI scanner? (6 marks)

> Use only MR safe monitoring equipment or MR conditional that has been deemed appropriate to use in that scanner.
> Check all equipment prior to use, that it is intact, that there is no breach in any insulating surfaces that might risk metal touching skin.
> Fibreoptic cables for ECG and pulse oximeter eliminate use of electrical current, which may result in induction currents and burns to underlying skin.
> Telemetric monitor to eliminate the risk of induction currents in connecting leads.
> ECG leads should be high impedance, braided and short to minimise risk of induction currents.
> ECG electrodes must be MR safe.
> Do not allow any cables to coil or cross each other as induction of current can result from capacitance coupling.
> Ensure leads are positioned to exit the scanner down the centre rather than at the side of the patient, close to the radiofrequency (RF) coils.
> Separate leads from patient's skin with e.g. foam insulating padding.

c) List other precautions you would take to minimise the risks associated with MRI. (7 marks)

> Equipment check: ensure all equipment to be used is MR safe or MR conditional and has been checked as safe to use on that scanner.
> Checklist: all staff and patients to complete checklist to ensure no contraindications to entering MRI scanner (see answer to d for more detail).
> Ferromagnetic objects:
  • Staff and patient to remove all ferromagnetic objects from clothes/ pockets to avoid the possibility of them becoming projectiles.
  • Ensure all equipment, e.g. trolley, is non-ferromagnetic, remove oxygen cylinders etc.
  • Some clothes, e.g. sportswear, contain silver fibres – cotton hospital gown to be worn.
  • Drug delivery patches may contain metal – remove due to risk of burns.

> Padding over RF coils: ensure padding intact to prevent direct contact between patient and coils.
> Ear protection: for all patients, anaesthetised or not, due to high noise levels in scanner.
> Monitoring equipment and breathing circuit: check that there is sufficient length by checking planned range of movement of MRI stretcher before leaving the scanning room.
> Inaccessibility of airway: meticulous securing of airway to ensure it does not become dislodged as difficult to access once in scanner.
> Monitoring: telemetric monitoring to facilitate the presence of monitoring screen in control room, reduces risk of failing to notice abnormalities.
> Remote site anaesthesia: ensure senior support available, ensure orientation with equipment/location/emergency kit prior to commencement, especially as some equipment will be unfamiliar as it is MR safe and therefore different to that used elsewhere. Ensure identical monitoring standards to those used elsewhere can be achieved; awareness of low light levels often used in radiology.
> Risks of gadolinium-based contrast agents:
>   • Avoid contrast if eGFR is less than 30 ml/min – risk of nephrogenic systemic fibrosis.
>   • Do not repeat contrast within seven days.
>   • Avoid in pregnancy unless absolutely necessary.
>   • Drugs to manage anaphylaxis to be readily available.

d) What are the contraindications to an MRI scan? (5 marks)

There are few absolute contraindications – most situations need further evaluation.

> Recent surgery involving ferromagnetic clips or implants.
> Ferromagnetic material in eye.
> Ferromagnetic cochlear implants.
> Ferromagnetic neurosurgical clips.
> Intra-aortic balloon pumps, ventricular assist devices.
> Ferromagnetic cardiac occluder devices within six weeks of implantation.
> Neurostimulators: some are safe for use in MRI.
> Programmable shunts/drug pumps: check for compatibility and check that exposure to MRI will not reprogram it.
> Pacemaker or ICD: risks of device failure, dislodgement and burns. However, some newer devices are MRI-compatible.
> Some aortic stent grafts.

References

Association of Anaesthetists of Great Britain and Ireland. *Safety in Magnetic Resonance Units: An Update*. London; 2010.

Reddy U, White M, Wilson S. Anaesthesia for magnetic resonance imaging. *Contin Educ Anaesth Crit Care Pain*. 2012; 12 (3): 140–144.

10. ORTHOPAEDIC SURGERY

An 80-year-old patient is to undergo second stage revision of a total hip arthroplasty for treated deep joint infection.

a) Which specific preoperative considerations are relevant to this patient? (5 marks)

b) Describe the important features of the intraoperative anaesthetic management of this case. (7 marks)

c) List the patient risk factors for bone cement implantation syndrome (4 marks) and the steps that can be taken to prevent or minimise its effect. (4 marks)

March 2015

Chairman's Report

46.8% pass rate; 17.7% of candidates received a poor fail.

Examiners felt that this question should have proved relatively easy, so the pass and poor fail rates are surprising. Inexperience probably accounts for these results. Strong candidates considered issues such as anticipated blood loss and analgesia. Weak candidates focused on infection control issues and ignored the information that the patient had been treated. This question had a very strong correlation with overall candidate scores.

The subject of BCIS was very topical leading up to the publication of the new guideline, again highlighting the importance of keeping up to date with current issues and guidance.

a) Which specific preoperative considerations are relevant to this patient? (5 marks)

Treatment of infection:
> Ensure adequacy of treatment by assessment of symptoms and signs of patient and by white cell count and CRP level.
> Plan for perioperative antibiotics. Consider recent antibiotic treatment and causative agent. Liaise with microbiology.

Effects of chronic infection:
> Check for anaemia and treat if necessary to reduce risk of need for perioperative blood transfusion.
> Reduced mobility may have resulted in deconditioning. Early physiotherapy input should be planned.
> Dietician input for nutritional assessment and management if weight loss has occurred or appetite compromised.

Advanced age of patient:
> Increased risk of comorbidities that will require assessment and management. Specifically assess for comorbidities such as respiratory disease, ischaemic heart disease, and valvular heart disease, which will influence choice of anaesthesia.

Plan for postoperative care:
> Location dependent on discussion with surgeon regarding complexity of surgery, likelihood of blood loss, presence of comorbidities.

b) Describe the important features of the intraoperative anaesthetic management of this case. (7 marks)

In attempting to come up with a suitable list of important features, I have followed the alphabet again. It helped organise my thoughts in the absence of a more obvious way of addressing this question.

Risk of BCIS:
> Increased risk due to age and gender. Take steps to mitigate its effects, see section (c).

Postoperative delirium:
> Increased risk due to patient age. Avoid long-acting sedative drugs. Neuraxial or other regional techniques reduce need for long-acting opioid use.

Deep vein thrombosis prophylaxis:
> Risks: elderly patient, lower limb orthopaedic surgery, prolonged duration of surgery. Mechanical prophylaxis intraoperatively and plan for mechanical and pharmacological prophylaxis postoperatively. Ensure adequate hydration.

Blood loss:
> Ensure cross matched blood available.
> Use cell salvage.
> Ensure adequate starting haemoglobin.
> Neuraxial technique.
> Consider tranexamic acid use.
> Invasive monitoring: arterial line and cardiac output monitoring.

Further risk of joint infection:
> Antibiotic prophylaxis as discussed in part (a).
> Maintain normothermia.

Patient positioning:
> Elderly patient and prolonged surgery. Optimise pressure area care, padding of supports.

Risk of renal dysfunction:
> Risks: hypotension associated with blood loss and neuraxial techniques, as well as advanced age. Maintain adequate volume status, use vasopressor as directed by flow monitoring, avoid nephrotoxic drugs including NSAIDs.

Duration of surgery:
> Spinal anaesthesia is commonly used for primary joint replacements but is unlikely to offer sufficient duration of anaesthesia for this operation.
> Prolonged period in lateral position may not be tolerated with combined spinal and epidural with sedation.
> A combination of general anaesthesia, sedation, combined spinal and epidural, and nerve blocks may be used.

c) List the patient risk factors for bone cement implantation syndrome (4 marks) and the steps that can be taken to prevent or minimise its effect. (4 marks)

Patient risk factors
> Increasing age.
> Significant cardiopulmonary disease.
> Diuretic treatment.
> Male gender.

Steps that can prevent or minimise the effect of BCIS:

> Avoid use of cement where surgically appropriate or where patient's physiological status dictates.
> Communication: preoperative assignation of roles in the event of BCIS, surgeon to inform anaesthetist before applying cement, anaesthetist to acknowledge.
> Surgical management:
  • Wash and dry femoral canal.
  • Apply cement in retrograde fashion using cement gun with a suction catheter and intramedullary plug in the femoral shaft.
  • Avoid vigorous pressurisation of cement in at risk patients.
> Anaesthetic management:
  • Ensure adequate resuscitation pre- and intraoperatively – aim for blood pressure within 20% of pre-induction value.
  • Monitor for cardiorespiratory compromise: blood pressure and $etCO_2$ (if general anaesthesia).
  • Prepare vasopressors in case of cardiovascular collapse.

Reference

Association of Anaesthetists of Great Britain and Ireland. Safety guideline: Reducing the risk from cemented hemiarthroplasty for hip fracture 2015. *Anaesthesia* 2015; 70: 623–626.

11. PERIOPERATIVE MEDICINE

---

a) List the commonest causes of chronic liver disease in adults. (15%)

b) Outline the effects of chronic liver disease on organ systems. (60%)

c) What elements constitute the Child–Pugh scoring system? (25%)

September 2011

a) List the commonest causes of chronic liver disease in adults. (15%)

I think that three causes would probably gain you the full 15%, but my list is longer than that.

Most common:
> Alcoholic liver disease.
> Non-alcoholic fatty liver disease (caused by obesity, diabetes).
> Viral hepatitis, B and C.

Also:
> Autoimmune causes: primary biliary cholangitis, sclerosing cholangitis.
> Metabolic disease: Wilson's, haemochromatosis, alpha-1-antitrypsin deficiency.
> Toxins, drugs.
> Right heart failure.

b) Outline the effects of chronic liver disease on organ systems. (60%)

Straight into my alphabet classification for this. It asks for an 'outline'. Liver disease is a massive topic, and a thorough explanation of every possible systemic change would take too long for you to write. Stick to the core issues.

Airway:
> Risk of reflux due to raised intra-abdominal pressure due to ascites.

Respiratory:
> Diaphragmatic splinting due to ascites, resulting in basal atelectasis, V/Q mismatch, reduced functional residual capacity.
> Pleural effusions.
> Hepatopulmonary syndrome: pulmonary arteriovenous malformations causing right to left shunt. Causes platypnoea (shortness of breath relieved by lying down) and orthodeoxia (decreased oxygen saturations on sitting up).

Cardiac:
> Hyperdynamic circulation with high cardiac output, low blood pressure, and low systemic vascular resistance (SVR) (portal hypertension triggers excessive vasodilatory mediator action in peripheral and splanchnic circulation).
> Portopulmonary hypertension.
> Cirrhotic cardiomyopathy.
> Low SVR may mask underlying coronary artery disease.
> Pericardial effusion.

Neurological:
> Hepatic encephalopathy. May be precipitated by gastrointestinal bleed, infection, sedative drugs, hypoglycaemia, excessive protein intake, hypotension, hypoxia.
> Wernicke's encephalopathy due to thiamine deficiency associated with alcoholic liver disease.

Gastrointestinal:
> Delayed gastric emptying in the presence of raised intra-abdominal pressure due to ascites.
> Risk of varices and gastric erosions, associated with blood loss.

Haematological:
> Anaemia due to chronic blood loss from gastrointestinal tract, hypersplenism-induced haemolysis, chronic illness, malnutrition.
> Coagulopathy due to failure to synthesise clotting factors.
> Thrombocytopaenia and platelet dysfunction.

Immune, infection:
> Reduced immune function, infection prone.

Renal:
> Hepatorenal syndrome (renal dysfunction occurring as a result of chronic poor perfusion due to the disproportionately low SVR in relation to circulating volume. Renal arteries vasoconstrict in response to the activation of the renin–angiotensin–aldosterone system and sympathetic nervous system, but renal perfusion remains inadequate nonetheless).
> Secondary hyperaldosteronism contributes to ascites, effusions and peripheral oedema.

Metabolic:
> Depletion of hepatic and muscle glycogen stores increases risk of hypoglycaemia.

c) What elements constitute the Child–Pugh scoring system? (25%)

It is not very clear what this question wants from you. If it really does just want 'the elements', then the answer is bilirubin, albumin, prothrombin time, encephalopathy and ascites. I suspect that it wants more, as 25% of the marks are for this section, and when the question was repeated in March 2015, they changed the wording. Look at the question from March 2015 for more detail.

Reference
Vaja R, McNicol L, Sisley I. Anaesthesia for patients with liver disease. *Contin Educ Anaesth Crit Care Pain.* 2010; 10 (1): 15–19.

You are asked to anaesthetise a patient with chronic kidney disease (CKD; stage ≥4).

a) List organ system effects that must be considered. (40%)

b) Outline pharmacological factors that must be considered. (30%)

c) What problems may occur with postoperative pain management in this patient? (30%)

March 2012

Chairman's Report

59% pass rate.

Many candidates listed specific drugs that they would or would not use in patients with CKD but failed to comment on general issues such as alterations of protein binding, volume of distribution, excretion of drugs, antihypertensive medication and accumulation of active metabolites.

This question is very similar to those concerning anaesthesia for cadaveric renal transplant in September 2014 and March 2017 (see General, Urological and Gynaecological Surgery chapter). The main difference is section (b) addressed here: the rest of the topics are covered in the questions from 2014 and 2017.

b) Outline pharmacological factors that must be considered. (30%)

> Hypoalbuminaemia and acidosis increase free drug availability and volume of distribution: reduce benzodiazepine, barbiturate and propofol doses. Reduce local anaesthetic dose by 25%.

> Elimination of highly ionised lipid insoluble drugs dependent on renal excretion (but single-dose duration limited by redistribution). Affects penicillin, cephalosporins, neostigmine, salicylates.

> Morphine, pethidine and benzodiazepines are hepatically metabolised to a water soluble form for excretion by kidneys. Active metabolites may accumulate with repeated dosing (such as morphine-6-glucaronide and norpethidine) with consequent respiratory depression and reduced consciousness. Remifentanil and fentanyl may be safely used.

> Metabolism of sevoflurane and enflurane – theoretical risk from nephrotoxic fluoride ion production. Only a consideration if anaesthesia very prolonged.

> Vecuronium and rocuronium (partially) renally excreted. Duration of action not increased with single dose but prolonged neuromuscular blockade may occur with repeated or very large doses.

> Hyperkalaemia may contraindicate suxamethonium use.

> Avoid nephrotoxins, especially in the perioperative period, when the patient may be exposed to other factors such as hypotension and dehydration that cause renal damage: angiotensin converting enzyme inhibitors, angiotensin II receptor antagonists, gentamicin, NSAIDs, contrast media.

> Patient is likely to be on multiple medications, the effects of which must be considered: antihypertensives, diuretics, insulin or other hypoglycaemic agents.

> If the patient has had a previous transplant (now failing), may be taking steroids and other immunosuppressive drugs (e.g. tacrolimus, cyclosporin). These drugs need to remain therapeutic to avoid rejection, so seek advice from renal physicians regarding dosing perioperatively, whilst nil by mouth.

> May require steroid supplementation due to previous or current steroid treatment.

> Patient may be anticoagulated due to recent heparin administration for haemodialysis.

Reference

Mayhew D, Ridgway D, Hunter J. Update on the intraoperative management of adult cadaveric renal transplantation. *BJA Educ.* 2016; 16 (2): 53–57.

A 57-year-old patient is scheduled for resection of a colonic carcinoma in 3 weeks' time. The haemoglobin is 10.1 g/dl at time of referral to the pre-assessment clinic.

a) What intraoperative methods can be used to minimise allogeneic blood transfusion? (35%)

b) What steps constitute the final check required by the National Patient Safety Agency's 'Right Patient, Right Blood' guideline? (25%)

c) What are the additional preoperative preparations that must be made if this patient is a Jehovah's Witness. (40%)

March 2012

Chairman's Report

45.2% pass rate.

A routine question on core knowledge not answered well. The knowledge of blood checking procedure was particularly disappointing. Very few candidates failed to mention the need to check with the patient, the ID band and the blood form. Very few stated that the personal [sic] responsible for the transfusion should check.

a) What intraoperative methods can be used to minimise allogeneic blood transfusion? (35%)

The intraoperative period can be subclassified into the alphabet classification, or surgical, patient and anaesthetic factors. In this situation, the patient factors have already been given to you in the question, and I have added a section called pharmacological (which would normally be encompassed by anaesthetic factors), as there is quite a bit to talk about under that heading.

Surgical:
> Senior surgical team.
> (Staged) laparoscopic surgery.
> Meticulous haemostasis, diathermy.
> Biological haemostats, e.g. Kaltostat (cellulose), fibrin glues (Tisseel).
> Cell salvage (leucocyte depletion filter in view of malignancy).

(In other types of surgery, the use of a tourniquet and positioning to avoid venous stasis will also help minimise blood loss).

Anaesthetic:
> Senior anaesthetic team.
> Avoid venous congestion: adequate relaxation, avoid high intrathoracic pressures, avoid hypercapnia.
> Patient warming: avoid the coagulopathy associated with hypothermia.
> Flow monitoring: optimise tissue oxygen delivery by appropriate fluid and vasopressor use.
> Regional anaesthesia.
> Keep blood pressure low – depends on comorbidities.
> Near patient monitoring of coagulation.

Pharmacological:
> Recombinant clotting factors VIII, IX, VIIa.
> Antifibrinolytics, e.g. tranexamic acid.
> Desmopressin promotes von Willebrand's factor release.

b) What steps constitute the final check required by the National Patient Safety Agency's 'Right Patient, Right Blood' guideline? (25%)

The NPSA no longer exists. However, like with all guidelines, if you haven't read it, don't panic. Think of what you do normally and write down something sensible.

At the patient's bedside, the person responsible for transfusion must:
> Ask the patient to state name, surname and date of birth (if able).
> Check those details against identity wristband.
> Check those details against label/tag on blood unit.

c) What are the additional preoperative preparations that must be made if this patient is a Jehovah's Witness? (40%)

Preoperative:

> Advance decision: full discussion with patient (in absence of family, with time for the patient to make decisions) regarding what, if any, blood components are acceptable. Check acceptability of cell salvage. Discussion about increased risk of morbidity and mortality if blood transfusion refused. Appreciation that there are no true blood alternatives. Understanding that the patient is free to change mind until they are unable to do so due to anaesthesia, and that no one else is able to change the directive on their behalf. Can have another conversation in the presence of family/member of Hospital Liaison Team if desired.

> Haematology advice: consideration of preoperative erythropoietin, iron (may be intravenous), folate, B12 (effect likely to be limited by the existence of malignancy and short time available).

> Stop anticoagulants and antiplatelets if possible.

> Plan for intraoperative care to ensure that senior teams (who are willing to comply with the patient's refusal of blood products), cell salvage etc. are all available on day of surgery.

> Plan for postoperative care and discuss rationale with the patient:
  - Higher dependency postoperative care, possibly ventilation on ICU depending on blood loss.
  - Supplemental oxygen.
  - Careful monitoring to optimise cardiac output and, therefore, oxygen delivery, but also to check for postoperative bleeding.
  - Consideration of hyperbaric oxygen if haemoglobin very low and facility permits.

References

Association of Anaesthetists of Great Britain and Ireland. *Management of Anaesthesia for Jehovah's Witnesses*. London: AAGBI; 2005.

National Patient Safety Agency. Right Patient, Right Blood: Advice for safer blood transfusions. http://www.nrls.npsa.nhs.uk/resources/collections/right-patient -right-blood/ [Accessed 10th July 2017].

A 74-year-old patient is scheduled for a primary total hip replacement.

a) What are the potential benefits of an enhanced recovery ('fast-track') programme for this type of surgery? (20%)

b) List the preoperative (30%), intraoperative (35%) and postoperative (15%) factors necessary for a 'fast-track' programme in this patient.

September 2013

Chairman's Report

49.9% pass rate.

A question on enhanced recovery after colorectal surgery featured in the May 2011 paper. Many of the principles of 'fast-track' status are now being applied to hip and knee replacement surgery. Some candidates misread the question and focused on anaesthesia for surgery on fractured neck of femur.

To pass the question a very generic answer would have sufficed. Excluding the specific details specific to hip replacement surgery, the following basic principles of enhanced recovery formed part of the model answer.

a) Potential benefits:

    Early mobilisation (operative day if possible)

    Decreased postoperative complications esp. cardiopulmonary

    Decreased length of hospital stay

    Cost reduction/theatre efficiency

b) Preoperative factors

    Appropriate patient selection

    Patient education and motivation delivered by multi-disciplinary team

    Preoperative optimisation

    Admit on the day of surgery (staggered admissions if possible)

    Use of carbohydrate loading (clear complex carbohydrate drinks) NB care with diabetics

Intraoperative factors:

    Surgical technique: minimise operative time, avoidance of drains

    Fluid management: targeted fluid replacement

    Tranexamic acid intraoperatively

    Prevention of PONV, e.g. avoidance of nitrous oxide, use of TIVA, routine anti-emetics

    Use long-acting opioids sparingly

    Maintenance of normothermia

    Use of quick offset anaesthetic agents to allow rapid recovery

Postoperative factors:

    Use of multimodal analgesia/oral opioids (avoid PCA)

    Encourage oral fluids early and early nutrition (energy drinks)

    Planned mobilisation and physiotherapy

The board of examiners felt that the pass mark should be high, a designated 'easy question'. The question was a strong discriminator.

You need 14/20 points to pass a question that has been designated 'easy'. The chairman's report on this question is fantastically useful in showing how most of the points are available for writing down things you will know from experience of a few elective joint replacement lists, rather than facts gleaned from textbooks. Intraoperatively, I would have added the following: avoidance of urinary catheter where possible; neuraxial block (using intrathecal opioid) with sedation to reduce long-acting opioid use and to avoid general anaesthesia; local anaesthetic infiltration to reduce long-acting opioid use; avoidance of nerve blocks that may result in prolonged motor block and delay mobilisation. Postoperatively, I would have included post-discharge community support or helpline.

If the question were to recur for colorectal surgery (as featured in the March 2011 paper), factors to consider (in addition to the ones above that are not specific to joint replacement surgery) would include the following:

a) Potential benefits

Early recovery of bowel function/decreased duration of ileus.

b) Preoperative

Avoidance of bowel preparation.

Intraoperative

Surgical technique: transverse incision, minilaparotomy incision, laparoscopic approach in selected patients.

Avoid routine nasogastric tubes and drains.

Anaesthetic technique should aim to optimise pain control with minimal opioid use (consideration of regional technique including spinal anaesthesia and rectus sheath catheters), facilitate return to eating and drinking as rapidly as possible postoperatively (consideration of total intravenous anaesthesia, adequate provision for antiemesis) and ensure appropriate fluid therapy (optimised with cardiac output monitoring).

Postoperative

Prokinetics, e.g. metoclopramide.

Acute pain team involvement: multimodal analgesia.

Community support, helpline.

Reference

Kitching A, O'Neill S. Fast-track surgery and anaesthesia. *Contin Educ Anaesth Crit Care Pain.* 2009; 9 (2): 39–43.

A 72-year-old patient with longstanding severe rheumatoid arthritis (RhA) presents for total knee replacement.

a) Which joints may be affected in RhA and indicate why this involvement is of relevance to anaesthesia. (4 marks)

b) Which systemic features of RhA may be elicited during preoperative assessment? (10 marks)

c) Outline the preoperative investigations that are specifically indicated in this patient and the derangements that each may show. (6 marks)

September 2014

Chairman's Report

41.9% pass rate.

This question was one of the easiest on the paper. The overall pass rate for this question seems very low given that patients with rheumatoid arthritis are regularly encountered in daily practice, particularly for arthroplasty procedures. The answers given by most candidates reveal a poor understanding of important factors in the preoperative assessment of these patients. Many scripts demonstrated a 'medical student' level of appreciation of the topic, e.g. writing 'the neck' in response to the first question on joints affected by the disease. A 'scattergun approach' was taken by weaker candidates, who wrote down all the preoperative investigations they could recall despite the question asking for specific examples.

There was a similar question in 2008. Every time you write down an investigation that you would like, qualify why in this particular patient. Every time you state that you would ask something in the history or examine some aspect of the patient, state why in this particular circumstance. Every time you say that you would do this or that monitoring, state why in this particular patient. It is no good just to say 'I would take an anaesthetic history, examine the airway and cardiorespiratory systems and order an FBC and ECG'. Finally, remember ABCDEFGHIJKLMNOP and you will have a structured answer that will help you dredge knowledge from your brain.

a) Which joints may be affected in RhA and indicate why this involvement is of relevance to anaesthesia. (4 marks)

> RhA is characterised by a chronic symmetrical polyarthritis of (mainly) peripheral joints, especially the fingers, elbows, ankles, but also more proximal joints, shoulders, neck, knees, hips. Any of these may be relevant to anaesthesia as they may be the focus of an operation and so dictate the choices of anaesthetic technique. Also, the involvement of any joint may make positioning for regional anaesthesia problematic.
> Temporomandibular joint: may impact on mouth opening and, hence, ease of intubation. May necessitate fibreoptic intubation.
> Cricoarytenoid joint fixation: may cause preoperative hoarseness. Minimal oedema may therefore cause airway obstruction postoperatively.
> Atlantoaxial subluxation: assess range of movement and symptoms whilst the patient is awake. Excessive movement (such as with airway management) can cause cord compression. May necessitate fibreoptic intubation.
> Cervical ankylosis: causing limited neck extension, difficult airway.
> Costovertebral and costotransverse joints: restrictive lung defect.
> Small joints of hand: limited ability to manage PCA.

b) Which systemic features of RhA may be elicited during preoperative assessment? (10 marks)

Airway:
> Difficult airway for reasons detailed in part (a).

Respiratory:
> Fibrosing alveolitis causing restrictive defect.
> Pleurisy with effusion.
> Nodules.
> Costochondral disease causing reduced chest wall compliance.

Cardiovascular:

> Pericarditis and pericardial effusions, rarely leading to tamponade, usually gradually restrictive and requiring pericardectomy.
> Rheumatoid nodules in any layer of the heart, damaging valve function, causing conduction defects, rarely congestive cardiac failure.
> Increased atherosclerosis and coronary artery disease.

Neurological:

> Peripheral neuropathy due to:
  • Peripheral nerve entrapment (carpal tunnel, ulnar, lateral popliteal).
  • Mononeuritis multiplex due to vasculitis.
  • Drug treatment.
> Autonomic dysfunction: blood pressure and heart rate lability, gastric paresis.
> Compression of nerve roots due to spinal involvement (especially cervical spine).

Endocrine:

> Chronic steroid use: compromises glucose tolerance, may ultimately result in diabetes. Consider the need for perioperative replacement, effect on immune function, skin fragility.

Haematology:

> Normochromic, normocytic anaemia of chronic disease.
> Iron deficiency anaemia due to chronic gastrointestinal losses with NSAID treatment.
> Thrombocytosis due to inflammation.
> Bone marrow depression due to disease-modifying anti-rheumatic drugs (DMARDs).

Immune, infection:

> Increased susceptibility to infection due to DMARDs or TNF inhibitors.

Cutaneoumusculoskeletal:

> Friable skin (due to chronic steroid loss), risk of damage with dressings for cannulae, handling.
> Fixed joint deformities – care with positioning.

Renal:

> Chronic inflammation may cause amyloidosis.
> Drug treatments may cause CKD.
> CKD affects metabolism of drugs used perioperatively.

Hepatic:

> Methotrexate may cause liver cirrhosis, which will impact on drug metabolism.

c) Outline the preoperative investigations that are specifically indicated in this patient and the derangements that each may show. (6 marks)

Full blood count:

> Neutropaenia: should not continue with elective surgery if the patient is currently neutropaenic.
> Anaemia: further investigations may be indicated to determine the underlying cause. Efforts should be made to correct anaemia before major surgery.
> Platelet level: impacts on feasibility of neuraxial technique.

Renal function:

> Elevated urea, creatinine, reduced glomerular filtration rate – chronic kidney disease may occur due to drugs or the disease itself.

Liver function tests:

> Transaminases and alkaline phosphatase may rise in active disease.
> Derangements in all liver function tests may occur due to liver cirrhosis caused by methotrexate.

ECG:
> Conduction disorders.
> Left ventricular hypertrophy.

Chest x-ray:
> Indicated if there are respiratory symptoms. May reveal pleural effusions, infection, fibrotic lung disease, nodulosis.

Lung function tests:
> If respiratory symptoms. Usually reveals a restrictive pattern.

Echocardiogram:
> If a murmur is noted or there are symptoms or signs to suggest poor cardiac function. Regurgitant valves may be due to nodulosis or pericardial fibrosis.

24-hour ECG tape:
> If the patient has palpitations that cannot be diagnosed on resting ECG alone. Arrhythmias may be due to nodulosis of the conduction pathways.

Nasendoscopy and ENT assessment:
> If there is preoperative hoarseness of the voice or other indicator of airway limitation.

Flexion/extension x-rays or MRI of the cervical spine:
> If the patient has pain or neurological symptoms on neck extension or flexion.

Reference

Fombon F, Thompson J. Anaesthesia for the adult patient with rheumatoid arthritis. *Contin Educ Anaesth Crit Care Pain*. 2006; 6 (6): 235–239.

A 35-year-old man presents for a laparoscopic cholecystectomy. He was diagnosed with myotonic dystrophy 10 years ago.

a) What is myotonic dystrophy and how is it inherited? (2 marks)

b) What are the problems of myotonic dystrophy relevant to anaesthesia? (10 marks)

c) Outline the important aspects of preoperative assessment and intraoperative management that are specific to myotonic dystrophy. (8 marks)

September 2014

Chairman's Report

6.5% pass rate.

The prevalence of myotonic dystrophy is comparatively high, and anaesthetists are much more likely to encounter a patient with this condition than one with malignant hyperthermia risk. Poorly applied general anaesthesia causes significant morbidity and mortality in myotonic patients, and the disease is rightly considered an 'old chestnut', which all clinicians should be able to manage appropriately. Most candidates had very poor knowledge of this subject confusing myotonia with forms of muscular dystrophy whose prevalence is rarer. However strong candidates scored significantly in excess of the pass mark which suggests their preparation for the Final FRCA examination was better. Most weak individuals thought incorrectly that suxamethonium was contraindicated due to a risk of hyperkalaemia, and failed to mention the importance of preoperative echocardiography in detecting any associated cardiomyopathy. This question was a poor discriminator as so many candidates scored very poorly, and remedial reading on the topic is recommended for the majority of this cohort.

a) What is myotonic dystrophy and how is it inherited? (2 marks)

> Disorder of chloride conductance affecting skeletal, smooth and cardiac muscle resulting in myotonia (delayed relaxation of muscle contraction).
> Associated multisystem features.
> Autosomal dominance. May demonstrate anticipation, i.e. worsening of disease with successive generations.

b) What are the problems of myotonic dystrophy relevant to anaesthesia? (10 marks)

Airway:
> Delayed gastric emptying and pharyngeal muscle wasting increases risk of aspiration.

Respiratory:
> Restrictive lung defect due to progressive spinal deformity.
> Central and obstructive sleep apnoea.
> Risk of aspiration and pneumonia.
> Exaggerated respiratory depressant effect of opioids and intravenous anaesthetic agents.

Cardiovascular:
> Conduction defects (risk of sudden death).
> Cardiomyopathy.
> Hypotensive and myocardial depressant effects of anaesthetic agents may be exaggerated.

Neurological:
> Can result in reduced intelligence, may lead to problems with capacity and consent.
> Early cataracts affect vision.
> Myotonia results from shivering (avoid hypothermia) or suxamethonium.

Endocrine:
> Increased risk of type 2 diabetes mellitus.
> Increased risk of hypothyroidism.

Pharmacological:

> Suxamethonium causes myotonia, which may make intubation difficult.
> Non-depolarising neuromuscular blocking agents may have prolonged action in the presence of muscle wasting and reversal may cause myotonia. Ideally use short-acting agents, e.g. atracurium, cis-atracurium.

Gastrointestinal:

> Delayed gastric emptying, risk of reflux.

Cutaneomusculoskeletal:

> Muscle wasting. Care with padding. Care to avoid precipitating myotonia.

c) Outline the important aspects of preoperative assessment and intraoperative management that are specific to myotonic dystrophy. (8 marks)

I struggled to answer this without repeating aspects of (b)....

	Preoperative	Intraoperative
Airway	Assess the safety of airway: history of poor swallow, recurrent aspiration pneumonia.	Consider the need for a modified rapid sequence induction.
Respiratory	Assess for evidence of obstructive sleep apnoea, restrictive lung defect, active pneumonia. Consideration of need for formal lung function testing.	Positive pressure ventilation.
Cardiovascular	Assess with history and examination for the possibility of heart failure associated with cardiomyopathy, arrhythmias. Preoperative ECG required, preoperative echocardiogram if indicated.	ECG monitoring: monitor for arrhythmia. Blood pressure monitoring: maintain vigilance for hypotension. Consider intra-arterial blood pressure monitoring.
Neurological	Assess capacity for consent.	
Endocrine	Diabetic management depends on usual diabetic regimen and on the duration of starvation.	VRIII if indicated, or just regular CBG checks.
Pharmacology	Avoid sedative premedication to which the patient may have an exaggerated response.	Use short-acting neuromuscular blocking agents; do not use suxamethonium.
Gastrointestinal	H_2 receptor antagonist or proton pump inhibitor premedication in view of increased risk of reflux.	
Metabolic	Check electrolytes and correct if necessary to reduce intraoperative risk of arrhythmia.	Ensure the patient is warmed to normothermia with forced air warmer and warmed fluids.

References

Marsh S, Ross N, Pittard A. Neuromuscular disorders and anaesthesia. Part 1: Generic anaesthetic management. *Contin Educ Anaesth Crit Care Pain*. 2011; 11 (4): 115–118.

Marsh S, Pittard A. Neuromuscular disorders and anaesthesia. Part 2: specific neuromuscular disorders. *Contin Educ Anaesth Crit Care Pain*. 2011; 11 (4): 119–123.

A patient with end-stage chronic liver disease is listed for elective surgery under general anaesthesia.

a) List the common causes of chronic liver disease. (3 marks)

b) Explain which systemic effects of chronic liver disease are of importance to the anaesthetist and why. (9 marks)

c) Outline the Child–Pugh scoring system and explain how this may be used to stratify mortality risk for this patient. (8 marks)

March 2015

Chairman's Report

54.0% pass rate; 35.8% of candidates received a poor fail.

This question proved the most discriminatory question of the paper. Many candidates showed poor general knowledge of liver disease. Weak candidates were unable to associate the effects of chronic liver disease with the consequences for anaesthesia, which raises concerns for safe practice. Few understood how the Child–Pugh score allowed stratification of risk.

This question is virtually identical to that from September 2011, with a few noteworthy changes.

a) List the common causes of chronic liver disease. (3 marks)

As for September 2011.

b) Explain which systemic effects of chronic liver disease are of importance to the anaesthetist and why. (9 marks)

On this occasion, they have asked for an explanation of <u>why</u> the listed systemic effects are of importance to the anaesthetist.

Airway:
> Risk of reflux due to raised intra-abdominal pressure due to ascites. Rapid sequence induction and premedication with proton pump inhibitor required.

Respiratory:
> Diaphragmatic splinting due to ascites, resulting in basal atelectasis, V/Q mismatch, reduced functional residual capacity. May require paracentesis, sodium and water restriction preoperatively in order to improve ventilatory mechanics.
> Pleural effusions can impact on lung expansion, impairing gas exchange. May need to be drained preoperatively.
> Hepatopulmonary syndrome: pulmonary arteriovenous malformations causing right-to-left shunt. Results in hypoxia that cannot be corrected by administration of oxygen.

Cardiac:
> Hyperdynamic circulation with high cardiac output, low blood pressure and low systemic vascular resistance (SVR) (portal hypertension triggers excessive vasodilatory mediator action in peripheral and splanchnic circulation).
> Portopulmonary hypertension, cirrhotic cardiomyopathy and pericardial effusion may all increase cardiovascular instability under anaesthesia.
> Low SVR may mask underlying coronary artery disease.
> Echocardiogram useful in demonstrating effects of cirrhotic cardiomyopathy, portopulmonary hypertension and pericardial effusion. Cardiological input may be required preoperatively.
> Invasive blood pressure and cardiac output monitoring can help optimise fluid and vasopressor use.

Neurological:
> Hepatic encephalopathy. May be precipitated by gastrointestinal bleed, infection, sedative drugs, hypoglycaemia, excessive protein intake, hypotension, hypoxia. Ensure gas exchange is monitored and hypoxia appropriately managed; avoid long-acting sedative drugs.

> Wernicke's encephalopathy due to thiamine deficiency associated with alcoholic liver disease. Ensure thiamine supplementation from the time of admission, intravenously if necessary.

Gastrointestinal:

> Risk of varices and gastric erosions, associated with blood loss. Ensure full blood count checked; oesophageal Doppler contraindicated in the presence of varices.

Haematological:

> Anaemia due to chronic blood loss from gastrointestinal tract, hypersplenism-induced haemolysis, chronic illness, malnutrition. Check full blood count and haematinics if indicated. Ensure anaemia is adequately treated preoperatively.
> Coagulopathy due to failure to synthesise clotting factors. Regional anaesthesia may be contraindicated. Clotting factor supplementation may be required; seek senior haematological advice.
> Thrombocytopaenia and platelet dysfunction. May contraindicate regional anaesthesia. Platelet supplementation may be required to facilitate surgery.

Immune, infection:

> Reduced immune function, infection prone. Assess for the presence of infection by checking for symptoms, check white cell count, investigate as appropriate.

Renal:

> Hepatorenal syndrome. Avoid other renal insults in the perioperative period such as hypotension, dehydration, nephrotoxic drugs.
> Secondary hyperaldosteronism contributes to ascites, effusions and peripheral oedema. Patient may already be taking aldosterone antagonists.

Metabolic:

> Depletion of hepatic and muscle glycogen stores increases the risk of hypoglycaemia. Blood glucose must be monitored perioperatively, especially when under general anaesthesia, to avoid dangerously low glucose level. Supplementation may be required.

Ultimately, a risk benefit assessment must be made in conjunction with the patient, liver specialist and surgeon to determine whether proceeding with elective surgery is warranted if the degree of liver impairment is significant and risks of morbidity and mortality are judged to be high.

c) Outline the Child–Pugh scoring system and explain how this may be used to stratify mortality risk for this patient. (8 marks)

The word 'outline' suggests that the College just wants a descriptive explanation, along the lines of:

Five variables (bilirubin, albumin, prothrombin time, encephalopathy and ascites) are quantified and given a score from 1 (least severe) to 3. The numbers are added up to give a total. Based on the total, the patient is classified as Child's A, B or C (A being least severe). Based on population studies, an individual's Child's category can be used to predict their overall survival and also their likely mortality associated with surgery.

Here it is in more detail:

	1	2	3
Bilirubin (mcg/l)	<34	34–50	>50
Albumin (g/l)	>35	28–35	<28
Prothrombin time (s>control)	<4	4–6	>6
Encephalopathy	None	Mild (Grades I–II)	Marked (Grades III–IV)
Ascites	None	Mild	Marked

Used as a risk prediction tool for patients undergoing abdominal surgery:

<7 = Child's A, <5% mortality

7–9 = Child's B, 25% mortality

>9 = Child's C, 50% mortality

Or just for assessing overall mortality risk:

One-year survival

A: 100%

B: 80%

C: 45%

Reference

Vaja R, McNicol L, Sisley I. Anaesthesia for patients with liver disease. *Contin Educ Anaesth Crit Care Pain*. 2010; 10 (1): 15–19.

A 74-year-old patient is scheduled for a primary total hip replacement.

a) What are the potential benefits of an enhanced recovery ('fast-track') programme for this type of surgery? (4 marks)

b) List the preoperative (6 marks), intraoperative (7 marks) and postoperative (3 marks) measures that should be included in the enhanced recovery programme for this patient.

September 2016

Chairman's Report

59.4% pass rate.

This was predicted to be an easy question, and whilst most candidates answered it well, some did not appear to know the reasons for having an enhanced recovery program nor what the elements of it would be. This is surprising given that most hospitals now run such programs for their patients in various surgical areas.

It is even more surprising that this was not well answered when you consider that a virtually identical question (with the Chairman's Report offering a really detailed explanation of what was required to pass) appeared just a few years earlier.

A patient scheduled for primary elective total knee replacement is found to be anaemic, with a haemoglobin level of 90 g/litre.

a) What perioperative consequences may be associated with preoperative anaemia? (5 marks)

b) What physiological adaptations occur to offset the effects of anaemia? (6 marks)

c) Describe perioperative events that may worsen the effects of the anaemia. (4 marks)

d) What further blood tests may help in the classification of this anaemia? (5 marks)

March 2017

Chairman's Report

29.5% pass rate.

Detailed knowledge of the consequences of anaemia and the physiological adaptations accompanying it were lacking. In particular candidates scored poorly in part (d) which asked about blood tests used to help classify anaemia.

a) What perioperative consequences may be associated with preoperative anaemia? (5 marks)

> Cancellation and, therefore, delayed treatment.
> Increased length of hospital stay, increased length of ICU stay, increased all-cause morbidity and mortality.
> Increased risk of cardiac events, including myocardial infarction.
> Increased risk of respiratory, urinary and wound infections.
> Increased risk of thromboembolic events.
> Delayed wound healing.
> Increased need for autologous blood transfusion and its risks.

b) What physiological adaptations occur to offset the effects of anaemia? (6 marks)

> Increased oxygen extraction by tissues thus reducing SvO_2. Brain and heart already have high extraction ratios and so are unable to compensate further.
> Increased cardiac output: as a response to reduced systemic vascular resistance due to decreased blood viscosity, and also sympathetic response to hypoxia.
> Redistribution of cardiac output to areas of high demand such as brain and heart.
> Rightward shift of oxygen dissociation curve due to increased 2,3DPG, thus reducing the affinity of haemoglobin for oxygen, favouring oxygen offloading at tissues.

c) Describe perioperative events that may worsen the effect of the anaemia. (4 marks)

Increased oxygen requirement:
> Shivering.
> Pain.
> Stress response.
> Fever.

Reduced oxygen delivery:
> Hypoxaemia due to inadequate oxygen therapy, failure to adequately manage the airway, basal atelectasis, thromboembolic event, hypoventilation due to drug effects.
> Reduced cardiac output due to anaesthetic agents.
> Blood loss due to surgery.
> Reduced erythropoiesis due to inflammatory response.
> Hypothermia causing leftward shift of oxygen dissociation curve.

d) What further blood tests may help in the classification of this anaemia? (5 marks)

What follows is a fairly exhaustive list of blood tests that could be used to investigate anaemia. I don't know which ones the College would have awarded points for and how many they would have wanted to see documented.

> Iron. Lack causes microcytic anaemia.
> Folate. Lack causes macrocytic anaemia.
> B12. Lack causes macrocytic anaemia.

> Reticulocyte count. Low count may indicate problem with bone marrow, whereas high number may indicate premature haemolysis of red blood cells.
> Red cell distribution. Represents a variety in red blood cell sizes due to a range of different causes of anaemia.
> Iron concentration.
> Total iron binding capacity. An indirect measure of the amount of transferrin present in the blood. Will be raised in iron deficiency anaemia, low in anaemia of chronic disease.
> Transferrin saturation. Will be low in iron deficiency anaemia but high in anaemia of chronic disease.
> Serum ferritin. Deficiency indicates lack of iron.
> Urea and electrolytes. May indicate an underlying cause such as renal dysfunction.
> Liver function tests.
> Inflammatory markers. May support a diagnosis of anaemia of chronic disease.
> Haptoglobin levels. Reduced level suggests intravascular haemolysis.
> Lactate dehydrogenase. Released with cell breakdown; therefore an indicator of haemolysis.
> Free plasma haemoglobin. Indicative of intravascular haemolysis.
> Tests for haemoglobinopathies.

References

Clevenger B, Richards T. Pre-operative anaemia. *Anaesthesia*. 2015; 70 (Suppl 1): 20–28.

Hans G, Jones M. Preoperative anaemia. *Contin Educ Anaesth Crit Care Pain*. 2013; 13 (3): 71–74.

a) List the main measures of fitness that are obtained by a cardio-pulmonary exercise test (CPET). (4 marks)

b) What abnormalities seen at the time of testing in a CPET may suggest cardiorespiratory disease? (4 marks)

c) When might CPET, using a bike, be impractical (3 marks) and how else can patients' functional capacity be assessed? (3 marks)

d) What scoring systems can help predict perioperative risk before major (non-cardiac) surgery? (6 marks)

September 2017

Chairman's Report

24.3% pass rate.

This question was not well answered, which is surprising given the widespread use of cardiopulmonary exercise testing. The inclusion of perioperative medicine in the curriculum will hopefully lead to more exposure to this and other preoperative testing methods and to a greater understanding of risk assessment in general.

a) List the main measures of fitness that are obtained by a cardiopulmonary exercise test (CPET). (4 marks)

The question has asked for a list, not an explanation. It has also asked for the 'main' measures of fitness. It seems that 4 marks is a lot for three measures, but all of the other measures feature in the answer to section (b), and the College repeatedly warns that the Final SAQ paper never asks for repetition.

> Anaerobic threshold (AT): the level of oxygen delivery (VO_2) at which anaerobic metabolism starts to occur.
> Peak oxygen delivery (VO_2 peak).
> Workload achieved.

b) What abnormalities seen at the time of testing in a CPET may suggest cardiorespiratory disease? (4 marks)

Cardiac:
> Rapid rise in heart rate, especially at low levels of work.
> Reduced heart rate reserve.
> Reduced peak oxygen pulse (reflects stroke volume).
> Pathologically altered ECG with exercise (e.g. ST segment elevation or depression, arrhythmia, left bundle branch block).
> Reduction in blood pressure with exercise.

Respiratory:
> Raised ventilatory equivalent for carbon dioxide or oxygen.
> Spirometry abnormalities such as significant reductions in FVC, FEV1 or both.
> Significantly reduced oxygen saturations at peak exercise.

c) When might CPET, using a bike, be impractical (3 marks) and how else can patients' functional capacity be assessed? (3 marks)

There is a list of situations where CPET is contraindicated (severe aortic stenosis, recent myocardial infarction, respiratory failure etc.), but this question is asking about situations where it may be impractical.

Situations where CPET is impractical:
> History of amputation that has compromised ability to use a bicycle.
> Severe peripheral vascular disease.
> Severe arthritis, some patients awaiting lower limb joint replacements.
> Balance or coordination problems.
> Inability to tolerate face mask/mouth piece due to e.g. claustrophobia.
> Lack of motivation.

Other methods of assessing patients' functional capacity:
> Questionnaire-based approaches such as the Duke Activity Status Index.
> Six-minute walk test.
> Incremental shuttle walk test.

> CPET using a hand crank. Results not comparable to results from bike CPET due to different muscle groups and size of muscles involved.

d) What scoring systems can help predict perioperative risk before major (non-cardiac) surgery? (6 marks)

Generic scoring systems:
> American Society of Anesthesiologists Physical Status Score (ASA).
> Physiological and Operative Severity Score for the enUmeration of Mortality and Morbidity (POSSUM). Limited by the need to include a prediction of intraoperative issues.
> Surgical Outcome Risk Tool (SORT).
> American College of Surgeons Surgical Risk Calculator (ACS NSQIP).
> Charlson Age Comorbidity Index (CACI).

Scores for cardiac risk:
> Revised Cardiac Risk Index (RCRI).

Scores for respiratory comorbidity:
> Arozullah Respiratory Failure Index.
> Gupta calculators for postoperative respiratory failure and pneumonia.
> ARISCAT Risk Index.

Scores for specific operations or operation types:
> Nottingham hip fracture score.
> POSSUM for vascular surgery (V-POSSUM).
> Carlisle risk calculator for survival after elective AAA repair.

References

Agnew N. Preoperative cardiopulmonary exercise testing. *Contin Educ Anaesth Crit Care Pain*. 2010; 10 (2): 33–37.

Albouaini K et al. Cardiopulmonary exercise testing and its application. *Heart*. 2007; 93: 1285–1292.

Barnett S, Moonesinghe S. Clinical risk scores to guide perioperative management. *Postgrad Med J*. 2011; 87: 535–541.

Minto G, Biccard B. Assessment of the high-risk perioperative patient. *Contin Educ Anaesth Crit Care Pain*. 2014; 14 (1): 12–17.

12. REGIONAL ANAESTHESIA

a) Describe the innervation of the anterior abdominal wall. (20%)

b) In which types of surgery would a transversus abdominus plane (TAP) block be used and what are the potential benefits? (25%)

c) Outline how you would perform a TAP block. (40%)

d) What are the specific complications of a TAP block? (15%)

September 2012

Chairman's Report

67.4% pass rate.

The question was relevant and topical. Many candidates had poor knowledge of the innervation of the anterior abdominal wall. Overall was answered well.

Regional nerve blocks have peaks of popularity and interest – make sure you know about the current hot favourites.

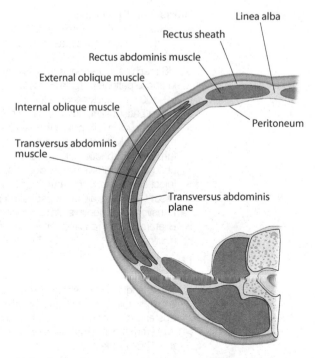

Abdominal wall

a) Describe the innervation of the anterior abdominal wall. (20%)

The anterior rami of T7–T12 and L1 lie between internal oblique and transversus abdominus and supply the anterior abdominal wall. Cutaneous branches of these then pierce the rectus sheath to supply overlying skin.

> T7–9 supply superior to the umbilicus.
> T10 supplies the periumbilcal area.
> T11–12 with iliohypogastric and ilioinguinal nerves supply the area inferior to the umbilicus.
> Iliohypogastric: L1 origin. Supplies the inguinal region.
> Ilioinguinal: L1 origin. Supplies the inguinal hernia sac as well as scrotum/labia and medial aspect of thigh.

b) In which types of surgery would a transversus abdominus plane (TAP) block be used and what are the potential benefits? (25%)

TAP block provides pain relief to the anterior abdominal wall (not effective for visceral pain) from T7 to L1 level. Spread above the umbilical level is unreliable, so it is useful for any surgery involving anterior abdominal wall where the incision is below the level of the umbilicus:

> Abdominal hysterectomy.
> Caesarean section.
> Retropubic prostatectomy.
> Inguinal hernia repair (will not cover areas supplied by ilioinguinal and iliohypogastric nerves).
> Appendicectomy.
> Lower abdominal open colorectal surgery.
> Laparoscopic surgery.

Potential benefits:
> Part of a multimodal analgesia approach, reducing dependence on other modes of analgesia and their associated adverse effects.
> Reduced opioid requirement, useful in patients for whom opioids may be undesirable, for example those with respiratory disease.
> May avoid the need for neuraxial technique in patients in whom this is contraindicated, e.g. patients with coagulopathy (however, unlikely to be as effective as neuraxial technique).
> Offers pain relief after emergency caesarean, where urgency has not permitted neuraxial technique.

c) Outline how you would perform a TAP block. (40%)

Ultrasound (US) guided:
> Consent, assess for contraindications, skilled assistant, resuscitation drugs, venous access, assemble equipment, aseptic technique, full monitoring.
> US machine, high-frequency linear array probe (curvilinear may be required in obese patients), sterile cover, 0.5% chlorhexidine spray, sterile US gel, 50–100 mm block needle, 20–40 ml local anaesthetic (LA), 10 ml saline.
> Clean patient skin; allow to air dry.
> Patient supine. US probe transverse to the orientation of the patient, in midaxillary line between the ribs and iliac crest.
> In-plane introduction of needle to reach the space between the internal oblique and transversus abdominis.
> Inject saline to confirm that the needle is in the correct plane, then inject LA in 5-ml aliquots, aspirating prior to each injection, watching transversus abdominis plane expand with injection.
> Bilateral blocks required for midline incisions and incisions that cross the midline.

Landmark:
> Preparation as for ultrasound-guided technique.
> The Triangle of Petit should be identified by palpation of the iliac crest inferiorly, the anterior border of latissimus dorsi posteriorly and the posterior border of the external oblique anteriorly.
> A 50-mm block needle is usually sufficient as a more direct approach to the plane is taken.

> The needle is inserted perpendicularly to the skin in the Triangle of Petit just above the iliac crest in the posterior axillary line.
> Two pops are felt as the needle passes through the fascial extensions of the external and then internal oblique.
> Aspiration should be negative prior to injection.

d) What are the specific complications of a TAP block? (15%)

Don't just write 'nerve damage, bleeding, failure' – explain the issues associated with this particular block.

> Failure – there is significant variation in degree of local anaesthetic spread with TAP block.
> Local anaesthetic toxicity – large volumes of local anaesthetic are used, especially if bilateral block.
> Risks of incorrect site of injection much reduced with the use of ultrasound but include intraperitoneal injection, intrahepatic injection, bowel perforation or haematoma.
> Transient femoral nerve block.

References

Yarwood J, Berrill A. Nerve blocks of the anterior abdominal wall. *Contin Educ Anaesth Crit Care Pain*. 2010; 10 (6): 182–186.

Townsley P, French J. Transversus Abdominus Plane Block. Anaesthesia Tutorial of the Week. 239: 2011.

a) Which specific nerves must be blocked to achieve effective local anaesthesia for shoulder surgery? (6 marks)

b) What are the possible neurological complications of an interscalene block? (6 marks)

c) Outline the measures available to reduce all types of neurological damage during shoulder surgery. (8 marks)

March 2013

Chairman's Report

69.2% pass rate.

This question was answered well. If an open question is asked on the possible neurological complications of a block, then this will include damage to both the peripheral and central nervous system. Some candidates focused on the peripheral nerves only. The answer to part (c) required an account of both anaesthetic and surgical factors that would reduce neurological damage. This included 'avoiding interscalene block' in the first place. The question was a very good discriminator.

a) Which specific nerves must be blocked to achieve effective local anaesthesia for shoulder surgery? (6 marks)

It would seem that to get the six points, you need only list the nerves. I have included more detail in (in italics) as it is useful information for the sake of the viva.

Nerve	Area supplied
Supraclavicular nerve *(C3,4)* *(for awake surgery, would either need to perform superficial cervical plexus block OR infiltrate around posterior port site).*	Skin above clavicle, shoulder tip and first two intercostal spaces anteriorly.
Upper lateral cutaneous nerve of arm, *branch of axillary nerve (C5,6).*	Skin over deltoid.
Medial cutaneous nerve of arm, *medial cord of brachial plexus (C8, T1).*	Skin of medial arm and axilla.
Suprascapular nerve *(C4–6).*	Acromioclavicular joint, capsule, glenohumeral joint.
Axillary nerve *(C5,6).*	Inferior aspect of capsule and glenohumeral joint.
Musculocutaneous nerve *(C5–7).*	Very variable input.

b) What are the possible neurological complications of an interscalene block? (6 marks)

> Phrenic nerve block or damage.
> Stellate ganglion block or damage leading to Horner's syndrome.
> Spinal anaesthesia.
> Epidural anaesthesia.
> Direct nerve damage of any of the nerves intended to be blocked, causing temporary or permanent neuropraxia.
> Syrinx or cavity formation in cervical cord due to injection into it resulting in paraplegia.

c) Outline the measures available to reduce all types of neurological damage during shoulder surgery. (8 marks)

Nerve damage is a risk during any operation and may occur in relation to nerve blocks, general anaesthesia, surgery and positioning. Be really careful when reading the questions to establish exactly what they are asking.

Nerve block:
> Adequate training and experience of the anaesthetist.
> Minimise risk of infection and neurotoxicity: full asepsis, use of 0.5% chlorhexidine spray, air dried.
> Minimise risk of neuropraxia: use of ultrasound, awake patient, appropriate needle length, low pressure injection.
> Avoid nerve blocks altogether.

General anaesthesia:
> Risk of hypotension causing reduced cerebral blood flow especially if deckchair position: ensure adequate filling, appropriate use of vasopressors and leg elevation, avoid excessive depth of anaesthesia.

Positioning:
> Risk of neuropraxias: careful positioning on table, padding to avoid peripheral nerve compression (ulnar and common peroneal at risk in lateral position), avoid excessive stretch on brachial plexus in deckchair or lateral position.

Surgery:
> Risk of contusion or traction (rarely laceration) of nerves (axillary nerve close to inferior shoulder capsule is particularly vulnerable): minimised by appropriate training, careful technique.
> Risk to brachial plexus by arm manipulation: minimise manipulation.

Reference
Beecroft C, Coventry D. Anaesthesia for shoulder surgery. *Contin Educ Anaesth Crit Care Pain*. 2008; 8 (6): 193–198.

a) List five nerves that can be blocked at ankle level for foot surgery. (5 marks)

b) For each of these nerves, describe the sensory distribution within the foot. (5 marks)

c) Give the anatomical landmarks for an ankle block which aid correct placement of local anaesthesia for each nerve. (5 marks)

d) What are the advantages and disadvantages of an ankle block? (5 marks)

You may use a table for this answer if you wish.

September 2014

Chairman's Report

65.9% pass rate.

Common clinical subjects tend to score well in the SAQ paper and discriminate between strong and weak candidates as was the case for this question. Weak candidates had poor anatomical knowledge or failed to list the advantages of this specific block, giving instead the features common to any local anaesthetic technique. Poor candidates tended to describe features of blocks at the popliteal level, perhaps due to failing to read the question thoroughly as ankle level was highlighted. The importance of candidates retaining knowledge of the basic sciences has been highlighted before.

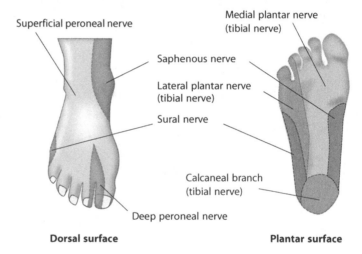

Dorsal surface   Plantar surface

Cutaneous innervation of the foot

a) List five nerves that can be blocked at ankle level for foot surgery. (5 marks)

b) For each of these nerves, describe the sensory distribution within the foot. (5 marks)

c) Give the anatomical landmarks for an ankle block which aid correct placement of local anaesthesia for each nerve. (5 marks)

A table is perfect – minimises arm fatigue.

Nerve	Sensory distribution	Anatomical landmarks
Tibial	Heel and plantar aspect of the foot.	Midway between medial malleolus and tip of calcaneum, inject posteriorly to the posterior tibial artery.
Deep peroneal	1st/2nd toe web space.	2–3 cm distal to the intermalleolar line, palpate extensor hallucis longus. Lateral to this is the dorsalis pedis artery: inject either side.
Superficial peroneal	Dorsum of the foot excluding 1st/2nd toe web space.	Find tibial ridge, insert needle and direct towards lateral malleolus raising a subcutaneous wheal.
Sural	Plantar aspect 4th/5th web space and 5th toe, and lateral aspect of the foot.	Infiltrate subcutaneously between lateral malleolus and Achilles tendon.
Saphenous	Medial aspect of the foot and ankle.	Find saphenous vein anterior to medial malleolus: inject subcutaneously from here posteriorly as far as the Achilles tendon.

d) What are the advantages and disadvantages of an ankle block? (5 marks)

Advantages	Disadvantages
Provides good postoperative analgesia.	Can be uncomfortable to perform in awake or unsedated patients.
May avoid general anaesthesia in high-risk patients.	Risk of vascular puncture causing haematoma. Saphenous vein particularly at risk.
Relatively simple technique with low risk of local anaesthetic toxicity.	If a tourniquet is to be used, does not alleviate tourniquet pain.
Minimal motor block; can therefore be used for bilateral procedures.	

Reference

Kopka A, Serpell M. Distal nerve blocks of the lower limb. *Contin Educ Anaesth Crit Care Pain*. 2005; 5 (5): 166–170.

a) Which specific nerves must be blocked to achieve effective local anaesthesia for shoulder surgery? (6 marks)

b) What are the possible neurological complications of an interscalene block? (6 marks)

c) Outline the measures available to reduce all types of neurological damage during shoulder surgery. (8 marks)

September 2015

Chairman's Report

48.3% pass rate.

This question also correlated well with overall performance. The anatomy was not well known to a lot of the candidates so quite a few marks were lost here. This is a recurring theme in the Final exam – remember that anatomy relevant to clinical practice is likely to be included. Failure to read the question again caused some candidates to lose marks. Part (b) asked specifically for possible neurological complications of an interscalene block and quite a few candidates wrote about non-neurological complications.

Recognise this question? It is identical to the one from March 2013. However, only 48% of candidates passed the question. Topics recur with regularity; if you do no other preparation for this exam, at least look at the past papers.

An 80-year-old woman is admitted to your hospital having sustained a proximal femoral (neck of femur) fracture in a fall.

a) How would you optimise this patient's pain preoperatively? (5 marks)

b) You decide to perform a fascia iliaca compartment block for analgesia. What are the borders of the fascia iliaca compartment (4 marks) and which nerves are you attempting to block? (1 mark)

c) Describe how you would perform this block using an ultrasound-guided technique. (10 marks)

NB consent has already been obtained; you also have adequate assistance, emergency equipment, monitoring and venous access.

March 2017

Chairman's Report

22.2% pass rate.

It is disappointing that this question, concerning a very commonly seen clinical scenario and accompanying anaesthetic technique, was answered so poorly. In part (a) many candidates failed to mention assessment of pain as part of preoperative optimization. There was general lack of knowledge of anatomy in part (b). In part (c) some candidates failed to read the question correctly and described a technique using a nerve stimulator rather than ultrasound, or described a femoral nerve block rather than a fascia iliaca block. Some candidates still wrote about assistance and emergency equipment despite being told in the question that this was unnecessary. Many of the answers were somewhat brief but it is unclear whether this reflects a lack of knowledge or a lack of time.

22.2%! What a shocker. If I were in charge of the exam, I would set this question again.

a) How would you optimise this patient's pain preoperatively? (5 marks)

If candidates had learnt from past questions, they could have at least gained themselves these 5 points. Two recent exams have asked about pain management of patients with fractured hips.

March 2012: (b) Outline the recommendations made by The National Institute for Health and Clinical Excellence (2011) for the management of acute pain in this patient. (30%)

March 2014: (b) Outline the recommendations of best practice for the management of pain in this patient. (30%)

> Assess pain:
  • Immediately on admission.
  • 30 minutes after analgesia given.
  • Hourly until settled on ward.
  • As part of routine observations thereafter.
> Analgesia to be given immediately on admission with suspected hip fracture, even if cognitively impaired.
> Pain control should be adequate to allow investigations.
> Step-wise, multimodal analgesia:
  • Paracetamol six hourly unless contraindicated.
  • Opioid as necessary.
  • Nerve block (e.g. fascia iliaca block) by trained personnel.
  • NSAID not recommended.

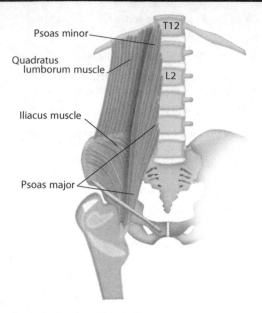

Posterior border of fascia iliaca compartment

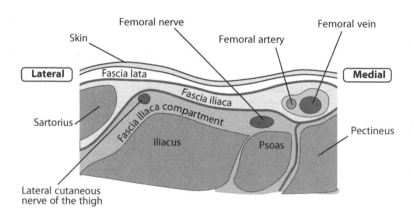

Fascia iliaca compartment

b) You decide to perform a fascia iliaca compartment block for analgesia. What are the borders of the fascia iliaca compartment (4 marks) and which nerves are you attempting to block? (1 mark)

> Anteriorly: posterior surface of fascia iliaca.
> Posteriorly: anterior surface of iliacus and psoas major muscles.
> Medially: origin of psoas major and vertebral column from which it originates.
> Laterally: origin of iliacus muscle along the inner aspect of the iliac crest.
> Nerves: femoral, lateral femoral cutaneous, obturator.

c) Describe how you would perform this block using an ultrasound-guided technique. (10 marks)

> Patient supine.
> Full asepsis: hat gown gloves mask, 0.5% chlorhexidine spray air dried, transducer sleeve, sterile ultrasound gel.
> 50-mm 22G block needle unless patient habitus dictates otherwise.
> High-frequency linear array probe, positioned transversely just below the inguinal ligament, lateral to the femoral artery. Identify the fascia iliaca, fascia lata and iliacus muscle.
> Inject a skin wheal of local anaesthetic above where sartorius is visualised.
> In plane needle insertion from lateral side, tip under fascia iliaca.

> Ensure negative aspiration then inject 1–2 ml local anaesthetic; ensure that the fascia iliaca is seen lifting from the muscle, spreading laterally and medially towards the femoral nerve.
> Continue to inject 30–40 ml dilute local anaesthetic (e.g. 40 ml 0.25% bupivacaine, ensure maximum of 2 mg/kg) with repeated negative aspiration.

Reference

New York School of Regional Anaesthesia. Ultrasound-Guided Fascia Iliaca Block. https://www.nysora.com/ultrasound-guided-fascia-iliaca-block [Accessed 12th January 2018].

13. SEDATION

You are asked to sedate a frightened adult patient for insertion of dental implants in an outpatient dental chair.

a) Complete the table in your answer booklet with the four levels of sedation in the American Society of Anesthesiologists (ASA) continuum of sedation (top row) and the clinical features seen at each level (columns below). (8 marks)

b) Outline drugs that may be used and their methods of administration, when providing sedation for this patient. (4 marks)

c) What are the best practice principles for providing safe sedation to this patient? (8 marks)

September 2015

Chairman's Report

62.1% pass rate.

This is an important topic and was generally well answered despite some confusion caused by the inclusion of a table that required completion. It had the highest pass rate of all the questions.

'Standards for Conscious Sedation in the Provision of Dental Care' was published in April 2015. In the following exam, there was a question based on sedation for dental care.

a) Complete the table in your answer booklet with the four levels of sedation in the American Society of Anesthesiologists (ASA) continuum of sedation (top row) and the clinical features seen at each level (columns below). (8 marks)

The clinical features follow the alphabet, A, B, C, D. Then remembering what goes into each box is straightforward.

	Minimal sedation: anxiolysis	Moderate sedation: conscious sedation	Deep sedation	General anaesthesia
Responsiveness	Normal response to verbal stimulation.	Purposeful response to verbal or light tactile stimulation.	Purposeful response to repeated or painful stimulation.	No response.
Airway	Unaffected.	No intervention required.	Intervention may be required.	Intervention usually required.
Spontaneous ventilation	Unaffected.	Adequate.	May be inadequate.	Frequently inadequate.
Cardiovascular function	Unaffected.	Usually maintained.	Usually maintained.	May be impaired.

b) Outline drugs that may be used and their methods of administration, when providing sedation for this patient. (4 marks)

> Nitrous oxide/oxygen 50:50 (entonox) via inhalation.
> Temazepam via oral route.
> Midazolam via intravenous, oral or intranasal route.
> Small, single dose of fentanyl via intravenous route, wait until peak effect. May be followed by cautious intravenous midazolam titration.

c) What are the best practice principles for providing safe sedation to this patient? (8 marks)

I have used the subheadings in the contents page of the 'Standards for Conscious Sedation in the Provision of Dental Care' report to guide this part of my answer. Part (c) is basically asking how you would run a safe service. Even if you haven't read the guideline, you still know what makes for safe provision of a sedation service. Don't forget the organisational aspects such as staff training and clinical governance.

> Environment: adequate monitoring, equipment, resuscitation facilities and drugs (checked and working), reversal agents, suitable area for patient recovery.
> Staffing: staff trained in adult life support (ALS), sufficient staff to monitor patient after procedure whilst recovering from sedation.
> Patient consent: written information detailing what conscious sedation is, options available, and associated risks.
> Patient selection/pre-procedure assessment: assessment for comorbidities, patient in agreement with plan.
> Peri-procedure management: monitoring (noninvasive blood pressure, capnography, oxygen saturations plus ECG if indicated by patient comorbidities), oxygen, minimum sedation necessary, ideally just entonox, careful titration of dose, allowing each dose to reach peak effect. Opioid administration only if pain likely to be a significant feature of the procedure that cannot be managed with local anaesthetic alone (discuss with dentist) and then only small dose of short-acting drug, i.e. fentanyl.
> Postprocedure care: suitable area for recovery with member of staff trained to care for and monitor such a patient (may be appropriate for anaesthetist to remain with patient), discharge to care of responsible adult who will escort patient home and remain with them for 24 hours. Discharge only to take place when patient orientated and observations stable. Written information to be provided regarding complications, advice to not drive/operate machinery/make important decisions for 24 hours, contact numbers for advice and what to do in an emergency.
> Clinical governance, audit, education and training: staff competencies in all areas of practice to be maintained (e.g. resuscitation, recovery etc.). Critical incident reporting and analysis.

References

American Society of Anaesthesiologists. Continuum of Depth of Sedation: Definition of General Anesthesia and Levels of Sedation/Analgesia. http://www.asahq.org/quality-and-practice-management/standards-and-guidelines [Accessed 4th July 2017].

Intercollegiate Advisory Committee for Sedation in Dentistry. *Standards for Conscious Sedation in the Provision of Dental Care*. The Dental Faculties of the Royal Colleges of Surgeons and the Royal College of Anaesthetists; 2015.

14. TRAUMA AND STABILISATION

A 90-year-old woman sustains a fractured neck of femur following a fall. She is scheduled for surgery.

a) What aspects of this patient's care will have the greatest impact on outcome? (45%)

b) Outline the recommendations made by the National Institute for Health and Clinical Excellence (2011) for the management of acute pain in this patient. (30%)

c) What causes of a fall in this patient might impact on the anaesthetic management? (25%)

March 2012

Chairman's Report

52.9% pass rate.

Significant number of candidates gave a generic answer without relating to the current NICE guidelines. A significant number of candidates in section (b) failed to concentrate on the management of pain and digressed to general aspects of care.

a) What aspects of this patient's care will have the greatest impact on outcome? (45%)

The NICE guidance was issued in 2011, thus making it very topical for the March 2012 paper. However, it was then updated in May 2017 and my answers here reflect the updated guidance.

1. Multidisciplinary care within a Hip Fracture Programme, to include the following:
   - Rapid optimisation of correctable conditions for surgery, e.g. anaemia, anticoagulation, volume depletion, electrolyte imbalance, uncontrolled diabetes, uncontrolled heart failure, correctable cardiac arrhythmia/ischaemia, acute chest infection, exacerbation of chronic chest conditions.
   - Orthogeriatrician input.
   - Individualised rehabilitation goals.
   - Liaison with related services (mental health, falls prevention, primary care, social services).

2. Surgery on planned trauma list on day of or day after admission. Team to include senior anaesthetist and surgeon.

3. Surgical approach:
   - Total hip replacement (rather than hemiarthroplasty) for displaced intracapsular fracture if the patient is previously fit, active and cognitively intact.

- Extramedullary implant for trochanteric fracture above and including the lesser trochanter (cheaper and less likely to be involved in periprosthetic fracture than intramedullary implant).
- Intramedullary nail for subtrochanteric fracture.

4. Rehabilitation: daily, to start no later than the day after surgery and to continue after hospital discharge.

b) Outline the recommendations made by the National Institute for Health and Clinical Excellence (2011) for the management of acute pain in this patient. (30%)

Even if you haven't read the guidance, you will still have had experience of managing such patients and will understand the need for an escalating, step-wise approach to pain relief. Don't forget to talk about the need for pain assessment.

> Assess pain:
  - Immediately on admission.
  - 30 minutes after analgesia given.
  - Hourly until settled on ward.
  - As part of routine observations thereafter.
> Analgesia to be given immediately on admission with suspected hip fracture, even if cognitively impaired.
> Pain control should be adequate to allow investigations.
> Step-wise, multimodal analgesia:
  - Paracetamol six hourly unless contraindicated.
  - Opioid as necessary.
  - Nerve block (e.g. fascia iliaca block) by trained personnel.
  - NSAIDs not recommended.

c) What causes of a fall in this patient might impact on the anaesthetic management? (25%)

Follow the alphabet to think of all possible causes of a fall that might impact on safety or manner of provision of general anaesthesia, neuraxial techniques or nerve blocks. The question has not specifically asked for an explanation of how those causes impact on anaesthetic management, so I have tried to be very brief in my explanations whilst being too nervous to leave out those explanations altogether.

> Respiratory: exacerbation of chronic obstructive pulmonary disease, pneumonia. Regional anaesthesia may be preferable to avoid interference with lung mechanics.
> Cardiovascular: brady- or tachyarrhythmias, myocardial infarction, valvular heart disease (e.g. aortic stenosis), structural abnormalities (e.g. hypertrophic obstructive cardiomyopathy). Higher levels of monitoring such as invasive blood pressure and cardiac output monitoring may be employed in the presence of significant comorbidities. Neuraxial techniques relatively contraindicated by left ventricular outflow-limiting disease.
> Neurological: stroke, peripheral neuropathy, dementia, Parkinson's. Confusion or other difficulty with positioning may cause problems complying with neuraxial approach. Pre-existing neuropathy should be documented prior to any form of anaesthesia.
> Endocrine: diabetes mellitus causing hypoglycaemia or diabetic ketoacidosis. Awake surgery would permit ongoing neurological monitoring (once fit for surgery).
> Pharmacology: polypharmacy in the elderly causes a multitude of side effects such as hypotension, bradycardia, electrolyte disturbance. More invasive monitoring and adjusted doses of drugs may be required.
> Infection, immune: sepsis causing confusion, hypoxia. Sepsis may contraindicate neuraxial technique.
> Cutaneoumusculoskeletal: arthritic conditions causing pain and deformity. May cause difficulty with positioning for regional or neuraxial techniques.

References

Maxwell L, White S. Anaesthetic management of patients with hip fractures: an update. *Contin Educ Anaesth Crit Care Pain*. 2013; 13 (5): 179–183.

National Institute for Health and Care Excellence. Management of Hip Fractures in Adults CG124. June 2011, updated May 2017.

National Institute for Health and Care Excellence. Hip Fracture in Adults Quality Standard [QS16]. March 2012, updated May 2017.

An elderly patient has sustained a fractured neck of femur following a fall and is scheduled for surgery.

a) Which aspects of this patient's care have a significant impact on outcome? (45%)

b) Outline the recommendations of best practice for the management of pain in this patient. (30%)

c) What causes of a fall in this patient might impact on the anaesthetic management? (25%)

March 2014

Chairman's Report

53.1% pass rate.

Management of a patient with a hip fracture is fundamental to anaesthetic practice and very topical. This question was straightforward for candidates who had read one of the recent guidelines published by NICE or the AAGBI, and a number of individuals gained maximum marks. The question proved highly discriminatory between generally strong and generally weak candidates.

Two years later, the question reappears with the wording changed ever so slightly and yet still only 53% of people pass it!

A 45-year-old man has a major haemorrhage following significant trauma and is admitted to your emergency department. He does <u>not</u> have a head injury.

a) Give one definition of major haemorrhage. (1 mark)

b) What are the principles of management of major haemorrhage in this patient? (11 marks)

c) What complications might follow a massive blood transfusion? (8 marks)

March 2016

Chairman's Report

85.3% pass rate.

This is an important topic and was generally well answered. It is reassuring that candidates have sound knowledge of the management of major haemorrhage and of the complications of massive transfusion.

The AAGBI 'glossy', 'The Use of Blood Components and Their Alternatives', brings together three previous AAGBI guidelines. It is clinically useful to read and also contains plenty of material that could be the basis of future questions.

a) Give one definition of major haemorrhage. (1 mark)

There are lots of definitions referred to in the guideline. Pick your favourite.

> Loss of more than one blood volume within 24 hours (70 ml/kg or 5 l in a 70 kg adult).
> 50% of total blood volume loss in less than three hours.
> Bleeding in excess of 150 ml/min.
> Bleeding that results in systolic blood pressure less than 90 mm Hg or heart rate greater than 110 bpm.

b) What are the principles of management of major haemorrhage in this patient? (11 marks)

You manage this situation commonly in the course of your normal working life. Think about the organisational aspects of managing major haemorrhage in addition to the more narrow focus of what you as an individual do. Stop haemorrhage, treat blood loss, treat related haematological disturbances.

This is a medical emergency. I would call for help and follow an ABCDE trauma team management approach to this patient, assessing and treating him simultaneously as issues are revealed.

Institute the major haemorrhage protocol:
> Immediate release of blood components (packed red cells and fresh frozen plasma) for initial resuscitation without prior approval by haematologist.
> Communication to key personnel: on-call anaesthetists, surgeons, portering staff, blood bank staff.
> Nominated individual to liaise with the laboratory.

Immediate patient management:
> Recognition of major haemorrhage: concealed or revealed, may have multiple sources, start to control.
> A and B:
  • 100% oxygen, definitive airway if indicated, cervical-spine control.
> C:
  • Early haemorrhage control: pressure, tourniquets, immobilisation and splinting until definitive intervention.
  • Large-bore intravenous access (intraosseous if intravenous not feasible).
  • Take blood for cross-match, coagulation, full blood count, urea and electrolytes, arterial blood gas. Repeat checks during resuscitation to guide ongoing management. Use point-of-care testing if available.
  • Use pressure infusers, blood warmers, cell salvage if applicable.
  • Do not give clear fluids unless profoundly hypotensive and no blood products imminently available.

- Allow permissive hypotension whilst the patient is actively haemorrhaging, avoid vasopressors.
- Follow protocol regarding patient identification prior to giving blood products.
- O negative should be immediately available in clinical area and can be used if there is a delay in blood issue from the blood bank. O positive may be used as patient is an adult male.
- Group specific blood should be ready in 15–20 minutes.
- Fresh frozen plasma should be given 1:1 with packed red cells to replace volume loss.
- Consider cryoprecipitate two pools and platelets one dose until bleeding is controlled and blood test results are available.
- Consider tranexamic acid 1 g.
- Establish whether the patient is taking drugs that interfere with coagulation. Discuss with haematologist and treat as indicated.
- Monitor resuscitation with point-of-care and laboratory tests:
  - Fresh frozen plasma if INR greater than 1.5.
  - Cryoprecipitate if fibrinogen less than 1.5 g/l.
  - Platelets if platelet count less than 75×10^9/l.
- Catheterise to help guide ongoing fluid management.

> D:
- The question states that there is no head injury. Monitor neurological status as another indicator of cardiovascular stability. Give paracetamol and cautious opioid-based pain relief as required.

> E:
- Full exposure to check for all sources of bleeding.
- Initiate patient warming.

c) What complications might follow a massive blood transfusion? (8 marks)

I have put in a few details of the mechanisms of some of these reactions because I find it easier to remember something when I understand it, but this is not actually asked for.

Early:
> Haemolytic reaction:
  - Immediate: ABO incompatibility due to error. Delayed: Rhesus, Kidd, other minor blood groupings.
> Non-haemolytic febrile reactions: reaction to donor leucocyte antigens.
> Allergic reaction: recipient immunoglobulin E versus donor proteins.
> Transfusion-related acute lung injury (TRALI): donor leucocyte antibodies reacting with human leucocyte antigens (HLA) and human neutrophil antigens (HNA) in the recipient.
> Reaction due to bacterial contamination.
> Transfusion-associated circulatory overload (TACO).
> Hyperkalaemia: potassium content in stored blood rises with time due to loss of activity of red blood cell Na/K ATPase pump.
> Citrate toxicity: large amounts of citrate in fresh frozen plasma and platelets, binds calcium resulting in hypocalcaemia, impacts on cardiac conduction and coagulation.
> Acid base disturbance: citric acid from anticoagulant and lactic acid from stored cells. Metabolism of both usually rapid so may result in alkalosis.
> Hypothermia.
> Air embolism.
> Thrombophlebitis.
> Coagulation abnormalities if other blood components not given appropriately.

Late:
> Infection:
  - Viral: Hepatitis A, B or C, HIV, CMV.
  - Bacterial.
  - Parasitic: malaria, toxoplasma.

- Prion: vCJD (risk reduced since universal leucodepletion of donated blood, exclusion of donors who have received blood transfusions in UK, sourcing of plasma for fractionation from abroad).
> Immune sensitisation, e.g. to rhesus.

Reference

Association of Anaesthetists of Great Britain and Ireland. AAGBI guidelines: the use of blood components and their alternatives 2016. *Anaesthesia*. 2016; 71: 829–842.

A 20-year-old man is brought to the emergency department having been pulled from a river where he got into difficulties whilst swimming.

a) Describe the <u>relevant</u> history (5 marks) and investigations (8 marks) for this patient who has suffered near-drowning.

b) He has a Glasgow Coma Score of 13 but is found to have an arterial oxygen partial pressure of 6 kPa (45 mm Hg) breathing 4 l of oxygen via a variable performance mask. Outline your initial management of this patient. (7 marks)

March 2016

Chairman's Report

57.9% pass rate.

Candidates who scored well in part (a) of this question presented well-organized answers. Examiners marking this question felt that candidates who scored poorly in part (b) did so because they tended to focus solely on airway management and did not mention other important measures in the resuscitation such as rewarming and fluid management. This part of the question asked for initial management, not just airway management.

a) Describe the <u>relevant</u> history (5 marks) and investigations (8 marks) for this patient who has suffered near-drowning.

Relevant history:
> Medical history: seek possible medical cause for near-drowning such as epilepsy, arrhythmia, cardiac history, uncontrolled diabetes.
> Toxins: drugs, alcohol ingestion.
> Trauma: may have associated injuries such as injury from a boat, diving, debris in water, foul play.
> Scene: timings, duration of submersion, contaminants in water, type of water (*this question says river*), ambient and water temperature. Witnesses useful.

Relevant investigations:
> Core body temperature.
> Capillary blood glucose:
  • Poor control of diabetes may be cause of events.
  • Target normal blood glucose to maximise neurological outcome.
> Arterial blood gases:
  • Likely hypoxic, hypercapnic, with lactic acidosis.
> Venous blood:
  • Urea, creatinine, creatine kinase. Acute kidney injury may develop from myoglobinuria, hypoxaemia, hypoperfusion, haemolysis.
  • Electrolytes. Occasionally, electrolyte changes from fluid shifts.
  • Full blood count and coagulation. Disseminated intravascular coagulation may occur.
  • Toxicological assays for drugs and alcohol.
> 12-lead ECG:
  • Risk of arrhythmias due to hypothermia, hypoxia, acid-base disturbance.
  • May identify underlying cardiac event.
> Chest x-ray:
  • Risk of ARDS.
> Transthoracic echo:
  • May help optimise cardiovascular management in the presence of instability.
> Trauma imaging:
  • Cervical spine imaging, CT head, as indicated by history and examination.
> Microbiology:
  • Sputum or tracheal aspirates once intubated. May help with antimicrobial management in the presence of developing sepsis.

b) He has a Glasgow Coma Score of 13 but is found to have an arterial oxygen partial pressure of 6 kPa (45 mm Hg) breathing 4 l of oxygen via a variable performance mask. Outline your initial management of this patient. (7 marks)

I would call for help and adopt an ABCDE trauma team management approach to this patient, assessing and treating him simultaneously as issues are revealed.

A:

> Assess airway patency, open airway.
> Prepare for rapid sequence induction (RSI) if patient unable to maintain own airway or does not respond rapidly to measures to improve breathing adequacy.
> Cervical spine control with all airway manoeuvres if there is any possibility of injury.

B:

> 100% oxygen by non-rebreathe bag, saturations monitoring, aim to rapidly improve PaO_2 as monitored by ABG. Need to resolve hypoxia to reduce risk of secondary brain injury. GCS may improve with better PaO_2. Move on to preoxygenation with a tight-fitting mask if insufficient improvement.
> Chest examination and auscultation may give evidence of associated injuries (including pneumothorax), developing ARDS, foreign body inhalation.
> If PaO_2 and GCS not rapidly improving with higher inhaled oxygen concentration, proceed with RSI (stomach likely full of water), intubate.
> Consider orogastric or nasogastric (if no associated head injury) tube to empty stomach of water and facilitate ventilation.
> Lung protective ventilation: 6 ml/kg, high PEEP, 100% oxygen initially.
> CXR may demonstrate ARDS, foreign body aspiration (e.g. sand – consider bronchoalveolar lavage).

C:

> Large-bore intravenous access.
> Intravascular depletion occurs due to pulmonary and systemic extravasation.
> Warmed intravenous fluids with cardiac output monitoring guidance.
> Arterial cannulation to monitor blood pressure and blood gases. Aim MAP greater than 80 mm Hg for neuroprotection.
> Inotropes or vasopressors may be required.
> Monitor for, and manage, arrhythmias caused by hypothermia or electrolyte disturbance.
> Catheterise. Monitor urine output as an indicator of end-organ perfusion.

D:

Manage secondary brain injury risks:

> Maintain glucose 5–10 mmol/l.
> Warm to 34°C only: warmed fluids, forced air warming, electrical warming pads for 24 hours (fully rewarm if patient is not intubated).
> Observe for seizures; treat with benzodiazepines as first line.
> 15–20 degree head-up tilt.
> Care with tube tie tightness – do not obstruct venous return.

E:

> Manage coexisting injuries, or precipitating causes.

Reference

Carter E, Sinclair R. Drowning. *Contin Educ Anaesth Crit Care Pain*. 2011; 11 (6): 210–213.

15. INTENSIVE CARE MEDICINE

a) What features are required to meet the American-European criteria for a diagnosis of acute respiratory distress syndrome (ARDS)? (20%)

b) List the clinical indices used to quantify and communicate problems with oxygenation in ARDS. (10%)

c) What tidal volume would you select for a patient that meets the criteria for ARDS? (10%)

d) List the ventilatory (30%) and non-ventilatory (30%) measures that can be taken to improve oxygenation or prevent further deterioration in a patient with ARDS.

September 2011

An almost identical question featured in the March 2017 paper. Definitions of ARDS changed between 2012 and 2017 and so I will address the topic in the later question.

You are asked to review an 18-year-old male in the emergency department who has been found obtunded at home. He is an insulin-dependent diabetic with a history of poor glycaemic control. Capillary blood glucose is 23.4 mmol/l.

a) List the clinical and biochemical findings that confirm severe diabetic ketoacidosis (DKA). (40%)

b) Outline the management plan for severe DKA within the first hour. (40%)

c) What are the serious complications that can follow the management of DKA? (20%)

March 2012

Chairman's Report

57.2% pass rate.

'The Management of Diabetic Ketoacidosis in Adults' was first published in 2010 and appeared in the exam two years later. It was then updated in September 2013 – time for a reappearance? I have answered this question based on the updated guidance. The guideline discusses management of diabetic ketoacidosis, broken down into actions to be performed within certain timescales. The answer to part (b) summarises their guidance for management over the first hour.

a) List the clinical and biochemical findings that confirm severe diabetic ketoacidosis (DKA). (40%)

The presence of any of the following indicates <u>severe</u> diabetic ketoacidosis, mandating consultant physician assessment and consideration of referral for level 2 care:

Clinical findings:
> GCS less than 12 or abnormal AVPU score.
> Oxygen saturation below 92% on air (assuming normal baseline respiratory function).
> Systolic BP below 90 mm Hg.
> Pulse over 100 or below 60 bpm.

Biochemical findings:
> Blood ketones over 6 mmol/l.
> Bicarbonate level below 5 mmol/l.
> Venous/arterial pH below 7.0.
> Hypokalaemia on admission (under 3.5 mmol/l).
> Anion gap above 16 (anion gap = $(Na^+ + K^+) - (Cl^- + HCO3^-)$).

b) Outline the management plan for severe DKA within the first hour. (40%)

Severe DKA is a medical emergency and I would seek senior help and diabetic team input and assess and manage the patient simultaneously adopting an ABC approach. DKA management guidance should be followed. Fluids followed by insulin treatment should be instituted without delay and so gaining intravenous access is a priority.

Airway:
> 15 l oxygen via non-rebreathe mask.
> Consider need for immediate intubation due to reduced conscious level or respiratory distress.

Respiratory:
> Monitor respiratory rate and continuous oxygen saturations.
> Auscultate chest, checking for evidence of underlying infection or heart failure.

Cardiovascular:
> Check pulse and establish monitoring: continuous ECG, blood pressure (initially noninvasive and then intra-arterial).
> Large bore cannulation.
> Fluid resuscitate:
  • 500 ml 0.9% sodium chloride/15 minutes if SBP less than 90 mm Hg.
  • Repeat if SBP remains below 90 mm Hg. If no improvement, consider other underlying causes and seek senior or critical care input.

- Once SBP greater than 90 mm Hg or if it is above this value on admission, 1000 ml 0.9% sodium chloride should be given over an hour.
- Give intravenous potassium if serum potassium is below the upper limit of normal range. If hypokalaemic on admission, seek senior assistance.

Neurological:
> Assess GCS.

Exposure:
> Full examination, seek underlying cause and manage appropriately.
> Check temperature.

Insulin:
> Fixed rate intravenous insulin infusion to start after commencement of fluids at 0.1 units/kg/h.
> Continue with the patient's usual long-acting insulin.

Investigations:
> Blood ketones.
> Capillary blood glucose.
> Venous plasma glucose.
> Urea and electrolytes.
> Venous blood gases.
> Full blood count.
> Blood cultures.
> 12-lead ECG.
> Chest radiograph if clinically indicated.
> Urinalysis and culture.
> Consider precipitating causes and investigate appropriately.
> Pregnancy test in women of childbearing age.

c) What are the serious complications that can follow the management of DKA? (20%)

> Hypo- or hyperkalaemia, with risk of cardiac arrhythmia.
> Acute pre-renal failure.
> Hypoglycaemia, risking cardiac arrhythmia, brain injury, death.
> Cerebral oedema (more likely in children) due to fluid shifts of DKA, exacerbated by rehydration.
> Pulmonary oedema, rarely, in susceptible patients such as the elderly or those with pre-existing cardiac disease.

Reference
Joint British Diabetes Societies Inpatient Care Group. *The Management of Diabetic Ketoacidosis in Adults*. 2nd Edition. September 2013.

A 54-year-old inpatient collapses in the toilet.

a) What symptoms (15%) and signs (15%) might suggest acute pulmonary thrombo-embolism (PTE) as the cause of this acute event?

b) List investigations and their characteristic findings that might be of further assistance in establishing the diagnosis of PTE. (40%)

c) What are the principles of management of a shocked patient resulting from massive acute PTE? (30%)

March 2012

Chairman's Report

77.5% pass rate.

a) What symptoms (15%) and signs (15%) might suggest acute pulmonary thrombo-embolism (PTE) as the cause of this acute event?

Symptoms:
> Sudden onset of dyspnoea.
> Pleuritic chest pain.
> Haemoptysis.
> Syncope.
> Anxiety.
> Light headedness.

Signs:
> Cyanosis.
> Pleural rub.
> Tachypnoea, increased work of breathing.
> Wheeze.
> Tachycardia.
> Hypotension.
> Signs of acute right ventricular dysfunction: distended neck veins, parasternal heave, accentuated P2, tricuspid regurgitation.
> Progression to cardiac arrest.
> Swollen, erythematous, tender calf.

b) List investigations and their characteristic findings that might be of further assistance in establishing the diagnosis of PTE. (40%)

You've been asked for a list, giving an indication of the level of detail required. It asks for those investigations that 'might be' useful and so the list is going to be fairly extensive. Whenever there is a question that requires you to list investigations, be systematic, start with the most basic and work onwards.

Test	Result	Limitations of test
D-dimer	Elevated	Very nonspecific
Arterial blood gas	Low PaO_2, low $PaCO_2$. High A-a gradient	Nonspecific
ECG	Tachycardia. Atrial fibrillation. Right axis deviation S1Q3T3 (less than 20% cases)	Poor specificity and sensitivity – may help exclude alternative cause
Chest radiograph	Hypovascularity, peripherally-located wedge-shaped area of consolidation	Nonspecific and non-sensitive – may help with alternative diagnosis
Ultrasound	Evidence of thrombus in leg veins	Supportive of diagnosis if present
Lung scintigraphy – V/Q scan	V/Q mismatch	High negative predictive value but frequently inconclusive
Computerised tomographic pulmonary angiography (CTPA)	Thrombus visualised in pulmonary artery. Will also give information about chronicity of clot, and consequences (right heart strain)	Highly specific and sensitive. Also useful to exclude alternate causes. Caution in renal impairment. Increased risk of consequences of ionising radiation in pregnant or recently post-partum women
Magnetic resonance angiography	Thrombus visualised in pulmonary artery	Diagnostic accuracy not as good as CT, and not as universally available
Echocardiography	Acute right heart strain: dilated right atrium and ventricle, impaired right ventricular function. Sometimes, thrombus can be visualised. Transoesophageal echo can detect intracardiac or pulmonary clot more reliably	Bedside test for unstable patient too unwell for transfer to radiology
Pulmonary angiography	Absence of blood flow in affected pulmonary artery	Invasive, rarely used for diagnosis

c) What are the principles of management of a shocked patient resulting from massive acute PTE? (30%)

PTE is classified as massive (hypotension and cardiogenic shock), submassive (haemodynamically stable but right heart strain evident on echo) and non-massive.

This is a medical emergency. I would call for help and assess and manage the patient simultaneously adopting an ABC approach.

Resuscitation:

> 100% oxygen, intubation likely to be required.
> Precise management depends on clinical situation.
> Intravenous access, cautious intravenous fluid (may exacerbate right heart failure) and inotropic support with phenylephrine or adrenaline, depends on patient condition.
> Prepare for possible cardiac arrest, call for drugs and defibrillator. Likely rhythm would be PEA and resuscitation efforts should be prolonged (if appropriate to the patient's overall condition) once thrombolysis is given.

Definitive management:

> Definitive treatment should not be delayed and is based on clinical findings and, if possible, bedside echo.
> Thrombolysis with alteplase. Assessment for contraindications but risk/benefit analysis in arrest or periarrest situations favours thrombolysis.
> Unfractionated heparin infusion to follow thrombolysis.
> Invasive techniques (thrombus fragmentation and IVC filter) should be considered in centres where expertise and facilities available.

References

British Thoracic Society Standards of Care Committee Pulmonary Embolism Guideline Development Group. British Thoracic Society guidelines for the management of suspected acute pulmonary embolism. *Thorax*. 2003; 58: 470–484.

Garner D, Pilcher D. The management of pulmonary embolism. *Anaesth Intensive Care Med*. 2010; 11 (12): 512–518.

You have been called urgently to attend a ventilated patient on the ICU who has become acutely agitated, hypertensive and profoundly hypoxic. A percutaneous tracheostomy was performed 18 hours ago and is being weaned from ventilatory support.

a) List possible causes for this patient's acute hypoxia. (25%)

b) What clinical features support an airway problem? (40%)

c) How would you manage an airway problem in this patient? (35%)

March 2012

Chairman's Report

76.6% pass rate.

In the main was a well-answered question.

This is one of the many questions that are based on the findings from NAP4. Please read it!

a) List possible causes for this patient's acute hypoxia. (25%)

They have said list – don't waste time on prose. And, the College has made it clear on many occasions that the use of tables is fine. I have tried to focus the answer on the issues that are most likely to affect the individual circumstances of this patient; don't just write a list of all known causes of hypoxia.

Patient problems	Equipment problems
Pneumothorax.	Tracheostomy tube blocked with secretions or blood.
Haemothorax.	Dislodged tube.
Pneumomediastinum.	Cuff puncture or deflation or herniation over end of tube.
Haemomediastinum.	Cuff inflated with speaking valve in situ.
Surgical emphysema.	Ventilator circuit blockage or disconnection.
Atelectasis, inadequate ventilation due to overly rapid weaning.	Inappropriate ventilator settings.
Aspiration.	Inappropriately low fraction of inspired oxygen.

b) What clinical features support an airway problem? (40%)

This is the second time I have underlined a word in this question – it really does help you focus your mind on what they are actually asking you. Again, this is suited to a list. The less you write, the less the examiner has to wade through your handwriting to find your answers.

> Acute desaturation.
> Obvious incorrect placement of tracheostomy.
> Paradoxical chest movement.
> Increased work of breathing and tachypnoea.
> Absence or abnormal morphology of capnography trace.
> Hypertension.
> Surgical emphysema.
> Neck swelling.
> In an awake patient, severe agitation and restlessness.

c) How would you manage an airway problem in this patient? (35%)

Tracheostomy dislodgement on ICU and failure to recognise or manage this eventuality contributed to ICU airway-related deaths reported to NAP4 (of 14 patients who had dislodgements, 7 died and 4 had hypoxic brain injury). NAP4 therefore produced a flowchart for management of this situation and many hospitals will have adapted these for their own use. You do not have to have memorised the guidelines for the purposes of the exam – if you are working at night, alone on an ICU, caring for patients with tracheostomy tubes, then you should have a mental plan for this issue anyway.

> Fast bleep for senior help/resuscitation team according to local protocols, and call for difficult airway trolley.
> 100% oxygen via Mapleson C to tracheostomy and over mouth.*
> Stop nasogastric feed.
> Assess:
  - Chest and Mapleson C bag movement.
  - Capnography waveform.
  - For obvious tube dislodgement, secretions, blood, neck swelling, surgical emphysema.
> In the absence of breathing or a normal capnography trace:
  - Attempt two ventilated breaths.
  - If unsuccessful, remove inner tube (if present) and pass suction tube through tracheostomy to clear any blood or secretions causing blockage (inner tube may need reinserting to reconnect to circuit).
  - If unsuccessful, deflate cuff and observe whether the patient now able to breathe around tracheostomy. Consider reinflating if condition improves (cuff may have herniated over end of tube).
> If no improvement, remove tracheostomy (occlude stoma with gauze and occlusive dressing), start 2 person face mask oxygenation with oropharyngeal airway, either spontaneous or manually assisted ventilation.
> If successful and oxygen saturations improving:
  - Continue whilst checking notes for previous ease of laryngoscopy, indication for percutaneous tracheostomy etc. (although laryngoscopy grade may have worsened).
  - Ensure emergency drugs, difficult airway trolley and senior help have arrived before attempting oral intubation.
> If unsuccessful try:
  - SAD.
  - Oral intubation (uncut tube to be advanced beyond stoma).
  - Intubation of stoma (size 6.0 COETT), although the tract will not have developed yet, and so mask ventilation via this route unlikely to be an option either.
> Once airway managed appropriately, move on to assess and manage cardiorespiratory stability.

There is a connection between the mouth and lungs in this patient – remember that this is not always the case.

Reference
4th National Audit Project of the Royal College of Anaesthetists and the Difficult Airway Society. Major complications of airway management in the United Kingdom. London 2011.

A 45-year-old man with a history of ulcerative colitis and alcohol abuse is admitted to the intensive care unit for inotropic and ventilatory support following a laparotomy to excise a toxic megacolon. His body mass index is 18 kg/m².

a) Why should this patient receive early nutritional support and what are the clinical benefits? (30%)

b) What is the specific composition of a nutritional regimen for this patient? (30%)

c) List the advantages and disadvantages of enteral nutrition. (40%)

September 2012

Chairman's Report

44.9% pass rate.

This question was answered poorly. The provision of enteral and parenteral nutrition in critically ill patients is very important and a detailed knowledge of the specific components of a feeding regimen is essential. The specific components required were:

> Water (ml/kg/day)
> Calories (kCal/kg/day)
> Protein, fat and carbohydrate (g/day)
> Na/K (mmol/kg/day) and minerals
> Vitamins
> Immunonutrition

Many candidates failed to be specific enough. Leaving the prescribing to the 'nutrition team' or 'intensive care dietician' are not appropriate answers.

a) Why should this patient receive early nutritional support and what are the clinical benefits? (30%)

Note two questions in one – make sure you answer both bits.

Need for early nutritional support:

> Existing malnourishment evidenced by low BMI.
> Chronic alcohol excess associated with malnutrition.
> Long-term gastrointestinal disease associated with malnutrition.
> Inflammatory condition, recent surgery, sepsis and critical illness all contribute to a catabolic state.
> Poor absorptive capacity.
> Unlikely to be able to re-establish normal oral feeding within the next five days so supplementation indicated.

Clinical benefits:
> Improved wound healing.
> Improved weaning from ventilator, reduced risk of respiratory infection, maintenance of respiratory muscle strength all contribute to fewer ventilator-dependent days.
> Improved immune function generally.
> Improved rehabilitation due to maintenance of skeletal muscle strength.
> Reduced ICU length of stay.
> Overall reduced mortality.

b) What is the specific composition of a nutritional regimen for this patient? (30%)

Assessment of this patient according to NICE guidelines indicates that he is at risk of refeeding syndrome. Risk factors include the following:

> *Low BMI with unintentional weight loss.*
> *Poor recent nutritional intake.*
> *Low serum potassium, magnesium or phosphate.*
> *History of alcohol abuse.*
> *Drugs including chemotherapy, insulin, antacids and diuretics.*

Chronic malnutrition causes depletion of electrolytes through reduced intake and utilisation for metabolism of fat and lipid stores. Serum electrolyte levels are maintained better than intracellular levels due to reduced energy for transmembrane pumping and reduced insulin-dependent pumping. Upon refeeding, there is a sudden insulin-driven uptake of glucose into cells and accompanying electrolytes. Serum levels of these ions, such as magnesium, phosphate, calcium and potassium, can drop precipitously. Also, cardiac muscle is weakened by chronic malnutrition. On refeeding, the circulating volume increases due to glucose-driven osmolality, risking heart failure. Weakened respiratory muscles must attempt to cope with increased carbon dioxide production as the body reverts to more carbohydrate-based metabolism (the respiratory quotient for a carbohydrate diet being 1, but 0.7 for fat- and 0.9 for protein-based diets, respectively). This may precipitate arrhythmias, seizures, respiratory failure, cardiac failure, coma, death.

> This patient is at risk of refeeding syndrome due to:
> * Low BMI.
> * Alcohol abuse.
> * Low recent oral intake likely due to illness.
> * Toxic megacolon and ulcerative colitis may have resulted in electrolyte imbalance.

> Water 30–35 ml/kg/day, but guided by fluid balance, abnormal losses and cardiac output monitoring. Avoid excessive fluid input in refeeding situation.

> The following are normal requirements, all of which should be cut to one-third for the first four to seven days of nutrition in a patient at risk of refeeding syndrome:
> * 30 kCal/kg/day.
> * 60% intake from carbohydrate so 4.8 g/kg/day.
> * 40% intake from fat so 1.3 g/kg/day.
> * Protein 0.8–1.5 g/kg/day.

> Electrolytes should be guided by frequent blood testing, and increased quantities likely to be needed in refeeding situation:
> * Sodium 1 mmol/kg/day.
> * Potassium 2–4 mmol/kg/day.
> * Phosphate 0.3–0.6 mmol/kg/day.
> * Magnesium 0.2 mmol/kg/day.

> Vitamins:
> * Intravenous thiamine and riboflavin: one to two pairs Pabrinex twice daily 30 minutes *before* starting feeding and continued for 10 days.
> * Supplement vitamins A, D, E, K, C.

> Trace elements:
> * Copper, zinc, selenium, manganese.

> Immunonutrition:
> * Glutamine 0.2 g/kg/day.

ICU dietician will work within the multidisciplinary team to optimise nutrition of this patient.

c) List the advantages and disadvantages of enteral nutrition. (40%)

Advantages	Disadvantages
Cheaper.	May not be absorbed.
Avoidance of line infections and the complications of line insertion.	May therefore result in malnutrition.
Reduced risk of stress ulceration.	Risk of aspiration and pneumonia.
Maintenance of gut integrity, absorptive and immune function.	Necrosis and bleeding of nose or small bowel due to erosion by feeding tube (nasogastric, PEG or PEJ).
Lower risk of hyperglycaemia.	
Reduced risk of abnormal liver function test results, hypertriglyceridaemia, metabolic acidosis, electrolyte imbalance and uraemia associated with parenteral feeding.	

References

Macdonald K, Page K, Brown L, Bryden D. Parenteral nutrition in critical care. *Contin Educ Anaesth Crit Care Pain*. 2013; 13 (1): 1–5.

National Institute for Health and Care Excellence. Nutrition support for adults: oral nutrition support, enteral tube feeding and parenteral nutrition CG32. 2006.

a) Outline the general principles in the management of poisoning by <u>oral ingestion</u>? (40%)

b) What are the mechanisms of toxicity of a tricyclic antidepressant (TCA) overdose? (10%)

c) List the clinical features of a TCA overdose (20%) and how the associated life threatening complications are managed. (30%)

March 2013

Chairman's Report

65% pass rate.

This question was also answered well. Some candidates failed to focus on the history of the overdose and risk assessments to attendants.

In section (b) on the mechanisms of toxicity of tricyclic antidepressants (TCA) the following points were required:

Decreased norepinephrine/serotonin reuptake

Anticholinergic effects

Direct alpha-adrenergic block

Na channel block

One mark for each mechanism (maximum of 2).

The management TCA overdose involved airway protection, gastric decontamination and the management of seizures. The model answer needed details of the treatment of hypotension, arrhythmias and acidaemia (fluids, sodium bicarbonate, vasopressors glucagon and magnesium).

The Chairman's Report on this question almost gives you a mark sheet, a really useful insight into the level of detail the examiners are looking for.

a) Outline the general principles in the management of poisoning by oral ingestion. (40%)

> This is a medical emergency. I would call for help and would assess and manage the patient simultaneously following an ABCDE approach.
> If there is any possibility of e.g. organophosphate poisoning, then staff protection should be considered.
> Airway:
>   • Oxygen 15 l/min via non-rebreathe bag.
>   • Intubate if unable to maintain own airway due to reduced or falling conscious level.
> Respiratory:
>   • Continuous oxygen saturations monitoring.
>   • Assess ventilatory adequacy and for signs of respiratory distress.
>   • Auscultate chest.
> Cardiovascular:
>   • Large-bore intravenous access.
>   • Continuous ECG and noninvasive blood pressure measurement.
>   • Intra-arterial blood pressure monitoring should be initiated as soon as possible.
> Neurological:
>   • Monitor GCS, which may deteriorate.
> Exposure:
>   • Full examination.
>   • Check capillary blood glucose.
> History:
>   • Ascertain likely poison (information from ambulance crew, family, empty packets or bottles found with patient, current prescriptions), quantity ingested and whether taken with alcohol.
>   • Attempt to establish likely interval between ingestion and presentation.
>   • Ascertain comorbidities and other regular medications that may cause interactions etc.

> Blood tests:
  - Arterial blood gas (pH, lactate, and to assess ventilatory adequacy), full blood count, urea and electrolytes, glucose, liver function tests, paracetamol levels (four hours post exposure, ideally), urine toxicology screen.
> Radiology:
  - Chest radiograph; pulmonary oedema may occur with salicylate or opiate poisoning.
  - Abdominal radiograph if considering body packing.
> Advice from Toxbase, National Poisons Information Service (NPIS) or Guy's and St Thomas' Poisons Unit (GTPU) re:
  - Specific antidotes.
  - Gastric decontamination.
  - Alkaline diuresis.
  - Haemodialysis.

b) What are the mechanisms of toxicity of a tricyclic antidepressant (TCA) overdose? (10%)

Sodium channel blockade	Cardiac depression, decrease in cardiac output, hypotension, arrhythmias, seizures.
Alpha adrenergic blockade	Hypotension.
Anticholinergic effects	Mydriasis, tachycardia, hypotension, ileus, irritability, confusion, seizures, coma, urinary retention, pyrexia.
Reduced norepinephrine and serotonin reuptake	Hypotension.

c) List the clinical features of a TCA overdose (20%) and how the associated life threatening complications are managed. (30%)

Clinical features	Management of associated life-threatening complications
• Respiratory depression, decreased level of consciousness, coma.	• Intubation, ventilation.
• Seizures.	• Benzodiazepines, anaesthesia.
• Acidosis, prolonged QRS.	• Sodium bicarbonate (increases sodium levels to compete with receptor blockade, alkalinises blood to reduce affinity of TCA for sodium channel).
• Arrhythmias.	• Magnesium, lidocaine, management of acidosis as previously.
• Hypotension.	• Intravenous fluid boluses. • Alpha agonists. • Glucagon (stimulates adenylate cyclase, which increases myocardial calcium causing increase in heart rate and contractility).
• Cardiac arrest.	• ALS guided resuscitation.
• All adverse reactions.	• Activated charcoal reduces absorption of TCA and so reduces all adverse effects.
• Life-threatening adverse neurological and cardiac symptoms, resistant to other treatments.	• Intralipid. • Consideration of ECMO.
• Pyrexia.	• Patient cooling.

References

Ozcan M, Weinberg G. Intravenous lipid emulsion for the treatment of drug toxicity. *J Intensive Care Med*. 2014; 29 (2): 59–70.

Penny L, Moriarty T. Poisoning in children. *Contin Educ Anaesth Crit Care Pain*. 2009; 9 (4): 109–113.

Ward C, Sair M. Oral poisoning: an update. *Contin Educ Anaesth Crit Care Pain*. 2010; 10 (1): 6–11.

a) What are the indications for renal replacement therapy (RRT) in the intensive care setting? (40%)

b) List the types of RRT available on intensive care. (30%)

c) Outline the principle mechanisms of solute and water removal by RRT. (30%)

September 2013

Chairman's Report

59.1% pass rate.

This was a relatively straightforward question that proved to be a very good discriminator. Sections (a) and (b) were answered well but section (c), on the description of the physical principles of filtration and dialysis were poor.

a) What are the indications for renal replacement therapy (RRT) in the intensive care setting? (40%)

> Acute kidney injury (AKI) with:
  • Refractory fluid overload.
  • Hyperkalaemia (greater than 6.5 mmol/l, failing to respond to medical management or rapidly rising).
  • Metabolic acidosis.
  • Rapidly increasing urea or creatinine.
  • Symptomatic uraemia: encephalopathy, pericarditis, bleeding, nausea.
  • Oliguria/anuria.
> Overdose with a dialysable drug or toxin.
> Severe sepsis.
> Management of pre-existing chronic kidney disease.

b) List the types of RRT available on intensive care. (30%)

Again, a list is required.

> Intermittent haemodialysis (cheaper, efficient, but more rapid fluid shifts may not be tolerated in cardiovascularly unstable or head injured patients. Not available in all ICUs).
> Continuous renal replacement therapies (CRRTs):
  • Continuous venovenous haemofiltration (CVVHF).
  • Continuous venovenous haemodialysis (CVVHD).
  • Continuous venovenous haemodiafiltration (CVVHDF).
> Peritoneal dialysis of a patient already using this form of RRT is feasible in the ICU but does not have the efficiency of haemodialysis, may cause problems with diaphragmatic splinting in ventilated patients, and is not appropriate in patients with intra-abdominal pathology.

c) Outline the principle mechanisms of solute and water removal by RRT. (30%)

Haemodialysis for removal of solutes:
> Blood pumped through an extracorporeal circuit that incorporates a dialyser (semipermeable membrane separating blood from crystalloid solution, the dialysate).
> Solutes move from high concentration to low according to Fick's laws of diffusion.
> To maintain concentration gradients, the dialysate flows countercurrent to the flow of the blood.

Haemofiltration for removal of water:
> Blood pumped through an extracorporeal system that incorporates a semipermeable membrane.
> Hydrostatic pressure drives plasma water across the membrane – this is ultrafiltration.
> Small molecules (less than 50 kDa) are dragged across the membrane with the water by convection.
> Ultrafiltrate is discarded and replacement fluid added according to desired fluid balance.

The following diagrams show the differences between haemodialysis and haemofiltration. You would not need to draw these to answer the question but they may help you to memorise the detail.

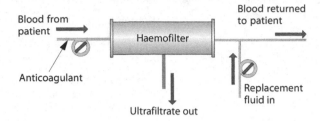

CVVHF

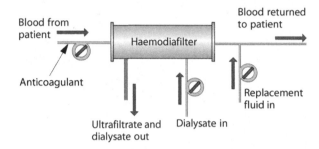

CVVHDF

References

Hall N, Fox A. Renal replacement therapies in critical care. *Contin Educ Anaesth Crit Care Pain*. 2006; 6 (5): 197–202.

Joannes-Boyau O et al. High-volume versus standard-volume haemofiltration for septic shock patients with acute kidney injury (IVOIRE study): a multicentre randomized controlled trial. *Intensive Care Med*. 2013; 39 (9): 1535–1546.

The RENAL Replacement Therapy Study Investigators. Intensity of continuous renal-replacement therapy in critically ill patients. *N Engl J Med*. 2009; 361: 1627–1638.

a) What are the indications for (20%) and possible contraindications to (25%) elective percutaneous tracheostomy (PCT)?

b) List the potential early (40%) and late (15%) patient complications of PCT.

March 2014

Chairman's Report

79.4% pass rate.

This question is highly relevant to modern critical care practice, and the involvement of trainees in PCT procedures is reflected by the very high pass rate. Most marks were lost in the section on complications but in general this question was well answered. It was obvious which candidates had observed or performed a significant numbers of PCTs and which had not.

Save your energy – this question is asking to be answered in bullet point or list form. Make sure you always leave space at the end of every subsection you answer in order to add another couple of points after you've moved on from the question.

a) What are the indications for (20%) and possible contraindications to (25%) elective percutaneous tracheostomy (PCT)?

Indications:
> For long-term ventilation or anticipated prolonged ventilatory wean.
> To avoid complications of long-term tracheal intubation (vocal cord damage, laryngeal damage and consequent stenosis).
> To allow sedation to be stopped whilst invasive ventilation is ongoing.
> To facilitate patient communication if patient is able, a tracheostomy with speaking valve is used.
> To reduce dead space.
> To facilitate tracheal suctioning.
> For airway protection in patient with poor airway reflexes, e.g. due to bulbar dysfunction.

Contraindications:

Absolute:
> Unstable cervical spine.
> Severe local infection of the anterior neck.
> Uncontrollable coagulopathy.

Relative:
> High PEEP or inspired oxygen requirements.
> Difficult anatomy (e.g. morbid obesity, short thick neck, reduced neck extension, excessive goitre, tracheal deviation, overlying blood vessels, extensive scarring).
> Proximity to extensive burns or surgical wounds.
> Haemodynamic instability.
> Previous neck radiotherapy.

b) List the potential early (40%) and late (15%) patient complications of PCT.

I have reverted to my alphabet approach here, in the absence of a better idea.

Early:
> Airway:
  • Loss of airway (with attendant risks of hypoxic brain damage and death).
  • Damage to airway: fracture of tracheal cartilages, damage to posterior wall of trachea, paratracheal placement.
  • Obstruction by blood, secretions, foreign body.
> Respiratory:
  • Derecruitment.
  • Pneumothorax.
  • Surgical emphysema.
> Cardiovascular:
  • Bleeding from any vessels of the neck.

> Neurological:
  • Damage to recurrent laryngeal nerve.

Late:
> Airway:
  • Displaced or blocked tube causing loss of airway (with attendant risks of hypoxic brain damage and death).
  • Tracheal stenosis and scarring (causing stridor, dyspnoea, poor cough, altered voice, dysphagia).
  • Tracheomalacia.
> Cardiovascular:
  • Erosion into blood vessels causing bleeding.
> Immune, infection:
  • Localised infection.
> Cutaneomusculoskeletal:
  • Scarring, persistent stoma.

Reference

Batuwitage B, Webber S, Glossop A. Percutaneous tracheostomy. *Contin Educ Anaesth Crit Care Pain*. 2014; 14 (6): 268–272.

a) What is Propofol-Related Infusion Syndrome (PRIS) and what are its clinical effects? (7 marks)

b) List the risk factors for PRIS. (5 marks)

c) What specific laboratory findings might be expected in a case of PRIS? (3 marks)

d) How may PRIS be prevented (3 marks) and managed? (2 marks)

September 2014

Chairman's Report

35.8% pass rate.

This question was felt to be hard to answer and was assigned a low pass mark after the Angoff process. It proved to be another very strong discriminator between candidates and was answered poorly in the main. Weak candidates had no real knowledge of the subject and did not appreciate that the cardiovascular consequences of the syndrome predominate. Many referred incorrectly to the precipitation of liver failure. Trainees undertaking a block of intensive care medicine will use propofol sedation for some patients so it is important that they understand any potential complications.

In each paper, there are '2 questions adjudged to be hard/difficult (pass mark 10–11/20),' and this was one of them. A CEACCP article about this topic was published in 2013. It really is common for questions to appear on topics that have been addressed in a CEACCP/BJA Education article within the previous two years.

a) What is propofol-related infusion syndrome (PRIS) and what are its clinical effects? (7 marks)

What is PRIS?

> Life-threatening syndrome associated with propofol use, usually at high doses for prolonged duration, in susceptible individuals.
> Propofol uncouples intracellular oxidative phosphorylation and inhibits electron flow through electron transport chain.
> Therefore, free fatty acids (which are an essential fuel for cardiac and skeletal myocytes) cannot be used for metabolism and reach elevated levels in the blood, risking arrhythmia and cardiac dysfunction.
> Cardiac and skeletal myocytes deprived of nutrition start to necrose.

Clinical effects?

> Cardiac dysfunction and arrhythmias: coved ST elevation in V1–V3 is characteristic, atrial or ventricular fibrillation, supraventricular tachycardia, bundle branch blocks, bradycardia, asystole.
> Rhabdomyolysis.
> Acute kidney injury.
> Lactic acidosis.
> Hypertryglyceridaemia.
> Hepatomegaly.
> Hyperkalaemia.
> Lipaemia.

b) List the risk factors for PRIS. (5 marks)

They have asked for a list, which makes life easier, but here is a bit of an explanation of why certain situations increase the risk as understanding the underlying reasons may help cement the list into your brain better:

> *Lipid overload from propofol or parenteral nutrition exacerbates accumulation of free fatty acids, which are proarrythmogenic. Adequate carbohydrate intake is required to suppress endogenous lipolysis in ill patients to reduce further increases in free fatty acid levels.*
> *Propofol antagonises β receptor and calcium channel binding, thus further depressing cardiac function whilst also reducing the effectiveness of inotropes to improve the situation.*
> *PRIS was first reported in children but is also seen in adults. Children may be more susceptible due to low glycogen stores causing increased endogenous lipolysis.*

> *Hyperdynamic circulation of sepsis or raised catecholamine levels of intracerebral lesions result in more rapid plasma clearance, insufficient sedation and, therefore, increased dose.*

> High infusion rates (greater than 4 mg/kg/h) for long duration (greater than 48 hours).
> Young age.
> Severe head injuries.
> Sepsis.
> High exogenous or endogenous catecholamines.
> High exogenous or endogenous glucocorticoids.
> Inborn errors of fatty acid oxidation.
> High ratio of lipid to carbohydrate intake.

c) What specific laboratory findings might be expected in a case of PRIS? (3 marks)

> Raised triglycerides.
> Raised creatinine kinase (CK).
> Raised lactate with accompanying acidosis.
> Evidence of acute kidney injury: elevated potassium, urea, creatinine.

d) How may PRIS be prevented (3 marks) and managed? (2 marks)

Prevention:
> Aim to keep infusion rates less than 4 mg/kg/h.
> If infusion rates are high, limit duration to less than 48 hours.
> Use alternative drugs for sedation.
> Ensure adequate carbohydrate supply (glucose infusion, ensuring parenteral nutrition offers adequate carbohydrate:lipid balance).
> Monitor markers of onset of syndrome: CK, lactate, triglycerides.

Management:
> Retain high index of suspicion for possibility of syndrome to facilitate timely management.
> Stop propofol, use alternative sedation.
> Pacing, inotropes, consideration of ECMO.
> Renal replacement therapy to manage lactic acidosis, acute kidney injury and to clear propofol and its metabolites.

Reference
Will Loh N, Nair P. Propofol infusion syndrome. *Contin Educ Anaesth Crit Care Pain*. 2013; 13 (6): 200–202.

a) Define critical illness weakness (CIW, 1 mark) and list the types that may occur. (3 marks)

b) List the risk factors for the development of weakness on the ICU. (6 marks)

c) What are the clinical features of CIW? (4 marks)

d) How may nerve conduction studies determine the type of CIW? (4 marks)

e) What are the options for the management of CIW? (2 marks)

March 2015

Chairman's Report

30.4% pass rate; 46.6% of candidates received a poor fail.

This question was anticipated to be difficult for the candidates, and the pass and poor fail rates reflect this expectation. The subject matter is topical and an important consideration in the management of critically ill patients. Many candidates had no idea that the definition excluded pre-existing pathology, and that the weakness was symmetrical with cranial nerves sparing. Few candidates had knowledge of the use of nerve conduction studies, and even fewer mentioned the MRC scale of scoring muscle power. The importance of preparing detailed notes on mandatory units of training when revising for the Final FRCA is exemplified by this question.

Did I mention how important CEACCP and BJA Education articles are? They are, basically, the College-approved opinion on a topic. Make use of them. An article on ICU-acquired weakness was published in 2012.

a) Define critical illness weakness (CIW, 1 mark) and list the types that may occur. (3 marks)

CIW definition:
> Clinically detectable, symmetrical, peripheral (not involving cranial nerves, thus facial sparing) weakness in critically ill patient that is not pre-existing.

CIW types:
(It can affect nerves, muscles or both).
> Critical illness polyneuropathy.
> Critical illness myopathy.
> Critical illness neuromyopathy.

b) List the risk factors for the development of weakness on the ICU. (6 marks)

Probable risk factors:
> Severe sepsis or septic shock, increased risk with increasing duration.
> Multiorgan failure, increased risk with increasing duration.
> Prolonged mechanical ventilation and bed rest.
> Hyperglycaemia.

Possible risk factors:
> Increasing age.
> Female gender.
> Severity of illness.
> Hypoalbuminaemia.
> Hyperosmolality.
> Parenteral nutrition.
> Renal replacement therapy.
> Vasopressors.
> Corticosteroids.
> Neuromuscular blocking agents.
> Aminoglycosides.

c) What are the clinical features of CIW? (4 marks)

Remember, this has been 'adjudged' as a difficult question. If you have got all the possible points so far, you only need one more point to pass.
> Weakness that has developed after onset of critical illness for a week or more, with exposure to risk factors as detailed earlier.
> Generalised, symmetrical, flaccid weakness, usually sparing cranial nerves (facial grimacing but no peripheral movement in response to painful stimulus).

> There may be associated sensory loss, but not autonomic involvement.
> Other causes excluded.
> Dependence on mechanical ventilation OR low muscle strength.

d) How may nerve conduction studies determine the type of CIW? (4 marks)

> Neuropathy: demonstrated by reduced amplitude of sensory nerve action potentials (SNAP) and compound motor action potentials (CMAP). Nerve conduction velocity normal/near normal.
> Myopathy: conduction velocity normal, SNAP normal, CMAP reduced (low amplitude motor unit potential on EMG).

e) What are the options for the management of CIW? (2 marks)

> Avoidance of risk factors.
> Blood glucose control.
> Early mobilisation.
> Physiotherapy from time of admission to ICU and during recovery.

Reference

Appleton R, Kinsella J. Intensive care unit-acquired weakness. *Contin Educ Anaesth Crit Care Pain*. 2012; 12 (2): 62–66.

a) What is meant by the term ventilator associated pneumonia (VAP)? (3 marks)

b) List the factors that increase the risk of the development of VAP. (10 marks)

c) What measures may reduce the risk of development of VAP? (7 marks)

September 2015

Chairman's Report

44.3% pass rate.

This is a common condition that candidates should have seen so it was surprising that it was quite poorly answered. Very few candidates were able to give a definition of VAP or to give details of the care bundles used in its prevention and treatment. Merely stating 'a care bundle would be used' suggests inadequate depth of knowledge.

a) What is meant by the term ventilator associated pneumonia (VAP)? (3 marks)	Nosocomial lung infection occurring more than 48 hours after commencement of ventilation via endotracheal tube. There are a range of different scoring systems to aid diagnosis that include clinical, microbiological and radiological factors.

The lack of a universally accepted diagnostic tool for VAP causes problems when comparing rates between units or evaluating interventions to reduce its incidence. The CDC (see reference at the end of this question) has produced an algorithm for diagnosing ventilator associated events for the purposes of surveillance. After a period of 48 hours of stability or improvement on ventilation, deterioration in oxygenation qualifies as a ventilator associated event. Further clinical and microbiological findings are then used to determine whether this is a ventilator-associated condition, infection-related ventilator-associated complication, or possible ventilator-associated pneumonia.

b) List the factors that increase the risk of the development of VAP. (10 marks)

> Endotracheal tube (loss of cough reflex, biofilm development on the inner surface of tube, pooling of secretions on top of cuff that then gain access via channels caused by folds in the cuff).
> Nasogastric tube (colonisation, predisposition to sinusitis and, therefore, a pool of infected secretions on cuff of tube).
> Nasal intubation (predisposition to sinusitis and therefore a pool of infected secretions).
> Positive pressure ventilation (forces bacteria to distal airways).
> Long duration of mechanical ventilation.
> Dysfunctions in immune response associated with critical illness, e.g. reduced level of salivary fibronectin, which normally protects against oropharyngeal colonisation with aerobic gram negative bacilli and Staphylococci.
> Severe burns.
> Supine position (risk of gastro-oesophageal reflux).
> Low GCS/excessive sedation.
> Enteral feeding (due to risk of aspiration, but for the purposes of overall morbidity and mortality, enteral feeding is still preferable overall to no/parenteral feeding).

c) What measures may reduce the risk of development of VAP? (7 marks)

> Avoidance of intubation, reducing the duration of intubation where feasible.
> Minimisation of risk of introduction of pathogens to breathing circuit:
  • Hand hygiene.
  • Closed suctioning.
  • Limit disconnections in circuit.
> Modifications to tube design:
  • Subglottic suction port.
  • Tapered cuff of ultra-thin polyurethane to avoid channelling.
  • Antimicrobial coating to discourage biofilm development.
> Ventilator care bundle checked at each shift change:
  • Nurse 30–45 degrees head up to reduce risk of aspiration.

- Daily sedation hold reduces overall number of ventilated days, facilitates more rapid wean, may help preserve some cough reflex.
- Histamine 2 receptor blocker is associated with reduced ICU complications and length of stay, therefore reduces number of ventilated days.
- Thromboprophylaxis – reduced complications reduces length of stay and ventilated days.
- Oral hygiene with chlorhexidine mouthwash.
- Cuff pressure check (20–30 cm H_2O or 2 cm H_2O above peak inflation pressure).

> Ensuring ventilator tubing positioned so that the condensate does not drain into the patient.

A care bundle is a group of evidence-based interventions that relate to a particular aspect of patient care. The strength of evidence supporting the individual components varies; some elements may just be accepted as good practice. Nonetheless, the aim of care bundle use is that the implementation of all of the components together should result in better patient outcomes. Care bundles are readily auditable. Think about the care bundles for sepsis management or reduction of surgical infection (part of the WHO checklist).

References

American Thoracic Society, Infectious Diseases Society of America: Guidelines for the management of adults with hospital-acquired, ventilator-associated, and healthcare-associated pneumonia. *Am J Respir Crit Care Med*. 2005; 171: 388–416.

Centers for Disease Control and Prevention. Ventilator-Associated Event (VAE) Protocol. January 2018. https://www.cdc.gov/nhsn/pdfs/pscmanual/10 -vae_final.pdf [Accessed 31st January 2018].

Gunasekera P, Gratrix A. Ventilator-associated pneumonia. *BJA Educ*. 2016; 16 (6): 198–202.

a) List <u>common</u> causes of acute pancreatitis in the United Kingdom. (3 marks)

b) How is acute pancreatitis diagnosed? (3 marks)

c) <u>Describe</u> the classification of severity of acute pancreatitis. (3 marks)

d) What are the <u>specific</u> principles of managing severe acute pancreatitis in a critical care environment? (11 marks)

March 2016

Chairman's Report

53.6% pass rate.

This is a condition seen commonly in intensive care. Many candidates did not mention alcohol as a cause in part (a). Few candidates could describe the classification of severity of acute pancreatitis as asked for in part (b). Also, some candidates tended to give a generic answer to part (d) describing the management of sepsis, rather than the specific management of acute pancreatitis as asked. This resulted in them losing marks in this section.

a) List 3 <u>common</u> causes of acute pancreatitis in the United Kingdom. (3 marks)

> Gall stones.
> Excessive alcohol intake (causes thick, proteinaceous secretions resulting in obstruction).
> Neoplasm resulting in obstruction (head of pancreas or periampullary primary, or metastasis from breast, renal gastric, ovarian, lung).

Other common causes include autoimmune diseases such as sclerosing cholangitis, viral infections such as CMV and the hepatitides, trauma following surgery or ERCP and idiopathic, but not scorpion bites.

b) How is acute pancreatitis diagnosed? (3 marks)

Diagnosis and classification are based on the revised Atlanta classification.

Two of the following three features:

> Abdominal pain consistent with acute pancreatitis (acute onset, persistent, severe, epigastric pain, often radiating to the back).
> Serum lipase (or amylase) at least three times greater than the upper limit of normal.
> Characteristic radiological findings, usually CT.

c) <u>Describe</u> the classification of severity of acute pancreatitis. (3 marks)

> Mild acute pancreatitis:
  • No organ failure.
  • No local or systemic complications.
> Moderately severe acute pancreatitis:
  • Organ failure that resolves within 48 hours and/or
  • Local or systemic complications.
> Severe acute pancreatitis
  • Organ failure persisting more than 48 hours.

d) What are the <u>specific</u> principles of managing severe acute pancreatitis in a critical care environment? (11 marks)

Following the alphabet helps to structure a coherent plan for the management of a patient in the ICU with severe acute pancreatitis.

Airway, respiratory:

> Supplemental oxygen, keep oxygen saturations above 95%.
> May require noninvasive ventilation or intubation and positive pressure ventilation due to ARDS, diaphragmatic splinting (pain, intra-abdominal oedema or fluid collections) or pleural effusions.

Cardiovascular:

> Targeted fluid therapy (loss due to reduced oral intake, vomiting, extravasation, hypoalbuminaemia) with intra-arterial blood pressure and cardiac output monitoring.
> Inotropic support as required.

Neurological:
> Sedation for invasive ventilation.
> Pain control – consider organ dysfunctions in evaluating choices.

Endocrine:
> Blood glucose management.

Gastrointestinal:
> Enteric nutrition (better outcome and cheaper), jejunal if gastric not tolerated.
> Parenteral nutrition if intolerant of any enteric feeding.
> Stress ulcer prophylaxis.

Haematological:
> Thromboprophylaxis: thromboembolic deterrent stockings or pneumatic compression devices. Low-molecular-weight heparin if no evidence of haemorrhage, unfractionated if evidence of acute kidney injury.
> Need for thromboprophylaxis must be balanced against risk of massive haemorrhage in acute severe pancreatitis due to pseudoaneurysm development (often splenic). Radiological management may be definitive or temporise for surgical management: balloon tamponade or coil embolisation.

Infection, immune:
> Antimicrobials if infected pancreatic necrosis suspected, or other associated sepsis. Ensure causative agent sought: radiologically guided aspiration of pancreatic or peripancreatic tissue if indicated. Treatment should target gram negative and fungal infection.

Renal:
> Minimise risk of acute kidney injury by optimising fluid status with cardiac output monitoring and by avoiding nephrotoxins. Target urine output greater than 0.5 ml/kg/h.
> Renal replacement therapy may be required.

Surgical Input:
> Acute pancreatitis secondary to gallstones may require ERCP or endoscopic sphincterotomy.
> Necrosectomy if necrosed areas are infected. May require repeat laparotomies or laparostomy for ongoing lavage.

References

Banks P, Bollen T, Dervenis C et al. Classification of acute pancreatitis – 2012: revision of the Atlanta classification and definitions by international consensus. *Gut*. 2013; 62: 102–111.

Young S, Thompson J. Severe acute pancreatitis. *Contin Educ Anaesth Crit Care Pain* 2008; 8 (4): 125–128.

A 20-year-old patient who satisfies the criteria for brainstem death has been accepted as an organ donor.

a) List the main adverse cardiovascular changes associated with brainstem death. (5 marks)

b) What are the physiological goals (with values) required to ensure optimisation of this donor? (7 marks)

c) Outline the measures and drugs that may be used to achieve these goals. (8 marks)

September 2016

Chairman's Report

68.8% pass rate.

Examiners anticipated that candidates would find this question difficult but gratifyingly most achieved enough marks to pass and demonstrated good knowledge of this important topic.

a) List the main adverse cardiovascular changes associated with brainstem death. (5 marks)

Sequentially:
> Brainstem ischaemia.
> Catecholamine release causing hypertension; tachycardia; increased systemic vascular resistance and pulmonary vascular resistance (causing pulmonary oedema); myocardial ischaemic damage and necrosis; other organ vasoconstriction and consequent damage.
> Reflex baroreceptor-mediated bradycardia.
> Progression of brainstem ischaemia and infarction and foramen magnum herniation results in loss of vasomotor centres and spinal cord sympathetic outflow.
> Ischaemia of the pituitary results in diabetes insipidus. Intravascular depletion contributes to cardiovascular instability.
> Vasodilatation, bradycardia, asystole.

A very similar question came up in 2008 asking about all systemic changes associated with brainstem death.

b) What are the physiological goals (with values) required to ensure optimisation of this donor? (7 marks)

NHS Blood and Transplant has an extended care bundle for management of patients who are to be donors after brainstem death. All of the physiological goals and the measures and drugs to achieve them are included in it.

> PaO_2 greater than 10 kPa.
> $PaCO_2$ 5–6.5 kPa.
> pH greater than 7.25.
> MAP 60–80 mm Hg.
> CVP 4–10 mm Hg.
> Cardiac index greater than 2.1 l/min/m².
> Central venous oxygen saturation greater than 60%.
> SVRI 1800–2400 dyne s/cm⁵/m².
> Temperature 36–37.5°C.
> Blood glucose 4–10 mmol/l.
> Plasma sodium less than 150 mmol/l.
> Urine output 0.5–2 ml/kg/h.

c) Outline the measures and drugs that may be used to achieve these goals. (8 marks)

Respiratory:
> Recruitment manoeuvres.
> Lung protective ventilation strategy (PEEP 5–10 cm H_2O, peak inspiratory pressure 25 cm H_2O, tidal volume 6–8 ml/kg).
> Keep fraction of inspired oxygen ideally below 0.4.
> 30–45 degree head-up positioning ensure adequate cuff inflation; continue airway suctioning, regular position changing and physiotherapy.

Cardiovascular:
> Site central venous catheter (ideally right side) and arterial line (ideally left side) for monitoring and therapy.
> Cardiac output and urine output monitoring to direct fluid management – excess fluid to be avoided.

> Commence vasopressin infusion if vasopressor required, wean off catecholamine infusions.
> Commence dopamine or dobutamine if goals not met with vasopressin.

Endocrine:
> Methylprednisolone.
> Insulin infusion.
> DDAVP or vasopressin if excessive urine output due to diabetes insipidus.

Haematological:
> Physical and pharmacological prophylaxis of thromboembolism.

Metabolic:
> Maintain normothermia using active warming if necessary.

Reference

NHS Blood and Transplant. Donation After Brainstem Death Donor Optimisation Extended Care Bundle. https://nhsbtdbe.blob.core.windows.net/umbraco -assets-corp/3654/dbd_care_bundle.pdf [Accessed 31st January 2018].

a) List criteria for a diagnosis of acute respiratory distress syndrome (ARDS)? (3 marks)

b) Which clinical indices are used to quantify oxygenation in ARDS? (3 marks)

c) What tidal volume would you select for a patient that meets the criteria for ARDS, using the ARDSNet protocol? (2 marks)

d) What are the ventilatory (6 marks) and non-ventilatory (6 marks) measures that can be taken to improve oxygenation or prevent further deterioration in a patient with ARDS.

March 2017

Chairman's Report

57.3% pass rate.

ARDS is a clinical condition which is seen commonly on ITU and of which candidates should have a thorough understanding. Whilst the definition was well known, the majority of candidates did not know the clinical indices used to assess oxygenation. Part (d) was on the whole well answered but those candidates who lost marks tended to write about general ITU care rather than the specifics of care for patients with ARDS.

The definitions of ARDS have changed since the time of the similar question in 2012, and this may have been what prompted its reappearance in the SAQ. Given the frequency with which questions recur, it is a shame that only 57.3% of people achieved a pass in the question this time.

ARDS is a multifactorial inflammatory process that may be triggered by a direct or indirect cause. There is a genetic component, as different individuals respond very differently to the same triggers. Direct causes include aspiration, pneumonia, drowning, pulmonary embolus, pulmonary contusion, inhalational injury and reperfusion injury. Indirect causes include sepsis, blood transfusion, pancreatitis, trauma, burns and drugs.

a) List criteria for a diagnosis of acute respiratory distress syndrome (ARDS)? (3 marks)

> Onset within one week of known clinical insult.
> Bilateral opacities on CXR or CT consistent with pulmonary oedema.
> Respiratory failure not fully explained by cardiac failure or fluid overload. Need to objectively assess this with e.g. echo if there is no clear ARDS-trigger present.
> Hypoxaemia with PEEP 5 cm H_2O or more.

PaO_2/FiO_2:

Mild less than 39.9 kPa.

Moderate less than 26.6 kPa.

Severe less than 13.3 kPa.

It is easier to remember the definitions of mild, moderate and severe ARDS when using mm Hg: less than 300, less than 200 and less than 100 mm Hg, respectively. No doubt you will remember that 760 mm Hg equates to 101 kPa, give or take a few decimal places. The main changes in the definitions are that the acuteness of the onset has now been defined, opacities may be seen on CT as well as CXR, ARDS can now be recognised as occurring alongside heart failure, the definition of hypoxaemia requires a PEEP of 5 at the time of measurement, and acute lung injury (ALI) has been redefined as mild ARDS.

b) Which clinical indices are used to quantify oxygenation in ARDS. (3 marks)

Mean arterial pressure (MAP), fraction of inspired oxygen (FiO_2), and arterial partial pressure of oxygen (PaO_2) are used to calculate the oxygenation index:

$$Oxygenation\ index = MAP \times FiO_2 \times 100/PaO_2$$

c) What tidal volume would you select for a patient that meets the criteria for ARDS, using the ARDSNet protocol? (2 marks)

Initiate ventilation at 8 ml/kg of predicted body weight, and then reduce by 1 ml/kg every two hours or less until target of 6 ml/kg achieved.

Overinflation may directly damage (volutrauma and barotrauma) remaining healthy areas of lung (as their compliance is greater than diseased areas). Resulting cytokine release mediates "biotrauma" to lungs and distant organs.

d) What are the ventilatory (6 marks) and non-ventilatory, (6 marks) measures that can be taken to improve oxygenation or prevent further deterioration in a patient with ARDS.

Ventilatory: aim to maintain adequate gas exchange until cellular damage resolves without causing further lung injury due to baro-, volu-, atelec- and biotrauma:

> PEEP.
> Tidal volume 6 ml/kg.
> Permissive hypercapnia.
> Accept PaO_2 sufficient to adequately oxygenate tissues.
> Keep peak pressure under 30 cm H_2O.
> Minimise the difference between peak pressure and PEEP.
> Recruitment manoeuvres: no proven survival benefit.
> Prone positioning.

Non-ventilatory:
> Management of any diagnosed underlying cause e.g. sepsis.
> Conservative fluid management.
> Physiotherapy: removal of secretions, improvement of gas exchange.
> Early enteral feeding.
> Ventilator care bundle: 30–45 degrees head-up, daily sedation hold, stress ulcer prophylaxis, venous thromboembolism prophylaxis.
> ECMO.

References

McCormack V, Tolhurst-Cleaver S. Acute respiratory distress syndrome. *BJA Educ.* 2017; 17 (5): 161–165.

Peek G et al. Efficacy and economic assessment of conventional ventilatory support versus extracorporeal membrane oxygenation for severe adult respiratory failure (CESAR): a multicentre randomised controlled trial. *Lancet.* 2009; 374 (9698): 1351–1363.

The Acute Respiratory Distress Network. Ventilation with lower tidal volumes as compared to traditional tidal volumes for acute lung injury and the acute respiratory distress syndrome. *N Engl J Med.* 2000; 342: 1301–1308.

The ARDS Definition Task Force. Acute respiratory distress syndrome, the Berlin definition. *JAMA.* 2012; 307: 2526–2533.

You are asked to review a 27-year-old male who is a known epileptic in convulsive status epilepticus.

a) Define convulsive status epilepticus. (1 mark)

b) Outline your initial management of this patient, including the use of emergency antiepileptic drug therapy. (7 marks)

c) 60 minutes after your initial management, the patient continues in status epilepticus. What would be your further management? (5 marks)

d) What are the complications associated with refractory convulsive status epilepticus? (7 marks)

March 2017

Chairman's Report

47.1% pass rate.

This question was judged to be easy and is relevant to everyday practice as anaesthetists may encounter such patients in multiple areas including ITU, neurosurgery and the emergency department. Very few candidates were aware of the up-to-date definition of status epilepticus. In part (b), some candidates failed to give details of drug management despite this being specifically asked for in the question.

Easy questions need 14/20 points in order to pass.

a) Define convulsive status epilepticus. (1 mark)

The definition of status epilepticus has changed and is now defined at the five-minute mark, as per NICE guidelines. However, there is only 1 mark for this. Most of the marks are still available to you if you can give a good account of how you would manage a real life patient in status in your real practice.

> Seizure activity lasting more than five minutes, or more than three seizures in one hour.

b) Outline your initial management of this patient, including the use of emergency antiepileptic drug therapy. (7 marks)

The NICE guidance divides up the management of a patient in status into time periods. If you know the guidance, it can be reproduced here for parts (b) and (c). If you don't, you will have to document your common sense approach to such a situation.

Status epilepticus is a medical emergency and I would adopt an ABC approach, assessing and managing the patient simultaneously. Antiepileptic drugs must be given without delay.

> A and B: 15 l/min oxygen via non-rebreathe mask. Assess airway patency and proceed to RSI if patient unable to protect own airway. Continuous oxygen saturations monitoring.
> C: large-bore intravenous access, continuous ECG monitoring, noninvasive blood pressure monitoring until arterial line sited.
> Lorazepam 0.1 mg/kg IV (approximately 4 mg).
> Investigations: arterial blood gas, blood glucose, urea and electrolytes, calcium and magnesium, coagulation, full blood count, antiepileptic drug (AED) levels.
> Give usual AED if feasible.
> Repeat lorazepam after 10–20 minutes.
> Treat acidosis if severe.
> Consider pabrinex and glucose (50 ml 50%) if any possibility of alcohol excess or malnutrition.
> Phenytoin or fosphenytoin IV.

c) 60 minutes after your initial management the patient continues in status epilepticus. What would be your further management? (5 marks)

This is now refractory status:
> Rapid sequence induction using propofol or thiopentone bolus followed by infusion.
> ICU care with EEG monitoring.
> CXR to check intubation and to check for aspiration.
> Identify and treat medical complications of status.

> Consider possible non-epileptic underlying cause or trigger.
> Consider need for brain imaging or lumbar puncture.

d) What are the complications associated with refractory convulsive status epilepticus? (7 marks)

There are so many possible complications that I have reverted to using the alphabet to help me classify them.

Airway:
> Oral soft tissue injury or dental damage.
> Obstruction.

Respiratory:
> Aspiration.
> Pneumonia.
> Respiratory failure.
> Pulmonary oedema.

Cardiac:
> Myocardial infarction.
> Hyper- or hypotension.
> Arrhythmias.
> Cardiac arrest.
> Cardiogenic shock.

Neurological:
> Cerebral hypoxia.
> Cerebral oedema.
> Cerebral haemorrhage.
> Excitotoxic CNS injury.

Haematology:
> DIC.

Musculoskeletal:
> Fractures.
> Rhabdomyolysis.

Renal:
> Acute kidney injury.

Hepatic:
> Acute liver injury.

Metabolic:
> Hyponatraemia.
> Hypoglycaemia.
> Hyperkalaemia.
> Metabolic acidosis.
> Hyperthermia.

References

Carter E, Adapa R. Adult epilepsy and anaesthesia. *Contin Educ Anaesth Crit Care Pain*. 2015; 15 (3): 111–117.

National Institute for Health and Care Excellence. Epilepsies: Diagnosis and Management CG137. January 2012, last updated February 2016.

a) What are the indications for renal replacement therapy (RRT) in the intensive care setting? (8 marks)

b) List the types of RRT available in intensive care. (6 marks)

c) Outline the principle mechanisms of solute and water removal by filtration (3 marks) and dialysis (3 marks) during RRT.

September 2017

Chairman's Report

84.9% pass rate.

This question had the highest pass rate in the paper. The topic is relevant to everyday practice in intensive care so it was reassuring to see that knowledge of it was generally excellent. However, a number of candidates still gave incomplete accounts of the differences between dialysis and filtration.

This question is identical to that from September 2013. RRT is a core area of knowledge for intensive care medicine.

16. OBSTETRICS

a) Amniotic fluid embolism (AFE) is one of four major direct causes of maternal mortality in the 2006–2008 report from Centre for Maternal and Child Enquiries (CMACE).

State the other three major causes. (15%)

b) How does AFE present clinically? (25%)

c) What are the differential diagnoses of AFE? (40%)

d) Describe two possible theories on the pathophysiology of AFE. (20%)

September 2011

a) Amniotic fluid embolism (AFE) is one of four major direct causes of maternal mortality in the 2006–2008 report from Centre for Maternal and Child Enquiries (CMACE). State the other three major causes. (15%)

The confidential enquiries into maternal death are now run by the collaboration MBRRACE-UK. For the sake of your obstetric practice and also your exams, make sure you have looked at their website, which contains links to all of their publications. AFE was number 4 and anaesthesia number 7 of the ranked causes of maternal death in the report that this question focuses on. A future question may be based on the current trends in leading causes of maternal death.

1. Genital tract sepsis.

2. Pre-eclampsia and eclampsia.

3. Thromboembolism.

b) How does AFE present clinically? (25%)

Sudden, profound, catastrophic maternal collapse usually during labour but also during caesarean section or after delivery (also, rarely, occurs with amniocentesis, abdominal injury in pregnancy or in early pregnancy).

> Cardiovascular and respiratory collapse: raised pulmonary vascular resistance, acute right heart failure, hypoxaemia. Direct myocardial depression from humoral factors and also from hypoxaemia. Left heart failure, pulmonary oedema, hypotension. ARDS may result in survivors.
> Disseminated intravascular coagulation. Massive haemorrhage may contribute to cardiovascular collapse.
> Neurological: seizures and loss of consciousness.

c) What are the differential diagnoses of AFE? (40%)

Depends on the stage in the time course of the process and the current features seen, but includes the following:

> Pulmonary embolism.
> Eclampsia.
> Sepsis.
> Anaphylaxis.
> Local anaesthetic toxicity.
> Myocardial infarction.

d) Describe two possible theories on the pathophysiology of AFE. (20%)

Entry of amniotic fluid containing fetal material into maternal circulation via small tears in lower uterine segment, endocervix or site of placental implantation.

> Embolic theory: fetal tissue or/and amniotic fluid forcibly entering maternal circulation causes transient pulmonary vasospasm, cardiac failure, hypoxaemia.
> Immune theory: biochemical mediators in solution in amniotic fluid trigger anaphylactoid reaction.

Likely to be a combination of both.

References

Centre for Maternal and Child Enquiries (CMACE). Saving Mothers' Lives: reviewing maternal deaths to make motherhood safer: 2006–08. The Eighth Report on Confidential Enquiries into Maternal Deaths in the United Kingdom. *BJOG*. 2011; 118 (1): 1–203.

Dedhia J, Mushambi M. Amniotic fluid embolism. *Contin Educ Anaesth Crit Care Pain*. 2007; 7 (5): 152–156.

a) Which dermatomes should be blocked prior to an elective caesarean section (CS) and how may the adequacy of the block be tested? (30%)

b) How might an initially inadequate block be improved sufficiently to allow surgery to proceed? (30%)

c) How could you manage a patient who complains of pain during a spinal CS? (40%)

March 2012

Chairman's Report

45.7% pass rate.

Most candidates knew the dermatome levels and how to test the level of a block, however section (b) was less well answered. Some candidates did not read the question carefully enough or appreciated that they were required to improve the block itself rather than provide supplementary analgesia. It was good to see that many candidates understood the importance of patient reassurance and how to manage pain during CS under spinal anaesthesia.

Like many of the obstetric questions in the Final SAQ, familiarity with your hospital's obstetric anaesthesia guidelines will make this a straightforward question for you.

a) Which dermatomes should be blocked prior to an elective caesarean section (CS) and how may the adequacy of the block be tested? (30%)

There is a lack of consensus on dermatome level that the upper extent of block should reach in the different testing modalities. The levels written here are commonly, but not universally, accepted.

> Upper level T4 bilaterally to cold: with ethyl chloride spray, demonstrate sensation on unblocked skin. Then spray on blocked skin moving in a cephalad direction until cold sensation perceived. Repeat on contralateral side.
> Upper level T5 bilaterally to light touch (when intrathecal opioid is given): testing as above with cotton wool or touch of spray on skin.
> Upper level T5 bilaterally to pain: testing as above with Neurotip.
> Lower level S5 bilaterally: check the lower extent of block to cold or light touch – can check S2 at sole of foot. Lack of awareness of urinary catheter insertion indicates loss of touch sensation at sacral level.
> Motor block: Bromage 3 (unable to flex knees) or 4 (unable to move legs or feet) is required.

b) How might an initially inadequate block be improved sufficiently to allow surgery to proceed? (30%)

Note that they have not specified what sort of regional anaesthesia has been used, so make sure your answer includes options for spinal and epidural.

> Positioning: flex hips to flatten lumbar lordosis, cautious head down tilt or lateral tilt if block inadequate on one side (remember need to avoid aortocaval compression).
> Epidural: if using epidural or combined spinal and epidural, top up the epidural. If using spinal only, consider inserting an epidural in order to raise the height of the block.
> Repeat spinal: consider reducing overall dose if some block is present. Good attention to patient positioning should help prevent high spinal.

c) How could you manage a patient who complains of pain during a spinal CS? (40%)

Communication:
> Ask obstetricians to stop surgery whilst establishing pain control (depends on stage of surgery – not feasible after uterine incision and before delivery of baby).
> Ask obstetricians to handle tissues as carefully as possible, avoid exteriorisation of uterus, large paracolic gutter packs etc.
> Ask the woman to describe the sensations felt. Determine whether it is true sharp pain or the normal tugging sensations that are to be expected. Reassurance often helps, but even if they are the 'normal sensations', if the woman remains distressed, then it should be addressed in the same manner as 'true' pain.

Options for pain relief:

> If surgeons have only just started skin incision, consider covering the wound, turning patient on their side, repeating spinal.
> Entonox.
> Alfentanil 50 mcg aliquots intravenously. Give oxygen, request the presence of paediatrician if before delivery, and inform them that opioids have been given. Morphine may then be given after delivery.
> Ketamine 5–10 mg boluses if familiar with its use.
> Local anaesthetic infiltration by surgeons if baby delivered and starting to close.
> General anaesthetic must be offered regardless of stage of surgery if the woman remains uncomfortable.

Postoperatively:

> Documentation of woman's experiences, stage of surgery and action undertaken. Include offers of options that the woman may have declined.
> Ensure adequate postoperative analgesia if the block has failed – sufficient opioids, transverse abdominis plane blocks.
> Debrief with the woman postoperatively once pain is controlled, after returning to ward, consultant involvement if necessary. Offer anaesthetic clinic appointment after discharge if the patient would like further conversations.

References

Chestnut D, Polley L, Tsen L, Wong C (eds.). *Chestnut's Obstetric Anesthesia Principles and Practice*. 4th edition. Philadelphia: Mosby Elsevier; 2009.

Hoyle J, Yentis, S. Assessing the height of block for caesarean section over the past three decades: trends from the literature. *Anaesthesia*. 2015; 70: 421–428.

a) What are the implications of managing a patient with an intrauterine fetal death (IUFD) at 36-weeks gestation? (55%)

b) How does the presence of an IUFD influence the choice in the method of pain relief in labour? (20%)

c) Which abnormal haematological results would contraindicate epidural analgesia? (25%)

September 2012

Chairman's Report

The question was written because the anaesthetist is often involved with the provision of analgesia for labour in these circumstances.

Section (a) was specifically asking about the implications of intrauterine fetal death (IUFD). The implications of IUFD focused on:

Psychological distress

Method of delivery

Mandatory level 1 care (MEOWS) and possible transfer to level 2 care

Exclude possible causes

Provide effective analgesia

Consider sedation

Section (a) was answered poorly but fared better in sections (b) choice of pain relief and (c) haematological results that might contraindicate epidural analgesia.

a) What are the implications of managing a patient with an intrauterine fetal death (IUFD) at 36-weeks gestation? (55%)

I am surprised by the inclusion of consideration of sedation in the Chairman's report, as this is not something that I would use in obstetric practice.

> Delivery decision: induction, expectant or occasionally caesarean due to previous obstetric history or patient preference or because underlying cause necessitates this (e.g. uterine rupture).
> Psychological: senior midwife experienced in caring for women with IUFD, early conversation with obstetric anaesthetist, dedicated room for care of women experiencing fetal loss away from the noise of labour ward but still with the facilities to provide level of care required. Good communication among all involved healthcare professionals to avoid the possibility of lack of awareness of the situation and subsequent insensitivity.
> Pain relief options: more detail in (b)
> Level of care: complications may have caused the IUFD or result from it. Obstetrician-led management and one-to-one midwifery care, MEOWS charting. Delivery suite is level 1 care, ward is level 0. May need to stay in level 1 care post-delivery. May require level 2 or even 3 care, depending on circumstances.
> Implications of underlying cause: may remain occult, may have major implications on delivery management. Abruption, pre-eclampsia, uterine rupture, thrombophilia, sepsis, maternal diabetes will all impact on intrapartum care and delivery mode.

b) How does the presence of an IUFD influence the choice in the method of pain relief in labour? (20%)

> Early consultation with the obstetric anaesthetist should be facilitated to discuss expectations and wishes.
> Maternal pain experience might be greater due to psychological distress and also if induction is necessary. There is therefore greater need for effective pain relief, and epidural may be optimal.
> Need not consider uteroplacental transfer: better pain-relieving opioids such as morphine and diamorphine may therefore be used instead of pethidine. May be given as PCA.
> Cause or consequence of IUFD may contraindicate regional technique: sepsis; pre-eclampsia with deranged clotting or thrombocytopaenia; haemorrhage or IUFD resulting in DIC.

> Remifentanil PCA contraindicated according to protocols, lack of experience and recent adverse incidents associated with use in presence of IUFD.

c) Which abnormal haematological results would contraindicate epidural analgesia? (25%)

> Raised white cell count:
  • Maternal sepsis (cause or effect of the IUFD).
> Low platelets:
  • May be present in severe pre-eclampsia or HELLP syndrome.
> Deranged coagulation, low fibrinogen:
  • May accompany low platelets in the presence of DIC due to abruption, uterine rupture or occasionally as a result of the IUFD itself.
  • May also occur in pre-eclampsia or HELLP syndrome.
  • Abnormal coagulation may also be present in maternal thrombophilias.

References

Marr R, Hyams J, Bythell V. Cardiac arrest in an obstetric patient using remifentanil patient-controlled analgesia. *Anaesthesia*. 2013; 68 (3): 283–287.

The Royal College of Obstetricians and Gynaecologists. Late Intrauterine Fetal Death and Stillbirth. Greentop Guideline No. 55. October 2010.

A woman experiences a headache 24 hours after delivery having had epidural analgesia for labour.

a) List the clinical features of a post-dural puncture headache (PDPH). (25%)

b) What is the differential diagnosis of PDPH? (30%)

c) Outline the conservative treatment options for PDPH. (15%)

d) How is an epidural blood patch performed? (30%)

March 2013

Chairman's Report

59.0% pass rate.

A very basic but and relevant question [sic] that was reasonably well answered. This question was the least discriminatory.

a) List the clinical features of a post-dural puncture headache (PDPH). (25%)

History:

> Known/suspected dural puncture, difficulty with insertion, multiple attempts, junior anaesthetist.
> Fronto-occipital headache developing within five days of puncture.
> Worse on standing or sitting, improves on lying flat.
> Accompanied by one or more of the following:
>   • Neck stiffness.
>   • Tinnitus.
>   • Hypacusia.
>   • Photophobia.
>   • Nausea.

Examination:

> Mainly to rule out other causes.
> Temperature normal.
> Cardiovascular examination, especially blood pressure, normal.
> Neurological examination usually normal, BUT neurological symptoms may occur with PDPH:
>   • Blindness cranial nerve II.
>   • Diplopia cranial nerves III, IV, VI.
>   • Tinnitus, hearing loss cranial nerve VIII.
>   • Head and facial pain cranial nerve V.
>   • Neck pain upper cervical nerves.
> Rarely, leak from the puncture site on the back.

b) What is the differential diagnosis of PDPH? (30%)

Infective	Meningitis. Encephalitis. Sinusitis.
Metabolic	Dehydration. Caffeine withdrawal.
Vascular	Migraine. Cerebral vein thrombosis. Cerebral infarction. Subdural haematoma. Subarachnoid haemorrhage. Posterior reversible leucoencephalopathy syndrome.
Obstetric-related	Pre-eclampsia. Lactation headache.
Neoplastic	Primary or secondary.
Other	Tension headache. Benign intracranial hypertension. Pneumocephalus.

c) Outline the conservative treatment options for PDPH. (15%)

> Adequate oral (or intravenous) hydration.
> Simple analgesia: regular paracetamol and NSAID.
> Antiemetics if required.
> Stool softeners to avoid straining.
> Encourage mobilisation; thromboembolic deterrent stockings and consideration of low-molecular-weight heparin prophylaxis if immobile.
> Regular reassessment, communication with woman and community midwifery team if discharged. Written discharge paperwork to accompany the woman.

d) How is an epidural blood patch performed? (30%)

> Patient suitability: afebrile, no contraindication for epidural, more than 24 hours since puncture, and other causes for headache ruled out.
> Consent:
>   • Local bruising on the back.
>   • Backache and stiffness, which can last a few days (no risk of long-term back pain).
>   • Another accidental dural puncture.
>   • Nerve damage, infection or bleeding.
>   • Seizure at the time of performing the EBP.
>   • Failure to treat headache: 30%–40%.
> Two anaesthetists, ideally one should be a consultant.
> Theatre environment.
> Full asepsis for both anaesthetists.
> Consultant locates epidural space at or below space at which the puncture occurred (because the injected blood is thought to spread in a cephalad direction).
> Other anaesthetist contemporaneously withdraws 30 ml blood.
> Blood injected via Tuohy until pain in back or all 30 ml used.
> Flush Tuohy with saline before withdrawal.
> Ensure the patient lies flat for two hours.
> Advise no lifting of weight heavier than her own baby for two weeks.
> Written discharge summary for GP, community midwife and woman to include issues that should prompt re-attendance at the hospital and contact details of the anaesthesia team.

References

Royal College of Anaesthetists and Association of Anaesthetists of Great Britain and Ireland. Risks associated with your anaesthetic Section 10: Headache after a spinal or epidural injection. 2015. https://www.rcoa.ac.uk/system /files/10-HeadachesSpinalEpidural2015.pdf [Accessed 8th January 2017].

Sabharwal A, Stocks G. Postpartum headache: diagnosis and management. *Contin Educ Anaesth Crit Care Pain*. 2011; 11 (5): 181–185.

A primiparous patient with a booking BMI of 55 kg/m² presents in the high-risk obstetric anaesthetic assessment clinic at 32-weeks gestation. She is hoping for a vaginal delivery.

a) Which specific points do you need to elicit from the history and examination? (30%)

b) What do you need to communicate to the patient? (35%)

c) Document your plan for her management on the delivery suite. (35%)

September 2013

Chairman's Report

72.8% pass rate.

This question was a modified version from the May 2006 paper. The implications of morbid obesity on a parturient and the importance of forward planning were well appreciated by most candidates.

Look at this very similar question from May 2006:

'A consultant obstetrician has asked you to review a woman in her first pregnancy in the anaesthetic ante-natal assessment clinic. Her body mass index is 45 kg.m⁻². There are no other abnormalities and at 32 weeks gestation she is hoping for a vaginal delivery. Write a summary recording the details you would wish to cover during the appointment and your recommendations for her management when she is admitted in labour'.

The format of the exam changed between these two questions. The questions moved away from short essay style to more directed questions. However, important topics remain important topics and will continue to be so after the next exam format change. Also, consider the timing interval between the publication of the CMACE report 'Maternal Obesity in the UK' and this exam paper. Make sure that you are prepared for topical questions.

a) Which specific points do you need to elicit from the history and examination? (30%)

Follow the alphabet to dredge the points out of your brain in a systematic manner. Remember that they have specifically asked for history and examination.

Airway:
> History of difficult airway.
> History of problems with anaesthesia in the past.
> Perform airway assessment.

Respiratory:
> History of obstructive sleep apnoea.
> History of other respiratory symptoms such as dyspnoea or asthma.
> Check oxygen saturations when supine and auscultate chest.

Cardiovascular:
> Assess exercise tolerance.
> Check for history or symptoms of ischaemic heart disease.
> Check blood pressure.
> Assess for likely ease of cannulation.

Endocrine:
> Check for history of diabetes mellitus or gestational diabetes and check medications and control.

Pharmacology:
> Document all medications.
> May be taking low-molecular-weight heparin, which has impact on the timing of neuraxial techniques.

Gastrointestinal:
> History of reflux and medications to control this.

Cutaneomusculoskeletal:
> Check weight – consider impact on equipment, theatre table.
> Assess for ability of woman to position herself for neuraxial technique.

Obstetric:
> Check for problems with pregnancy.

b) What do you need to communicate to the patient? (35%)

The Obstetric Anaesthetists' Association has produced a leaflet called 'Why Do I Need to See an Anaesthetist during My Pregnancy? Information for Pregnant Women with a High Body Mass Index (BMI)'. This is another reminder to read and make use of the guidelines and publications in common use.

> Reason for referral: raised BMI increases likelihood of needing caesarean or instrumental delivery, and therefore, there is an increased likelihood of an anaesthetist being involved in their care.
> Recommendation to avoid eating and to drink only clear fluids in labour, in view of the increased risk of needing assistance with delivery and, therefore, some form of anaesthesia. This reduces the likelihood of aspiration of particulate stomach content.
> Regular antacid in labour for same reason as earlier, to reduce the risk of aspiration of highly acidic stomach content.
> Epidural and spinal may be more difficult to do and take longer.
> Consider early epidural, especially if labour is not progressing well: easier to perform in early rather than advanced labour and can be topped up for the purposes of caesarean or instrumental delivery, thus possibly reducing the need for general anaesthesia.
> General anaesthetic may be more difficult to perform and may have increased risks. Optimum care of mother and baby is for the mother to remain awake (with neuraxial anaesthesia if necessary) for delivery.

c) Document your plan for her management on the delivery suite. (35%)

My documentation would include the following points:
> BMI and weight.
> Outcomes from clinic meeting, including any issues elicited from history and examination.
> Airway assessment, predicted difficulty with neuraxial block and any predicted issues with cannulation.
> If woman currently taking low-molecular-weight heparin, give clear advice regarding omission of dose if any chance that she is in early labour, to consult delivery suite early for assessment and admission if indicated.
> Any specific equipment requirements.
> Instruction to alert anaesthetist on arrival in labour, junior anaesthetist to contact consultant.
> Early cannula? Depends on consultation with the woman and her individual risks.
> Early epidural? Depends on consultation with the woman.
> Instruction to restrict oral intake to clear fluids only in labour and regular ranitidine to be given.
> Thromboembolic deterrent stockings to be worn in labour, consideration of low-molecular-weight heparin prophylaxis afterwards as per guideline (ensure dose appropriate to patient weight).

References

Centre for Maternal and Child Enquiries (CMACE). *Maternal Obesity in the UK: Finding from a National Project.* London: CMACE; 2010.
Obstetric Anaesthetists' Association. Anaesthetics and pregnant women with a high BMI. http://www.labourpains.com/assets/_managed/cms/files/A4%20 High%20BMI%20LeLeafl.pdf [Accessed 8th January 2017].

A 27-year-old woman is 13 weeks pregnant. In the antenatal clinic, she is found to have an asymptomatic heart murmur. A subsequent echocardiogram shows moderate to severe mitral stenosis.

a) List the causes of mitral stenosis. (15%)

b) How do the cardiovascular changes in pregnancy exacerbate the pathophysiology of mitral stenosis? (45%)

c) Outline the specific management issues when she presents in established labour. (40%)

March 2014

Chairman's Report

65.5% pass rate.

Overall, there was a disappointing lack of knowledge of the pathology of mitral stenosis and some candidates had no understanding at all. The physiological and clinical aspects were more soundly addressed, and the question proved a very strong discriminator between strong and weak candidates.

There was a great BJA Education article on mitral stenosis in 2017 – time for this question to come up again?

a) List the causes of mitral stenosis. (15%)

> Rheumatic fever (commonest cause worldwide but less common in developed countries).
> Infective endocarditis.
> Degenerative calcification.

b) How do the cardiovascular changes in pregnancy exacerbate the pathophysiology of mitral stenosis? (45%)

> 45% increase in intravascular volume: the fixed output of the left atrium is unable to cope, resulting in pulmonary oedema. Increase in left atrial stretch predisposes to atrial fibrillation and decompensation.
> 20% increase in heart rate: shorter diastole so reduced time for flow across stenosed valve, reduces left ventricular filling, reduces cardiac output (CO).
> Normal pregnancy has 40% increase in CO to cope with the 40% increase in oxygen consumption caused by the fetus and raised maternal metabolism. This increase cannot be facilitated with a significantly stenosed valve, resulting in decreased exercise tolerance, dyspnoea, cyanosis.
> 20% reduction in systemic vascular resistance in pregnancy causes reduction in coronary artery perfusion, resulting in risk of ischaemia.

c) Outline the specific management issues when she presents in established labour. (40%)

> Decision regarding delivery mode and location should have been made antenatally (tertiary centre with capabilities of managing an urgent valvotomy/valve replacement) as she presented early in pregnancy.
> Early communication between senior anaesthetist, senior obstetrician, cardiologist, cardiothoracic surgeon, midwifery team.
> Ensure cross-matched blood available (she will tolerate volume loss poorly and need replacement with fluid that has oxygen-carrying capacity).

Vaginal delivery:
> Airway and respiratory:
  • Supplementary oxygen.
  • Oxygen saturations monitoring.
  • Avoid nitrous oxide or hypoxia, which could raise pulmonary vascular resistance.
> Cardiovascular:
  • Intra-arterial blood pressure monitoring (neuraxial analgesia-related hypotension should be managed promptly with α-agonist).
  • ECG monitoring (tachycardia and loss of sinus rhythm are deleterious to cardiac output).
  • Monitor for blood loss.

> - Cautious intravenous fluids if dehydrated due to poor intake in labour (maintain left atrial filling).
> - Left lateral tilt to ensure unobstructed venous return.
> - Monitor for effects of autotransfusion after delivery.

> **Neurological:**
> - Early epidural to avoid sympathetically mediated heart rate increases, cautious top-ups to avoid drop in systemic vascular resistance, α-agonist use as necessary.

> **Pharmacology:**
> - Syntocinon to be given as an infusion rather than as a bolus to avoid tachycardia and vasodilatation. Ergometrine contraindicated as will cause pulmonary vasoconstriction.

> **Obstetric:**
> - Continuous fetal monitoring: fetal distress may be an indicator of poor maternal haemodynamics.
> - Consideration of instrumental second stage to avoid maternal effort as the associated valsalva will reduce venous return.

Caesarean delivery:

> **Airway and respiratory:**
> - Supplementary oxygen.
> - Oxygen saturations monitoring.
> - Avoid nitrous oxide or hypoxia, which could raise pulmonary vascular resistance.

> **Cardiovascular:**
> - Intra-arterial blood pressure monitoring – reduced afterload must be promptly managed with vasoconstrictor.
> - ECG monitoring – increased heart rate or loss of sinus rhythm is deleterious to CO.
> - Intravenous fluids to counteract the effect of neuraxial block and to maintain preload, but avoid left atrial overload.
> - Replace blood with blood.
> - Left lateral tilt to ensure unobstructed venous return.
> - Monitor for the effects of autotransfusion post-delivery.

> **Neurological:**
> - Optimum mode of anaesthesia is slow epidural top-up, combined spinal and epidural with low dose spinal component, or spinal catheter to avoid sudden decrease in systemic vascular resistance.

> **Pharmacology:**
> - If general anaesthesia is necessary, ensure opioid at induction to obtund the pressor response and at a dose that obviates the need for high-dose (vasodilatory) induction agent ('cardiac induction'). Paediatricians to be alerted to this.
> - Phenylephrine infusion to maintain systemic vascular resistance without inducing tachycardia.
> - Avoid drugs that make tachycardia likely, e.g. atropine.
> - Short acting β-blockers if necessary.
> - Syntocinon as an infusion to avoid tachycardia and vasodilatation.

> **Obstetric:**
> - Early consideration of e.g. B-lynch suture, intra-uterine balloon or hysterectomy if excessive bleeding as blood loss poorly tolerated and pharmacological options limited (ergometrine causes pulmonary vasoconstriction and hypertension, prostaglandins cause bronchospasm and may precipitate pulmonary oedema).

Reference

Holme K, Gibbison B, Vohra H. Mitral valve and mitral valve disease. *BJA Educ*. 2017; 17 (1): 1–9.

A 28-year-old woman presents for acute appendicectomy – she is 22 weeks pregnant.

a) List the risks to the fetus during anaesthesia for the mother. (5 marks)

b) How can the risks to the fetus be minimised? (10 marks)

c) What additional pre- and intraoperative steps would you take to ensure fetal safety if she was 27 weeks pregnant? (5 marks)

September 2014

Chairman's Report

33% pass rate.

The poor pass rate for this important subject is of concern as similar clinical scenarios are commonly encountered. Many candidates wrote principally on the preparation of a pregnant woman for general anaesthesia or on the conduct of a rapid intubation sequence, ignoring the emphasis on the fetus in the question. Teratogenesis by anaesthetic agents was frequently listed as an important consideration although the patient was in the second trimester of pregnancy. Many candidates failed to consider that a fetus of twenty two weeks gestation is highly unlikely to be viable and concentrated on preparation for an unplanned delivery. A clue to this consideration was given in section (c) where the focus was changed to a scenario in which the fetus is potentially viable, but weak candidates ignored this prompt.

Some key anaesthesia-relevant timings in obstetrics:

> *Risk of teratogenesis in first trimester when main organ systems are being developed, especially 2–8/40.*
> *Consider need for antacid premedication and RSI from approximately 12/40.*
> *Risk of aortocaval compression from approximately 20/40.*
> *Surgery and anaesthesia confer increased risk of miscarriage in the middle trimester and increased risk of early labour later in pregnancy.*
> *The fetus is potentially viable from 24/40 onwards, sometimes earlier.*

a) List the risks to the fetus during anaesthesia for the mother. (5 marks)

> Hypoxia, hypercarbia: failure to adequately manage maternal airway and ventilation can result in uterine artery constriction, hypoxia, hypercarbia and myocardial depression of the fetus.
> Hyperventilation of mother causing hypocarbia can cause uterine artery vasoconstriction, poor perfusion and leftward shift of maternal oxyhaemaglobin dissociation curve.
> Hypoperfusion: fetoplacental unit entirely dependent on maternal perfusing pressure. Therefore, it is necessary to maintain maternal blood pressure and manage aortocaval compression.
> As yet unconfirmed/unquantified anaesthetic-induced neuronal apoptosis in developing brain.
> Risk of miscarriage – unquantified. Likely to have more to do with the disease process necessitating the surgery or the surgery itself.

b) How can the risks to the fetus be minimised? (10 marks)

> Defer surgery until after delivery unless absolutely necessary.
> Multidisciplinary approach, involve obstetricians in the assessment of pre- and postoperative maternal and fetal well-being.
> Airway and respiratory:
  • RSI after antacid premedication, rapid securing of airway. Extubate awake, sitting up.
  • Ventilation targeted to end-tidal carbon dioxide and oxygen saturations to reduce the possibility of hypoxia and hypercarbia in the fetus.
> Cardiovascular:
  • Left lateral tilt, adequate filling, and maintenance of maternal blood pressure at normal levels all help minimise risk of placental hypoperfusion.

- Ensure adequate analgesia as raised circulating catecholamines will compromise placental perfusion.

> Neurological:
- Shortest duration of anaesthesia possible reduces the exposure of fetal brain to anaesthetic agents.
- Avoidance of general anaesthesia through the use of regional or neuraxial technique, where possible. Not an option for appendicectomy.

c) What additional pre- and intraoperative steps would you take to ensure fetal safety if she was 27 weeks pregnant? (5 marks)

> Discussion with neonatologists preoperatively: fetus is now viable and preparations for consequences of premature labour are necessary. If NICU cot not available, consideration should be given to in utero transfer to hospital where cot is available, if maternal condition permits.
> Discussion with obstetricians regarding possible need for tocolysis and steroids for fetal lung maturation (urgency of surgery may not allow time for this to be fully effective).
> Pre-, intra- and postoperative cardiotocographic fetal monitoring.
> Ensure liaison between obstetricians and surgeons regarding planned surgical approach: open versus laparoscopic approach, consideration of site of laparoscope insertion.
> Avoid NSAIDs due to risk of premature closure of ductus arteriosus.

Reference

Nejdlova M, Johnson T. Anaesthesia for non-obstetric procedures during pregnancy. *Contin Educ Anaesth Crit Care Pain*. 2012; 12 (4): 203–206.

You are asked to review a woman in the anaesthetic antenatal clinic. She is 30 weeks pregnant and a Jehovah's Witness. She requires an elective caesarean section at 39 weeks due to a low-lying placenta and a fibroid uterus.

a) What specific issues should be discussed with this patient based on the history outlined above? (10 marks)

b) Give the advantages and disadvantages of using intra-operative cell salvage during caesarean section. (10 marks)

March 2015

Chairman's Report

44.6% pass rate; 22.5% of candidates received a poor fail.

This question was poorly attempted by many candidates. Examiners reported that answers reflected a lack of knowledge or inaccurate reading of the question. Many candidates described anaesthesia for a Jehovah's Witness patient with placenta praevia and fibroid uterus rather than addressing pre-operative discussions as was asked. Candidates omitted mention of important perioperative risks such as haemorrhage, hysterectomy and other significant morbidity and mortality. Some candidates demonstrated a worrying lack of knowledge of cell salvage and in particular the disadvantages of this technique.

You need to understand the process of cell salvage in order to explain it to a patient:

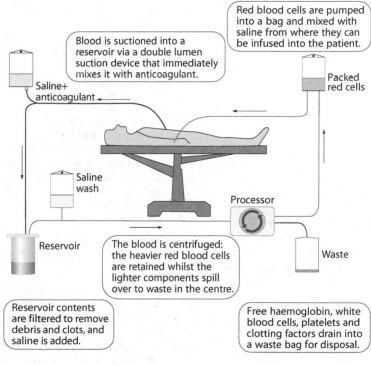

Cell salvage

a) What <u>specific</u> issues should be discussed with this patient based on the history outlined above? (10 marks)

> Ensure no coercion from family or fellow-witnesses.
> Discuss what advice the patient has received from fellow-witnesses, the hospital liaison team or other sources.
> Preoperative optimisation if necessary: check current haemoglobin and haematinics, liaise with haematologist if optimisation is required with iron (intravenous if rapid response required), folate, erythropoietin.
> Potential for bleeding: discuss the greatly increased risks due to fibroids AND placenta praevia.
> Risks of untreated haemorrhage: mortality and major morbidity, including prolonged ICU stay, prolonged ventilation and its complications, poor wound healing, infection, hysterectomy, consequent difficulties with caring for newborn.
> Specific wishes regarding blood products: whole blood, red blood cells, plasma and platelets are generally not acceptable to Jehovah's Witnesses, whereas albumin, immunoglobulins, individual clotting factors and anti-D are up to personal preference. Do not make assumptions – check the acceptability of all blood products and document.
> Appreciate that there are no true blood 'alternatives': Jehovah's Witnesses' website refers to blood substitutes. It is important that the woman understands that there are no true blood alternatives in existence.
> Understanding of techniques that can be employed to minimise risk of bleeding:
>   • Elective caesarean delivery.
>   • Consultant obstetrician and anaesthetist.
>   • Regional technique.
>   • Possibility of need for uterine artery catheters to be sited ready for deployment if excessive bleeding occurs.
>   • Use of oxytocics to minimise postpartum haemorrhage.
>   • Tranexamic acid use if bleeding occurs.
> Acceptability of cell salvage: description of process, up to the individual patient whether it complies with their beliefs and whether they can view the extracorporeal circuit as an extension of their own and 'uninterrupted'.
> Risks of cell salvage: see part (b).
> Advance decision: patient may have one already – ensure that it reflects the discussed wishes and copy taken for inclusion in patient's notes. Any hospital-specific paperwork must also be completed.
> Ability to change mind: free to reverse decision, including verbally, at any time. However, in an emergency, the patient may not be capable or conscious. No one else can change the patient's mind on her behalf in such a situation.

b) Give the advantages and disadvantages of using intraoperative cell salvage during caesarean section? (10 marks)

Notice that the focus is no longer on Jehovah's Witnesses, but on cell salvage during caesarean section generally.

Advantages:
> Avoidance of risks of allogenic transfusion: ABO incompatibility and other transfusion reactions, viral, bacterial and prion transmission, blood errors.
> Good value: consumables cost slightly more than one unit of donated blood.
> Blood reinfused at room temperature, reduces the risk of hypothermia associated with transfusion.
> Often acceptable to Jehovah's Witnesses.
> Useful in patients with atypical antibodies where cross-match may be difficult to achieve.
> Normal 2,3 DPG levels and, thus, oxygen-carrying behaviour.

Disadvantages:

> In the case of Rhesus-positive baby with Rhesus-negative mother, there is a risk of alloimunisation. However, this risk occurs in any delivery of positive baby to negative mother and anti-D administration is routine in such cases anyway.
> Leucodepletion filter may result in release of vasoactive substances causing hypotension.
> Air embolism.
> High cost per use in centres where cell salvage infrequently used.
> Staff training necessary, may be difficult to maintain staff competency if infrequently used.
> Risk of bacterial contamination.
> Risk of electrolyte imbalance.
> No platelets or coagulation factors so does not eliminate need for allogenic blood products in significant haemorrhage.
> Red cell lysis due to 'skimming' (suctioning of surface of shed blood) reduces the availability of whole cells for reinfusion and increases the quantity of free haemoglobin, which may cause renal damage.
> Slow flow rate through leucodepletion filter, may not be adequate during massive haemorrhage.
> Risk of circulatory overload.

References

www.jw.org

Association of Anaesthetists of Great Britain and Ireland (AAGBI). *Management of Anaesthesia for Jehovah's Witnesses*. AAGBI: London; 2005.

Kuppurao L, Wee M. Perioperative cell salvage. *Contin Educ Anaesth Crit Care Pain*. 2010; 10 (4): 104–108.

National Institute for Health and Care Excellence. Intraoperative Blood Cell Salvage in Obstetrics IPG 144. 2005.

A 25-year-old woman who is 37 weeks pregnant and known to have pre-eclampsia is admitted to your labour ward with a blood pressure of 160/110 mm Hg on several readings.

a) What is the definition of pre-eclampsia (1 mark) and which related symptoms should pregnant women be told to report immediately? (2 marks)

b) How should this patient be managed following admission to your labour ward? (12 marks)

c) What changes would you make to your usual general anaesthetic technique for a pregnant woman, if this woman needed a general anaesthetic for caesarean section? (5 marks)

September 2015

Chairman's Report

16.1% pass rate.

The poor pass rate for this important subject is of concern as pre-eclampsia is a common condition that all candidates should have encountered. Severe pre-eclampsia is an emergency for which the principles of management should be known. Surprisingly few candidates could give an acceptable definition of pre-eclampsia and even fewer knew that control of systolic hypertension is of prime importance in preventing intracerebral bleeding in women with severe pre-eclampsia. Again, as mentioned above, failure to read the question in part (c) meant that some candidates lost marks by not answering what was asked.

The abysmal pass rate makes me wonder if this is a question that will be repeated imminently.

a) What is the definition of pre-eclampsia (1 mark) and which related symptoms should pregnant women be told to report immediately? (2 marks)

Pre-eclampsia is new hypertension (systolic greater than 140 mm Hg, diastolic greater than 90 mm Hg) presenting after 20 weeks' gestation with significant proteinuria.

(Significant proteinuria: 24-hour urine collection greater than 300 mg protein OR urinary protein:creatinine ratio [PCR] greater than 30 mg/mmol).

Symptoms to report immediately:
> Severe headaches.
> Visual disturbance, blurred vision, flashing lights.
> Sudden swelling of hands, feet or face.
> Upper abdominal pain or vomiting.

b) How should this patient be managed following admission to your labour ward? (12 marks)

Multidisciplinary management is required of this obstetric emergency, with obstetric, midwifery, anaesthetic and intensive care input. Level 1 care as a minimum.

Assess and manage the patient simultaneously following a systems-based approach:

> Airway:
  • Airway assessment – anaesthesia for urgent delivery or airway support may be necessary.
  • Assess for voice change, hoarseness, facial oedema – laryngeal oedema and difficult intubation are more likely.
> Respiratory:
  • Pulmonary oedema may result in respiratory compromise.
  • Assess oxygen saturations, respiratory rate.
  • Auscultate chest.
  • Supplementary oxygen if required.
  • Consider fluid restriction to 1 ml/kg/h to a maximum of 80 ml/h (although may need extra bolus if hydralazine is commenced).
> Cardiovascular:
  • Cannulate. Start antihypertensive medication to target BP less than 150/100: first line oral or intravenous labetalol; second line intravenous hydralazine; third line oral nifedipine.
  • Monitor response with frequent blood pressure checks.

> Neurological:
>   • Assess for hyper-reflexia, severe headache, visual disturbance. May signify risk of eclampsia. Consideration of magnesium treatment if these symptoms are present or if there is significant proteinuria.
> Gastrointestinal:
>   • Keep nil by mouth and administer antacid in view of likely imminent delivery and possibility of seizure.
> Haematological:
>   • Check full blood count for platelet level and coagulation screen.
> Renal:
>   • Urinary protein:creatinine ratio and urine dip for protein to assess disease severity.
>   • Monitor urine output.
>   • Monitor renal function.
> Hepatic:
>   • Check transaminases and bilirubin.
> Obstetric:
>   • Continuous fetal monitoring with cardiotocograph, especially once antihypertensives are initiated.
>   • Uric acid is a marker of disease severity.
>   • Plan for delivery: baby is at term and ultimate cure for pre-eclampsia is delivery of the placenta.

c) What changes would you make to your usual general anaesthetic technique for a pregnant woman if this woman needed a general anaesthetic for caesarean section? (5 marks)

> Airway:
>   • Increased awareness of risk of and preparation for difficult airway: assess for upper body or facial oedema and hoarseness that may indicate oropharyngeal and laryngeal oedema.
>   • Airway oedema may worsen over duration of surgery: deflate endotracheal tube cuff to check for leak before extubation.
> Respiratory:
>   • Limit fluid input to 80 ml/h unless matching losses through e.g. haemorrhage.
>   • Higher airway pressures and PEEP may be required for oxygenation in the presence of pulmonary oedema – this may necessitate postoperative ventilation as well.
> Cardiovascular:
>   • Consideration of intra-arterial blood pressure monitoring.
>   • Mitigate pressor response of intubation with short-acting opioid, e.g. alfentanil 10 mcg/kg.
>   • Consider pressor response of extubation if blood pressure remains high and labile. Consider short-acting beta-blocker, e.g. labetalol 10–20 mg intravenously.
> Pharmacology:
>   • Caesarean section under general anaesthesia has an increased association with uterine atony. Ergometrine is contraindicated for this patient due to its hypertensive effect.
> Neurological:
>   • Even more important to ensure adequate pain relief before waking due to impact of circulating catecholamines on blood pressure. Consider transverse abdominis plane blocks and morphine.
>   • Magnesium prolongs the effect of depolarising and non-depolarising muscle relaxants: mandatory use of nerve stimulator, and anaesthesia may have to be prolonged to allow for this prolonged offset time.
> Renal:
>   • Avoid NSAIDs due to the effect of pre-eclampsia on kidney function.

Reference

National Institute for Health and Care Excellence. Hypertension in pregnancy: diagnosis and management NICE Clinical guideline CG107. 2010.

a) What factors may contribute to difficulties encountered when securing the airway under general anaesthesia in the pregnant patient? (9 marks)

b) What measures can be taken to reduce airway-related morbidity and mortality associated with general anaesthesia in a pregnant woman? (8 marks)

c) What are the recommendations in the 4th National Audit Project (Major Complications of Airway Management in the UK, NAP 4) regarding airway management in the pregnant woman? (3 marks)

March 2016

Chairman's Report

57.6% pass rate.

It is encouraging that the pass rate for the mandatory obstetric question was higher in this sitting of the SAQ than in the last several sittings. Knowledge of difficult airway management in the obstetric patient is fundamental to anaesthetic practice. It is disappointing, however, that the recommendations from NAP4 regarding the pregnant patient (part c) seemed very poorly known.

NAP4 has been the basis of numerous final SAQ questions. Its little vignettes make it quite readable, so give it a go. However, it is only part (c) that requires you to have to read anything; you could possibly answer the rest of the question by thinking about every suboptimal obstetric GA case you have experienced or heard about.

a) What factors may contribute to difficulties encountered when securing the airway under general anaesthesia in the pregnant patient? (9 marks)

Patient:
> Increased fatty tissue.
> Increased breast size.
> Increased tongue size.
> Pharyngeal or laryngeal oedema.
> Obesity (an increasing problem in the obstetric population generally).
> Active labour may make cooperation with pre-induction positioning difficult.

Circumstantial:
> Site of obstetric theatre often isolated, away from main theatres, without the second line airway equipment held in main theatres.
> Urgency resulting in failure to:
   • Assess airway.
   • Starve patient.
   • Premedicate the patient with antacid.
   • Position correctly.
   • Assess alternative modes of anaesthesia.
> Intraoperative conversion of regional to general anaesthesia may be challenging.

Staffing:
> Anaesthetist: commonly out-of-hours, therefore a trainee, low experience of general anaesthesia for obstetrics.
> Team: poor planning, poor communication, lack of awareness of other health care professionals about the potential difficulty with airway. Failure to warn, failure to assist.

b) What measures can be taken to reduce airway-related morbidity and mortality associated with general anaesthesia in a pregnant woman? (8 marks)

It is not clear whether they are asking purely about your anaesthetic practice in an individual case or more generally. So, to be safe, I have started with organisational factors.

Organisational:
> Locate labour ward theatre close to main theatres and delivery suite.
> Establish the personnel bleep list to be contacted in the event of need for general anaesthesia for pregnant woman – to include a second anaesthetist.

> Ensure adequate airway equipment, including immediate availability of difficult airway trolley.
> Staff training, skills and drills, implementation of DAS/OAA guidelines.
> Multidisciplinary protocols for antenatal assessment of high-risk parturients, and pathways for ensuring communication of a written management plan to staff on duty when parturient presents in labour.
> Guidance for handover between staff involved in obstetric care to include those at risk of airway issues such as those at risk of needing general anaesthesia and those known to have difficult or predicted difficult airway.

Prior to general anaesthesia:
> Outpatient antenatal assessment of high-risk women (obese, known previous difficult airway, regional likely to be difficult/unacceptable/contraindicated).
> Inpatient intrapartum assessment by anaesthetist of high-risk women.
> Junior anaesthetist to discuss likely problem patients with senior to assist in development of management plan.
> Regular ranitidine in labour for selected women according to protocol, oral or intravenous.
> Plans for likely difficult patients to be discussed with other staff, equipment readied.
> Anaesthetist to remain aware of efficacy of epidurals in situ on labour ward in order to increase chances of successful regional anaesthesia in an emergency, thus reducing need for general anaesthesia.

At the time of general anaesthesia:
> Planned, daytime delivery with senior staff for patients deemed very challenging.
> Team briefing of airway plan, second anaesthetist present.
> Suitable equipment ready, including full difficult airway kit.
> Confirmation of premedication with ranitidine and sodium citrate.
> Optimum patient positioning: ramping.
> Awareness of impact of left lateral tilt on anatomy.
> Adequate preoxygenation, cricoid pressure and auscultation of chest and check of capnography before cricoid pressure released.

After general anaesthesia:
> Same care with extubation as intubation: consider stomach emptying with orogastric tube, ensure the patient is wide awake, sitting up, fully reversed (use nerve stimulator).
> Awareness of impact of opioids on conscious level postoperatively (and use of opioid sparing techniques if suitable).
> Trained recovery staff, properly equipped recovery.

c) What are the recommendations in the 4th National Audit Project (Major Complications of Airway Management in the UK, NAP 4) regarding airway management in the pregnant woman? (3 marks)

> Difficult airway management and CICO skills must be kept up to date.
> Obstetric anaesthetists should be familiar with using second-generation SADs for airway rescue.
> Awake fibreoptic intubation should be available (skills and equipment) anywhere in the hospital.
> All recovery staff (including midwives working in recovery) should be properly trained and skills regularly updated.

Reference
Cook T, Woodall N, Frerk C (eds.). *4th National Audit Project of the Royal College of Anaesthetists and the Difficult Airway Society. Major Complications of Airway Management in the United Kingdom*. London: The Royal College of Anaesthetists and Association of Anaesthetists of Great Britain and Ireland; 2011.

a) Which methods of testing may be used to confirm the adequacy of a spinal (intrathecal) block for elective caesarean section? (4 marks)

b) Describe the actions you could take if your spinal block proves inadequate on testing <u>prior to starting</u> surgery for an <u>elective (category 4)</u> caesarean section. (3 marks)

c) What are the early symptoms and signs of a spinal block that is ascending too high? (5 marks)

d) How should you manage a patient who complains of pain during elective caesarean section under spinal anaesthesia? (8 marks)

September 2016

Chairman's Report

77.5% pass rate.

This was reassuringly well answered. Pain during caesarean section is an important topic as it is extremely unpleasant for patients and is one of the leading causes of litigation against anaesthetists. Most candidates knew the steps to take both when dealing with a poor spinal block identified before the start of surgery and when managing pain occurring during the procedure.

This question is very similar to that from March 2012, but there are differences. Questions often appear again with a few changes so be careful to answer the question in front of you, not the one that you have previously practiced.

a) Which methods of testing may be used to confirm the adequacy of a spinal (intrathecal) block for elective caesarean section? (4 marks)

As per the answer to the March 2012 question.

b) Describe the actions you could take if your spinal block proves inadequate on testing <u>prior to starting</u> surgery for an <u>elective (category 4)</u> caesarean section. (3 marks)

> Improve current block if close to adequate block on assessment:
  • Positioning; flex hips to flatten the lumbar lordosis, cautious head down tilt, tilt to suboptimal side (remember need to avoid aortocaval compression).
  • Ensure that adequate time has been allowed for block development.
> Further regional technique:
  • Repeat spinal – consider reducing overall dose if some block is present, good attention to patient positioning to help prevent high spinal.
  • Epidural – height of spinal block may be elevated by epidural injection, epidural component itself also provides anaesthesia.
> General anaesthetic:
  • If the patient does not want to consider further regional technique and there are no compelling contraindications to this.

c) What are the early symptoms and signs of a spinal block that is ascending too high? (5 marks)

Don't waste time with full sentences. The College has made it clear in numerous Chairman's Reports that lists are welcomed.

Symptoms:
> Difficulty breathing or taking a deep breath, difficulty speaking.
> Nausea and vomiting.
> Anxiety, feeling faint.
> Tingling and weakness of hands and arms.

Signs:
> Decreased respiratory effort, reduced saturations, weak cough.
> Cardiovascular instability: bradycardia and hypotension.
> Objective weakness of hands then arms then shoulders, high block on retesting.
> Sedation.

d) How should you manage a patient who complains of pain during elective caesarean section under spinal anaesthesia? (8 marks)

As per the answer to the March 2012 question.

The obstetric team tell you about a patient who is two days post-partum with what they suspect is a post-dural puncture headache (PDPH).

a) What is the differential diagnosis of post-partum headache? (8 marks)

b) What features in this patient would lead you to consider a serious underlying cause? (7 marks)

c) You diagnose a PDPH and arrange treatment by epidural blood patch (EBP). What are the described risks of EBP? (5 marks)

March 2017

Chairman's Report

Knowledge and management of post dural puncture headache (PDPH)

81.3% pass rate.

This question had the highest pass rate in the paper and also had the highest correlation with overall performance. PDPH is a common problem in obstetric anaesthesia so it is reassuring that the question was well answered and that candidates recognised possibly serious differential diagnoses.

This question is very similar to the obstetric question in March 2013. I hope you are convinced of the importance of looking at past papers and taking on board what is written in the Chairman's Reports.

a) What is the differential diagnosis of post-partum headache? (8 marks)

The answer to this is exactly the same as to part (b) of the March 2013 question except this time you must include post-dural puncture headache in your differential due to the slightly different way in which they have worded it.

b) What features in this patient would lead you to consider a serious underlying cause? (7 marks)

Essentially, think through your differential diagnoses and write their positive findings. Should I have included outcomes from simple investigations here? Is an investigation finding a 'feature?' I don't know, but I doubt marks would be lost for this.

History:
> Drowsiness, confusion, vomiting.
> Focal neurology.
> Seizures.
> Significant neck stiffness and photophobia (although photophobia may also be present in PDPH).

Examination:
> Focal neurology.
> Papilloedema.
> Hypertension.
> Hypotension and tachycardia.
> Fever.
> Reduced conscious level.
> Meningism: positive Kernig and Brudzinski's signs.
> Petechial rash.

Investigations (that may already be available):
> Features of infection: elevated CRP, raised or depressed white cell count. However, CRP and white cell count tend to be elevated after delivery anyway, so this must be viewed in the overall context.
> Features of pre-eclampsia: deranged transaminases and bilirubin, low platelets, haemolysis, elevated uric acid, proteinuria.

c) You diagnose a PDPH and arrange treatment by epidural blood patch (EBP). What are the described risks of EBP? (5 marks)

Again, be careful not to answer the question from March 2012: they want you to talk about the risks this time, not how you would perform an EBP. These are the risks as quoted by the RCoA's own leaflet about epidural blood patch.

> Local bruising on the back.
> Backache and stiffness, which can last a few days (no risk of long-term back pain).

> Another accidental dural puncture.
> Nerve damage, infection or bleeding.
> Seizure at the time of performing the EBP.
> Failure to treat headache: 30%–40%.

Reference

Royal College of Anaesthetists and Association of Anaesthetists of Great Britain and Ireland. Risks associated with your anaesthetic Section 10: Headache after a spinal or epidural injection. 2015. https://www.rcoa.ac.uk/system /files/10-HeadachesSpinalEpidural2015.pdf [Accessed 8th January 2017].

A woman who has had an intrauterine fetal death (IUFD) at 36 weeks' gestation in her first pregnancy is admitted to your delivery suite for induction of labour.

a) Describe the important non-clinical aspects of her management. (4 marks)

b) What are the considerations when providing pain relief for this woman? (13 marks)

c) If this patient requires a caesarean section, what are the advantages of using regional anaesthesia, other than the avoidance of the effects of general anaesthesia? (3 marks)

September 2017

Chairman's Report

Pass rate NA

This question was removed from the exam after marking but no candidates were disadvantaged by its removal. The reason for not including it in the final scores was that there was confusion amongst candidates about whether the intrauterine fetal death had occurred in the current, or a previous pregnancy. On reflection, the examiners agreed that the wording of the question did allow either interpretation. As has been outlined above, all the SAQs undergo rigorous scrutiny and are checked and rechecked for clarity and accuracy. Unfortunately, the alternative interpretation was not spotted in this case. The question will be reworded before being reused. Having said all of the above, the pass rate for this question was poor, with most marks being lost in section b where candidates were asked to discuss considerations for analgesia. Even those who had correctly interpreted the question tended to simply list methods of analgesia rather than outlining the advantages and disadvantages of each.

So this is reassuring: whilst you MUST read the questions carefully, you do not need to waste time agonising about what they mean if it isn't clear. If there is more than one way of interpreting the question, then there will probably be an even spread of approaches throughout the candidates which will highlight to the College the lack of clarity of the question. This question is similar to that from September 2012. It would be sensible to revise all aspects of management of IUFD as it would seem likely that a similar question will appear again soon.

a) Describe the important non-clinical aspects of her management. (4 marks)

> One-to-one senior midwifery care, trained in caring for women with IUFD.
> Good communication between all involved healthcare professionals to avoid possibility of lack of awareness of situation and subsequent insensitivity.
> Clear discussions with the woman regarding expectations and wishes for the delivery: pain relief, presence of friends or family, contact with the baby after birth, arrangement for mementoes to be created (photos, hair cuttings, footprints).
> Dedicated suite/room away from the noise of delivery suite, ideally with provision of non-clinical area where the woman may be with her birth partner/family/friends before delivery and may spend time with her baby, if desired, after birth. However, location for delivery is ultimately determined by maternal condition.

b) What are the considerations when providing pain relief for this woman? (13 marks)

This section holds the bulk of the marks, and asks for the same information as parts (b) and (c) in the September 2012 question.

c) If this patient requires a caesarean section what are the advantages of using regional anaesthesia, other than the avoidance of the effects of general anaesthesia? (3 marks)

> Offers optimum pain relief postoperatively.
> Facilitates early contact with the baby.
> Permits clearer recollection of events that may be important to the woman.
> Facilitates presence of partner at delivery.

17. PAEDIATRICS

A 9-year-old child with Down's syndrome is scheduled for an adenotonsillectomy.

a) List airway/respiratory (30%), cardiovascular (10%) and neurological (10%) features of the syndrome relevant to the anaesthetist.

b) What are the general principles involved in the preoperative (15%), intraoperative (25%) and postoperative (10%) management of this patient with Down's syndrome?

September 2011

a) List airway/respiratory (30%), cardiovascular (10%) and neurological (10%) features of the syndrome relevant to the anaesthetist.

You've been asked for a list – don't waste time and energy writing in prose. If you have started to organise your brain to think through issues alphabetically, this should be straightforward! Note that it has asked for features of the syndrome relevant to the anaesthetist, not features of this particular child.

Airway and respiratory:
> Subglottic or tracheal stenosis: may require smaller tube size.
> Atlantoaxial instability: care with neck manipulation, especially extension (this is an issue for positioning during tonsillectomy as well as during anaesthetic airway management).
> Cervical spine ankylosis (Klippel-Feil): limits neck extension, may make intubation difficult.
> Obstructive sleep apnoea (OSA) caused by craniofacial abnormalities (macroglossia, narrow midface, oropharyngeal hypotonia, micrognathia, small mouth, short neck, adenotonsillar hypertrophy): mask ventilation may be challenging.
> Predisposition to lower respiratory tract infection due to hypotonia, gastro-oesophageal reflux, reduced immunity.

Cardiovascular:
> Congenital heart disease: increased risk of atrioventricular canal defects, atrioseptal and ventriculoseptal defects, patent ductus arteriosus, tetralogy of Fallot.
> Pulmonary hypertension with or without associated cardiac lesions.
> Risk of conduction defects following repair of congenital lesions.
> Valve abnormalities in adulthood: mitral valve prolapse, aortic regurgitation.

Neurological:
> Hypotonia: care with positioning.
> Epilepsy.
> Intellectual impairment: consent, cooperation.
> Postoperative agitation.
> Reduced MAC requirement possibly due to reduced central catecholamine activity.
> Increased sensitivity to sedatives and anaesthetic agents.

b) What are the general principles involved in the preoperative (15%), intraoperative (25%) and postoperative (10%) management of this patient with Down's syndrome?

Preoperative:

> Full patient assessment involving parents or carers. Explanations and consent appropriate to patient's understanding and sensory function. Arrange ward visit and opportunity to meet staff to help manage anxiety.

> Airway: assess for difficulties associated with Down's syndrome, as detailed previously. Consider radiological assessment of cervical spine if atlantoaxial instability is likely.

> Respiratory: assess for possibility of OSA, especially considering that the patient is requiring an adenotonsillectomy. Assess for symptoms and signs of lower respiratory tract infection. Consider antisialagogue premedication with atropine.

> Cardiovascular: assess exercise capacity, history of cardiac defects and corrective surgery. Discuss with the cardiology or cardiothoracic team caring for the patient if necessary. Right heart strain on ECG may be indicative of pulmonary hypertension – investigate with echocardiogram. Topical local anaesthetic to be used in preparation for cannulation.

> Neurological: consider radiological assessment of cervical spine if atlantoaxial instability is likely.

> Endocrine: consideration of thyroid function testing and blood glucose, if diabetes is a possibility.

> Gastrointestinal: assess for presence of gastro-oesophageal reflux. Premedicate with proton-pump inhibitor and plan for rapid sequence induction if indicated.

Intraoperative:

> Ensure carer or parent accompanies child to theatre. Involve play specialist if required.

> Airway: intubate, possibly rapid sequence. Have range of tube sizes available, smaller tube may be required if subglottic stenosis (and children with Down's often smaller than other children of same age). Consideration of need for difficult intubation equipment. Oropharyngeal airway may be required to facilitate mask ventilation.

> Cardiovascular: cannulation may be challenging due to tendency to raised BMI. Prone to bradycardia after induction – ensure atropine and glycopyrrolate prepared according to child's weight. Avoid hypotension in order to preserve spinal cord perfusion. ECG monitoring due to possibility of arrhythmia.

> Neurological: care with positioning due to ligamentous laxity and atlantoaxial instability – care with all neck movement (even if radiographically normal), especially with the hyperextension normally required for tonsillectomy. Avoidance of long-acting opioids and consideration of lower MAC.

> Infection, immunology: scrupulous attention to asepsis due to increased risk of infection.

Postoperative:

> Risk of OSA. Patient may need CPAP, overnight oxygen saturations monitoring, and close nursing observation.

> Predisposed to postoperative agitation. Prolonged recovery stay and higher intensity nursing care on a higher dependency ward may be indicated.

> Postoperative pain relief. Consideration must be given to communication abilities. Parent or carer who knows child well may be required to assist in pain assessment. Avoid long-acting opioids especially if the patient has OSA.

> Monitor for signs of postoperative infection, especially lower respiratory tract infection. Alert parents/carers to signs to be aware of.

> Monitor for signs of spinal cord compromise and investigate promptly.

Reference

Allt J, Howell C. Down's syndrome. *BJA CEPD Rev*. 2003; 3 (3): 83–86.

A 4-year-old child is admitted to the emergency department with suspected meningococcal septicaemia. You are asked to help resuscitate the patient prior to transfer to a tertiary centre.

a) List the clinical features of meningococcal septicaemia. (35%)

b) Outline the initial management of this patient? (45%)

c) Which investigations will guide care? (20%)

September 2012

Chairman's Report

67.6% pass rate.

This paediatric emergency is commonly encountered both in secondary and tertiary centres. Although the question was answered satisfactorily, marks were lost by not calling for help and inappropriate fluid resuscitation. Many candidates failed to communicate with the tertiary centre for advice or to summon the paediatric retrieval team. This question was a very good discriminator.

Meningococcal disease may present as meningitis, septicaemia or (most commonly) as a combination of the two. NICE guidance on management of bacterial meningitis and meningococcal septicaemia was published in 2010, featured in this question in 2012 and was then updated in 2015 just in time for a slightly different version of this question to appear in the final.

a) List the clinical features of meningococcal septicaemia. (35%)

Nonspecific symptoms and signs:

Fever, nausea and vomiting, lethargy, irritable/unsettled, ill-looking, anorexia, headache, muscle ache/joint pain, respiratory symptoms and difficulty breathing, chills, shivering, rapid deterioration in illness.

More specific symptoms and signs:

Non-blanching rash, altered mental state, capillary refill time greater than two seconds, unusual skin colour, shock, hypotension, leg pain, cold hands/feet, unconsciousness, toxic/moribund state.

b) Outline the initial management of this patient? (45%)

Meningococcal septicaemia is a medical emergency and so I would assess and manage the patient simultaneously following an ABCDE approach.

Request senior help and give ceftriaxone 80 mg/kg intravenously without delay.

Initiate communication with paediatric retrieval service and download guidance to assist with drug dosing.

A: Assess airway patency – consider need for immediate intubation for either respiratory compromise or moribund state.

B: Assess respiratory rate, oxygen saturations, give 100% oxygen.

C: Intravenous access, ideally two cannulae. Obtain intraosseous access if intravenous access not immediately feasible. Assess for signs of shock:

> Capillary refill time greater than 2 seconds.
> Unusual skin colour.
> Tachycardia and/or hypotension.
> Cold hands/feet.
> Toxic/moribund state.
> Altered mental state/decreased conscious level.
> Poor urine output.

Treat shock with up to three boluses of 20 ml/kg 4.5% human albumin solution or 0.9% sodium chloride each over 5–10 minutes.

At the third bolus, intubate and ventilate the child, ensuring a cardiostable induction with ketamine (up to 2 mg/kg) and rocuronium (1 mg/kg). Ensure that emergency drugs are ready.

Further fluid boluses may be required: consider using blood.

Consider contributing causes to shock: acidosis, extravasation of fluids.

Initiate vasoactive support as per retrieval team guidance.

D: Continue to monitor the child's mental state (GCS or AVPU scoring) and need for intubation.

Assess for signs of meningism.

E: Examine child, look for rash, check capillary blood glucose.

Send investigations as detailed in section (c).

c) Which investigations will guide care? (20%)

For each investigation, I have stated how it would guide care. Some of the investigations that will guide care are very immediate, some have a delayed result.

> Full blood count: blood administration may be required especially after resuscitation with crystalloid. Elevated white cell count supports diagnosis of meningococcal disease, although may be normal or even low. Low platelets may contraindicate lumbar puncture.
> Coagulation screen: management of disseminated intravascular coagulation may be required. Results may contraindicate lumbar puncture.
> Glucose: hypoglycaemia may occur due to resuscitation with non-sugar fluids and critical illness, supplementation may be required.
> Electrolytes: must be managed due to administration of large quantities of intravenous fluids.
> CRP: usually elevated in meningococcal disease, supports diagnosis, but may be normal.
> Arterial blood gas: guides need for intubation and adequacy of ongoing ventilation. Acidosis may require treatment if shock is persistent despite fluids and vasoactive drugs.
> *Neisseria meningitidis* whole blood PCR: confirms diagnosis if positive. If negative, CSF should be tested for *N. meningitidis* and *Streptococcus pneumoniae* PCR.
> Blood culture: may confirm infective organism, therefore guiding antimicrobial treatment.
> CT brain: may indicate different diagnosis or may contraindicate lumbar puncture if features of raised intracranial pressure are present.
> CSF: PCR or culture may be diagnostic of underlying cause if negative for meningococcus. Causative bacteria determine the choice and duration of antibiotics.

Reference

National Institute for Health and Care Excellence. Meningitis (bacterial) and meningococcal septicaemia in under 16s: recognition, diagnosis and management CG102. February 2015.

An 8-year-old child with severe cerebral palsy is scheduled for an elective femoral osteotomy.

a) Define cerebral palsy. (15%)

b) List the clinical effects of cerebral palsy on the central nervous, gastrointestinal, respiratory and musculoskeletal systems with their associated anaesthetic implications. (50%)

c) What are the specific issues in managing postoperative pain in this patient? (35%)

March 2013

Chairman's Report

36.4% pass rate.

This question was poorly answered. Adult and paediatric patients with cerebral palsy presenting for surgery are not uncommon. Many examinees had little or no knowledge of the definition of cerebral palsy and could not put forward a coherent answered regarding the anaesthetic management. Awake-fibreoptic intubation was an inappropriate method of establishing the airway in this patient and the mention of sexual dysfunction was irrelevant.

A snapshot from the model answer below highlights the level of knowledge that was required.

Clinical Effects	Anaesthetic relevance
Flexion deformities/spasticity	Positioning problems; pressure sores; difficult IV access
Scoliosis	Restrictive respiratory pattern
Immobility	Unable to assess cardiopulmonary reserve
Low muscle bulk	Temperature control difficulties

Focusing on the gastrointestinal system involvement: one mark was available for each pair of answers (maximum 2)

a) Define cerebral palsy. (15%)

> Permanent damage to the developing brain in utero, at birth or in very early infancy.
> Primarily affects motor function, but may also impact on cognition, sensation and communication.
> Increased risk of epilepsy.
> Very variable presentation.

b) List the clinical effects of cerebral palsy on the central nervous, gastrointestinal, respiratory and musculoskeletal systems with their associated anaesthetic implications. (50%)

Notice that the College is asking you to order your knowledge according to systems here. Practising organising your thoughts according to the alphabet will put you in good stead.

	Clinical effects	Anaesthetic implications
Central nervous system	Epilepsy.	Ensure medication is not missed when nil by mouth. Ensure levels are checked if there is a recent change in seizure frequency. Consider the impact of enzyme inducers and enzyme inhibitors.
	Cognition or communication problems.	May increase child's anxiety. Involve carers, play specialist. Consider individual need for sedative/anxiolytic premedication but caution if child has respiratory compromise.
Gastrointestinal	Swallowing difficulties, oesophageal dysmotility, abnormal lower oesophageal sphincter tone.	Increased risk of reflux, consider need for rapid sequence induction.
	Swallowing difficulty.	Poor nutrition, low weight, need to calculate based on weight not age, consider the possibility of anaemia, dehydration or electrolyte disturbance and treat preoperatively (may have PEG), difficulty with oral medications.
	Risk of temporomandibular joint dislocation if affected by muscle spasticity.	Possibility of difficult intubation – difficult airway equipment, asleep fibreoptic or video laryngoscopy may be indicated.
	Poor dentition.	May complicate airway management. Loose or decayed teeth should be managed in advance.
Respiratory	History of premature birth and gastro-oesophageal reflux predispose to chronic lung disease.	Assess for acute infection. Consider need for respiratory assessment, physiotherapy. May still require long-term oxygen therapy or CPAP.
	Weak cough, respiratory muscle hypotonia, reduced immunity due to malnutrition.	Increased propensity to lung infection – check for acute infection preoperatively.
	Long term truncal spasticity results in scoliosis.	Restrictive defect, pulmonary hypertension, cor pulmonale, respiratory and cardiac failure.
Musculoskeletal	Spasticity causes fixed flexion deformities, joint dislocations.	Cannulation, monitoring and positioning problems.
	Thin skin, little subcutaneous fat, atrophic musculature (large surface-area-to-weight ratio).	Prone to pressure sores, poor heat conservation, poor wound healing. Need for careful padding and active warming at all times.
	Immobility.	Cannot assess cardiopulmonary reserve.
	Non-weight-bearing long bones become osteopenic.	Bone fragility, risk of fracture.

c) What are the specific issues in managing postoperative pain in this patient? (35%)

> Cognitive impairment or communication difficulties may make assessment of pain difficult.
> Muscle weakness and cognitive impairment may limit use of PCA.
> Opioid analgesia may further compromise lung function.
> Painful muscle spasms precipitated by cold, anxiety, pain. Consider epidural or regional nerve catheter to optimise pain relief. Continue regular antispasmodic medications. Epidural analgesia will necessitate escalated level of care postoperatively.
> NSAIDs may be contraindicated in the presence of renal impairment due to chronic neuropathic bladder or nephroureteric reflux.

Reference
Parry Prosser D, Sharma N. Cerebral palsy and anaesthesia. *Contin Educ Anaesth Crit Care Pain*. 2010; 10 (3); 72–76.

a) List the normal anatomical features of young children (<3 years old) which may adversely affect upper airway management. (35%)

b) Which airway problems may occur due to these anatomical features? (30%)

c) Outline how these problems are overcome in clinical practice. (35%)

September 2013

Chairman's Report

65.4% pass rate.

This question was a repeat from the May 2007 paper. Each anatomical feature was linked to an airway problem and how they might be overcome in clinical practice. It is quite acceptable to answer a question like this in the form of a table. Similarly, an 'advantages and disadvantages' question can be answered in this way and can avoid repetition of words and therefore save time.

Anatomical feature	Problem	Overcome by
Pliant sub-mental tissue	Easy obstruction by digital pressure	Ensure fingers applied to bony surfaces
Short trachea	High incidence of endobronchial intubation	High level of awareness, auscultate to check
Etc		

a) List the normal anatomical features of young children (<3 years old) which may adversely affect upper airway management. (35%)

b) Which airway problems may occur due to these anatomical features? (30%)

c) Outline how these problems are overcome in clinical practice. (35%)

As per the College's suggestion, I have put all of the information into one table. Be careful to read the question properly: it asks about airway problems that <u>affect upper airway management</u>, not a comparison of the whole respiratory system.

Anatomical feature	Problem	Overcome by
Large head with prominent occiput.	Tendency to flex neck.	Neutral position with e.g. folded towel under body.
Large tongue, pliant submental tissues.	Obstruction of airway by digital pressure.	Ensure fingers applied to bony surfaces.
Absence of teeth.	Difficulty maintaining face mask ventilation.	Use of appropriately sized guedel.
Long U shaped epiglottis, anterior larynx.	Difficulty with laryngoscopy, epiglottis flopping into visual field.	Straight blade.
Narrow trachea.	Flow proportional to radius to the power of 4. Small difference in radius due to trauma or oedema makes substantial difference to flow.	Careful handling of airway, select tube size carefully, minimise need for changes.
Airway narrowest at level of cricoid, not vocal cords.	Cricoid is a complete ring of non-compliant cartilage so pressure of tube may cause damage.	With uncuffed tubes, a leak should be ascertained. High volume, low pressure cuffed tubes (half a size smaller than uncuffed) are now used routinely except in neonates.
Short trachea.	Risk of endobronchial intubation.	Auscultate chest, vigilance.

Reference
Lawson T. *Paediatric Anaesthesia for Beginners*. London: Association of Paediatric Anaesthetists. 2011.

A 5-year-old patient presents for a myringotomy and grommet insertion as a day case. During your preoperative assessment, you notice that the patient has a nasal discharge.

a) Why would it be inappropriate to cancel the operation on the basis of this information alone? (25%)

b) List the features in the history (35%) and examination (25%) that might cause you to postpone the operation due to an increased risk of airway complications in this patient.

c) What social factors would preclude this child's treatment as a day case? (15%)

March 2014

Chairman's Report

44.7% pass rate.

This question was answered poorly considering the issue is 'meat and drink' to paediatric day case practice. The majority of candidates did not mention emotional aspects, financial losses, parental work absence, school absence and inefficient use of hospital resources in the answer. The history section was poorly answered although examination features were more typically known. Surprisingly, social factors were infrequently given, although these have a major impact on suitability as a daycase. Overall, there seem to be few candidates thinking about the organisational and logistical aspects of bringing a child in for daycase surgery.

a) Why would it be inappropriate to cancel the operation on the basis of this information alone? (25%)

There is not enough information so far to determine whether the operation should be cancelled – a runny nose alone is insufficient reason. It is very common in young children and more so in children awaiting this type of surgery.

There are consequences to such a cancellation:

> Inefficient list usage.
> Wasted time off school for child.
> Delayed surgery resulting in ongoing hearing issues in child. May impact on education.
> Wasted parent's time off work, financial loss.
> Loss of trust between parents/child and hospital, especially if surgery later takes place with runny nose still.

b) List the features in the history (35%) and examination (25%) that might cause you to postpone the operation due to an increased risk of airway complications in this patient.

History:
> Fever.
> Unwell in self, too unwell for school, parent states that child is unwell.
> Loss of appetite.
> Shortness of breath.
> Sore throat.
> Cough.
> Sputum production.
> Purulent nasal discharge.
> Significant comorbidities such as obstructive sleep apnoea, severe asthma, cardiac condition.

Examination:
> Fever.
> Listless, unwell.
> Tachypnoea or other signs of respiratory distress.
> Purulent nasal discharge.
> Crackles on auscultation.
> Tachycardia.
> Delayed capillary refill.

c) What social factors would preclude this child's treatment as a day case? (15%)

> No telephone.
> Poor housing conditions.
> No private transport.
> Distance more than one hour from hospital.
> Parents unable or unwilling to care for child postoperatively.

Reference

Bhatia N, Barber N. Dilemmas in the preoperative assessment of children. *Contin Educ Anaesth Crit Care Pain*. 2011; 11 (6): 214–218.

A 5-year-old child presenting for day case dental surgery under general anaesthesia is found to have a heart murmur that has not been documented previously.

a) What features of the history (5 marks) and examination (5 marks) might suggest that the child has a significant congenital heart disease (CHD)?

b) If the murmur is caused by an atrial septal defect (ASD), what ECG findings would you expect? (2 marks)

c) Which imaging modalities might be used in the assessment of the ASD (2 marks) and what specific additional information may be obtained? (2 marks)

d) List the current national guidelines regarding prophylaxis against infective endocarditis in children with CHD undergoing dental procedures. (4 marks)

September 2014

Chairman's Report

39.1% pass rate.

This question was poorly answered by many candidates who could not list the history and examination findings in such a patient. Many felt that congenital heart disease only caused left sided cardiac abnormalities and were ignorant of national guidelines on infective endocarditis prophylaxis, although the need for the latter must be encountered on a regular basis in adult subjects.

a) What features of the history (5 marks) and examination (5 marks) might suggest that the child has a significant congenital heart disease (CHD)?

The biggest chunk of the marks is here – the question is basically asking if you have a safe approach to dealing with a common finding at paediatric preassessment.

History:
> History suggestive of cardiac failure: failure to thrive, difficulty feeding as a neonate, recurrent chest infections, cough, poor exercise tolerance.
> Squatting, parental report of cyanosis.
> Family history of congenital cardiac disease.
> Syndrome known to be associated with congenital cardiac disease: Down's, VATER, Turner's.

Examination:
> Irregular pulse.
> Features of the murmur: innocent murmurs are either a continuous venous hum or early systolic. All others are likely to be pathological: harsh, variable sound, presence of a precordial thrill.
> Signs suggestive of cardiac failure: tachypnoea, accessory muscle use, crackles on auscultation, cool peripheries, sweating, tachycardia, hepatomegaly.
> Cyanosis.
> Features suggestive of a syndrome associated with congenital cardiac defects.

b) If the murmur is caused by an atrial septal defect (ASD), what ECG findings would you expect? (2 marks)

You either know it or you don't, but it is only 2 marks.

> Prolonged PR interval.
> Right bundle branch block.
> Left axis deviation if primum defect, right axis deviation if secundum defect.

c) Which imaging modalities might be used in the assessment of the ASD (2 marks) and what specific additional information may be obtained? (2 marks)

Echo (transthoracic or transoesophageal):
> To determine whether secundum or primum defect: assessment of involvement of tricuspid and mitral valves and shunt between ventricles.
> Assess the direction of the shunt.
> Assess for the presence of pulmonary hypertension.

Cardiac MRI:

> 3D structure of heart lesion, valvular involvement, shunt volume.

Cardiac CT:

> 3D structure of heart lesion, chamber size.

Chest x-ray:
> Assess for presence of pulmonary oedema.

d) List the current national guidelines regarding prophylaxis against infective endocarditis in children with CHD undergoing dental procedures. (4 marks)

> Be aware of the increased risk of infective endocarditis in these children.
> Explain to patients and/or their parents that risk of prophylaxis outweighs benefits.
> Do not give antibiotic prophylaxis.
> Do not give chlorhexidine mouthwash.
> Prompt treatment if infection does occur.

References

Bhatia N, Barber N. Dilemmas in the preoperative assessment of children. *Contin Educ Anaesth Crit Care Pain*. 2011; 11 (6): 214–218.

National Institute for Health and Care Excellence. Prophylaxis against infective endocarditis: antimicrobial prophylaxis against infective endocarditis in adults and children undergoing interventional procedures. Clinical guideline [CG64]. 2016.

A 5-year-old boy with autistic spectrum disorder (ASD) is listed for dental extractions as a day case.

a) What constitutes ASD (1 mark) and what are the key clinical features? (6 marks)

b) List the important issues when providing anaesthesia for dental extractions in children. (6 marks)

c) Give the specific problems of providing anaesthesia for children with ASD and outline possible solutions. (7 marks)

March 2015

Chairman's Report

46.2% pass rate; 22.1% of candidates received a poor fail.

It was anticipated that candidates would find this subject matter to be difficult and this was borne out by the pass and poor fail rates. Autistic spectrum disorder (ASD) is an important issue within paediatric anaesthetic practice, and this result suggests specific teaching on the topic needs to be undertaken in all Schools of Anaesthesia. Failure to read section (b) correctly led to low scores as candidates did not realise that the question referred to all children not just individuals with ASD.

In the last question, ASD is atrial septal defect. Now, ASD is autistic spectrum disorder. However, the College does not use abbreviations without defining them so read the question. Also, really properly reading the question would avoid the mistake of answering section (b) as if it were asking about children with autism only.

a) What constitutes ASD (1 mark) and what are the key clinical features? (6 marks)

7 marks in total here. Don't panic. You will all have interacted with children with autism – describe them.

ASD is a lifelong condition affecting brain development. It impacts on communication, social interaction and abstract thought. It may be associated with reduced IQ in approximately half of all cases.

Key clinical features:
> Communication problems: language delay, avoidance of conversation, failure to understand nuance, literal interpretation.
> Interaction: lack of eye contact, reduced interaction, low understanding of the usual rules of social interaction. Intolerance of people entering their personal space, minimal use of gestures.
> Abstract thought: inability to generalise information, unable to appreciate that different people have different thoughts, knowledge and beliefs. Inability to understand metaphorical explanations.
> Behaviours: routine (and distress if routines broken), repetitive behaviours, rigid food preferences, highly specific interest for particular subjects or activities.

b) List the important issues when providing anaesthesia for dental extractions in children. (6 marks)

Organisational:
> Proper hospital setting required offering the same standard of care as for other cases requiring general anaesthesia.
> Availability of paediatric anaesthetic equipment.
> Staff trained in care of paediatric patients including resuscitation.
> Facility for preoperative assessment in advance in selected cases.

Preoperative:
> Preoperative assessment will usually be done on day of admission so careful questioning to ensure fitness for procedure and good explanations for consent are required.
> Premedication including topical local anaesthesia for cannulation, consideration of antisialagogue.
> Play specialist/psychologist especially for children with special needs or specific fears.
> Well-managed induction to maximise cooperation of patient.
> Strategies for uncooperative child, parental presence.

Intraoperative:
> Shared (small) airway.
> Blood from extractions may result in blood inhalation or laryngospasm.
> Throat pack.
> Risk of dislodgement of airway with surgery/gag.
> Head-up positioning risks reduced cardiac output and cerebral perfusion pressure.

Postoperative:
> Management of pain – NSAIDs and paracetamol (which may be given preoperatively) usually sufficient.
> Some children resist taking oral medication, especially if there is oral pain following dental work.
> Management of nausea and swelling (dexamethasone plus ondansetron).
> Day-case procedure so antiemesis and analgesia must be sufficiently well managed to facilitate early postoperative eating and drinking and then discharge.
> Risk of laryngospasm in recovery due to blood in airway.

c) Give the specific problems of providing anaesthesia for children with ASD and outline possible solutions. (7 marks)

Problem	Possible solution
Distress due to unfamiliar hospital setting may make it difficult to perform preoperative assessment on day of admission.	May be necessary to do this in the community, including weight measurement. Quiet, separate waiting area.
Language issues may make it difficult for the child to comprehend what is to happen.	Use of appropriate visual information, play specialist or psychologist to enhance comprehension. Information provision in advance.
Lack of familiarity with environment, out of routine, may cause distress.	Maximise the familiarity of the environment, minimise the disruption to routine by allowing e.g. own clothes, familiar objects, parent/carer, minimise waiting time. Give clear timetable of day ahead and stick to it.
Preoperative starvation may be poorly tolerated as it breaks routine.	First on list, clear fluids until one hour before surgery.
May dislike physical contact.	Keep to a minimum, warn first.
Topical local anaesthetic may not be tolerated.	Consider inhalational induction, consider staffing requirements for this.
Lack of cooperation.	Discussion regarding physical restraint in advance. Consideration of cancelling and bringing back after premedication.
Dysphoric response to midazolam is possible in ASD.	Consider whether premedication is necessary. Consider combining midazolam and ketamine.
Inability of child to communicate likes and dislikes.	Utilise parents' knowledge of child to anticipate problems, communication passport.

References

Adewale L. Anaesthesia for paediatric dentistry. *Contin Educ Anaesth Crit Care Pain*. 2012; 12 (6): 288–294.
Association of Paediatric Anaesthetists of Great Britain and Ireland. APA Consensus Statement on Update Fluid Fasting Guidelines. https://apagbi.org.uk/node/199 [Accessed 30th May 2018].
Short J, Calder A. Anaesthesia for children with special needs, including autistic spectrum disorder. *Contin Educ Anaesth Crit Care Pain*. 2013; 13 (4): 107–112.

You are called to the emergency department to see a 2-year-old child who presents with a four-hour history of high temperature and drowsiness. On examination, there is prolonged capillary refill time and a non-blanching rash. A presumptive diagnosis of meningococcal septicaemia is made.

a) What are the normal weight, pulse rate, mean arterial blood pressure and capillary refill time for a child of this age? (4 marks)

b) Define appropriate resuscitation goals for this child (2 marks) and outline the management in the first 15 minutes after presentation. (7 marks)

c) After 15 minutes, the child remains shocked and is unresponsive to fluid. What is the most likely pathophysiological derangement in this child's circulation (2 marks) and what are the important further treatment options? (5 marks)

September 2015

Chairman's Report

56.9% pass rate.

The pass rate for this question was the second highest in the paper, but the examiners still felt that it was not particularly well answered. Many candidates lost marks because they wrote similar answers for parts (b) and (c), despite the fact that in part (c), they were asked to comment on what they would do if the measures used in (b) were not successful in resuscitating the child. Incorrect dosages of drugs, particularly antibiotics, were often quoted.

a) What are the normal weight, pulse rate, mean arterial blood pressure and capillary refill time for a child of this age? (4 marks)

It is difficult to give a definitive answer as there is such a variety of ranges and calculations in use. I would hope that the College would recognise a range of values. Also, average mean arterial blood pressure is very rarely quoted for children in the literature.

Weight	12–17 kg.	Traditionally, 2 (age in years + 4), but as this tends to underestimate weight, a newer calculation is 3 (age in years) + 7
Pulse rate	95–140 bpm.	
Mean arterial blood pressure	58 mm Hg.	(1.5 × age in years) + 55.
Capillary refill time	Less than two seconds.	

b) Define appropriate resuscitation goals for this child (2 marks) and outline the management in the first 15 minutes after presentation. (7 marks)

Resuscitation goals:
> Capillary refill time less than 2 seconds.
> Mean arterial pressure 58 mm Hg.
> Normal pulses with no differential between central and peripheral.
> Warm extremities.
> Urine output greater than 1 ml/kg/h.
> Normal mental status.

Management in the first 15 minutes after presentation:

The answer for this is as for part (b) of the September 2012 question, up to giving a second bolus of fluid and continuing with assessment of D and E whilst awaiting response to resuscitation efforts.

c) After 15 minutes, the child remains shocked and is unresponsive to fluid. What is the most likely pathophysiological derangement in this child's circulation (2 marks) and what are the important further treatment options? (5 marks)

The child has developed septic shock: in addition to the organ dysfunction occurring as a result of the child's physiological response to infection, shock has developed due to circulatory, cellular and metabolic dysfunction. Consequences include vasodilatation, activation of inflammatory and coagulation cascades, capillary leak and dysfunctional oxygen utilisation at cellular level.

The answer to the second part of this question is the management of the child from the third fluid bolus onwards, when intubation is recommended, as per the September 2012 answer.

References

Advanced Life Support Group. *Advanced Paediatric Life Support: A Practical Approach to Emergencies.* 6th Edition. Chichester, UK: Wiley Blackwell; 2016.

Dellinger R, Levy M, Rhodes A et al. Surviving Sepsis Campaign: International guidelines for management of severe sepsis and septic shock: 2012. *Crit Care Med.* 2013; 41: 580–637.

Haque I, Zaritsky A. Analysis of the evidence for the lower limit of systolic and mean arterial pressure in children. *Ped Crit Care Med.* 2007; 8 (2): 138–144.

Luscombe M, Owens B. Weight estimation in resuscitation: is the current formula still valid? *Arch Dis Child.* 2007; 92: 412–415.

You have anaesthetised a 5-year-old boy for manipulation of a forearm fracture. During the operation, you notice that he has multiple bruises on his upper arms and body that you think may indicate child abuse.

a) Which other types of physical injury should raise concerns of abuse in a child of this age? (6 marks)

b) What timely actions must be taken as a result of your concerns? (7 marks)

c) List parental factors (5 marks) and features of a child's past medical history (2 marks) that are known to increase the risk of child abuse.

March 2016

Chairman's Report

44.7% pass rate.

This is an important topic which is relevant to the practice of paediatric anaesthesia and forms part of mandatory training for all doctors. The question was not particularly well answered, with many candidates appearing not to have knowledge of the presenting signs and symptoms of child abuse. Candidates assumed that the parents were harming their child so missed important steps such as informing the senior paediatrician before contacting social services. The general lack of knowledge on this subject was reflected in the poor pass rate.

In March 2007, an intercollegiate document involving the RCoA was issued that detailed the manner in which anaesthetists may encounter child abuse and what actions should be taken in the event. Child abuse was then the focus of a question in the final written paper in October 2008. The document was updated and the new version issued in July 2014. 20 months later, this question appears. It really is important to keep an eye on the College website and be aware of topical publications and issues.

a) Which other types of physical injury should raise concerns of abuse in a child of this age? (6 marks)

> Unusual or excessive bruising.
> Cigarette burns, other thermal injury.
> Bite marks.
> Injuries in inaccessible places: neck, ear, feet, buttocks.
> Unexplained intra-oral injury.
> Ano-genital trauma or unusual ano-genital appearance.
> Trauma without adequate history, delayed presentation, inconsistent explanations, e.g. intra-abdominal, rib fractures.

b) What timely actions must be taken as a result of your concerns? (7 marks)

> Act in the best interests of the child.
> Respect child's right to confidentiality, although this is not always possible in cases concerning actual or possible abuse.
> Check hospital notes for known safeguarding issues, details regarding other members of family.
> Inform:
  • Anaesthetic consultant on call.
  • Child's paediatrician, on-call paediatric consultant if out of hours, or Safeguarding Team within hours.
  • Theatre team: surgeon, senior scrub, ODP.
> Ask the paediatrician to look at injuries as long as this does not excessively prolong anaesthesia – brief visual assessment only.
> Full documentation of findings and actions.
> Consultant paediatrician and anaesthetist to discuss the issue with parents and child after surgery (except in unusual circumstances where this may increase risk to child).
  • If there is a fully reasonable explanation, then no further action is taken.
  • If there is continued concern, then the consultant paediatrician should refer to social care, possibly involve police if there is risk to other children at home, take full history from child and carer and consider need for forensic examination, and decide whether it is appropriate for the child to go home.

c) List parental factors (5 marks) and features of a child's past medical history (2 marks) that are known to increase the risk of child abuse.

Parent-related factors:
> Step parents.
> Teenage parents.
> Substance abuse.
> Parent abused as a child.
> Disabled parent.
> Mental health problems.
> Single parent.
> Domestic violence.
> Social isolation.
> Unemployment.
> Poverty.

Child-related factors:
> Chronic physical or mental disability or illness.
> Prematurity or low birth weight.
> Unplanned or unwanted child.

References

National institute for Health and Care Excellence. Child maltreatment: when to suspect maltreatment in under 18s. Clinical guideline [CG89]. 2009.

Royal College of Anaesthetists, Association of Anaesthetists of Great Britain and Ireland, Association of Paediatric Anaesthetists of Great Britain and Ireland, Royal College of Paediatrics and Child Health. Child Protection and the Anaesthetist Safeguarding Children in the Operating Theatre. July 2014.

A 5-year-old child with Down's syndrome (trisomy 21) is scheduled for adenotonsillectomy.

a) List the cardiovascular (2 marks), airway/respiratory (5 marks) and neurological (3 marks) problems that are associated with this syndrome in children and are of relevance to the anaesthetist.

b) What are the potential problems during induction of anaesthesia and initial airway management in this patient? (6 marks)

c) What are the possible specific difficulties in the postoperative management of this child? (4 marks)

September 2016

Chairman's Report

62.1% pass rate.

Knowledge of this subject appeared to be good and the question was generally well answered. However, some candidates lost marks because they did not go into enough detail regarding airway difficulties. Simply stating 'difficult airway' was not sufficient as this does not describe the specific difficulties in this case. These could be divided into those related to the presence of enlarged adenoids and tonsils and those related to a child with Down's syndrome. Candidates who scored well mentioned the possibility of airway obstruction after induction of anaesthesia, the need for airway adjuncts, possible subglottic stenosis and/or atlanto-axial instability, amongst other things.

Part (a) is exactly as it was in the question concerning Down's syndrome in September 2011, although the weighting of the scores has changed slightly. The answers to parts (b) and (c) are all present in the answer to the September 2011 question, just in a slightly different format.

b) What are the potential problems during induction of anaesthesia and initial airway management in this patient? (6 marks)

Communication difficulties:

> It may be more challenging to establish good communication and rapport with this child. Parents, carer and/or play specialist may be required to assist.

Airway management:

> Increased risk of gastro-oesophageal reflux may dictate plan for airway management: intubation, possibly rapid sequence intubation.
> Increased likelihood of difficulty with mask ventilation due to craniofacial changes associated with Down's syndrome (as detailed above) and with adenotonsillar hypertrophy. May need oropharyngeal airway.
> Possibility of difficulty intubating due to subglottic stenosis – smaller tube sizes should be available.
> Neck extension may be limited by Klippel-Feil or by the presence of atlanto-axial instability – videolaryngoscopy or asleep fibreoptic intubation may be indicated.

A 12-week-old male baby presents for a unilateral inguinal hernia repair. He was born at 30 weeks gestation (30/40).

a) What are the specific perioperative concerns in this baby? (11 marks)

b) What are the options for anaesthesia? (4 marks)

c) Discuss the advantages and disadvantages of general anaesthesia for this baby. (5 marks)

March 2017

Chairman's Report

28.0% pass rate.

Knowledge of the anaesthetic issues surrounding prematurity and the very young is important. In part (a), candidates who organized their answer by systems tended to score well. Candidates who scored poorly tended to give generic answers about physiological problems in any paediatric patient rather than specific perioperative problems for this particular ex-premature neonate.

a) What are the specific perioperative concerns in this baby? (11 marks)

Apart from the fact that it was very preterm, you have no other information about the baby's condition or when it left the neonatal intensive care unit. Therefore, write down all of the issues that may affect a baby born this early. Keep asking yourself whether it is an issue that affects premature babies or a generic issue affecting all babies.

This baby was born at a stage when organogenesis was ongoing and is therefore at risk of immature physiology, the consequences of whatever treatment it had due to its prematurity and also issues associated with low birth weight. An assessment must be made as to whether it is appropriate to proceed with elective surgery at this stage or whether to defer until a later stage.

Airway:
> Complications of previous prolonged intubation: tracheomalacia or subglottic stenosis. Risk of difficult intubation or need for smaller tube diameter.

Respiratory:
> Bronchopulmonary dysplasia: alveoli and surfactant development still ongoing at the time of this baby's birth and he may therefore have required ventilatory support. More than four weeks ventilation/oxygen treatment results in risk of bronchopulmonary dysplasia due to volutrauma, barotrauma, oxygen toxicity. Outcome: reduced lung compliance, increased oxygen requirement, obstructive lung disease with a reactive component.
> Apnoeas: risk of obstructive, central and mixed apnoeas (cessation of breathing of more than 20 seconds or loss of effective breathing with bradycardia). Central apnoeas occur due to reduced chemoreceptor sensitivity, reduced central response to hypoxaemia and hypercapnia, and change in the response to hypoxaemia (apnoea only instead of the normal hyperventilation followed by apnoea). Perioperative factors such as anaesthetic agents, opioids and hypoxia increase the risk, as do stress and sepsis. Risk persists until 60 weeks post-conception. Common in the first 12 hours postoperatively, may continue up to 72 hours postoperatively. Necessitates overnight admission for observation.
> Respiratory fatigue: young babies can only increase minute ventilation by increasing respiratory rate. Hypoglycaemia and reduced proportion of type I muscle fibres in diaphragm make fatigue more likely.

Cardiovascular:
> Increased risk of all cardiac defects and delayed closure of ductus arteriosus.
> Difficulty cannulating due to multiple previous cannulations.

Neurological:
> Premature babies are at significant risk of intraventricular haemorrhage – this baby may suffer the consequences of this such as cerebral palsy or hydrocephalus.

Endocrine:
> Reduced glycogen stores in conjunction with preoperative starvation may result in hypoglycaemia. Excessive starvation must be avoided and consideration given to glucose supplementation.

Pharmacology:
> Altered liver and renal handling of drugs due to immaturity.

Gastrointestinal:
> Reflux is common due to underdevelopment of gastro-oesophageal sphincter, thus increasing the risk of aspiration and apnoeas.

Haematological:
> Risk of anaemia related to previous frequent blood sampling.

Metabolic:
> All babies have high risk of hypothermia, but an ex-premature baby is at even greater risk due to paucity of subcutaneous fat, immature thermogenesis due to reduced brown fat, and increased surface-area-to-volume ratio. The consequences may be greater, too, with risk of apnoeas and hypoglycaemia.

b) What are the options for anaesthesia? (4 marks)

General anaesthesia:
> Rapid sequence induction (rarely indicated) or standard intubation. Gas induction may offer better control and reduced risk of desaturation over intravenous induction. Positive pressure ventilation to reduce fatigue.
> Caudal analgesia or local infiltration by surgeons may reduce opioid requirements, thus reducing the risks of apnoeas and unpredictable effects due to immaturity of liver and kidneys.

Spinal anaesthesia:
> Caudal analgesia in addition may increase postoperative analgesia.
> Ideally, sedatives should be avoided.

Caudal anaesthesia:
> Rarely used alone, short duration of anaesthesia.

Aim to use short-acting drugs wherever possible, especially opioids. Consider liver and kidney immaturity when selecting drugs.

c) Discuss the advantages and disadvantages of general anaesthesia for this baby. (5 marks)

Advantages:
> Regional anaesthesia may produce suboptimal operating conditions in moving baby.
> Use of sedatives to improve operating conditions when using regional anaesthesia may increase the risk of postoperative apnoeas in an ex-premature baby.

Disadvantages:
> Possible difficult airway due to previous intubations.
> Increased risk of periods of desaturation such as at induction, with consequent risks of hypoxaemia.
> Ideally, general anaesthesia to be avoided in an oxygen-dependent baby with severe lung disease.
> General anaesthesia does not have the inherent postoperative analgesic effects of a regional technique.
> Some evidence suggests increased risk of postoperative apnoeas after general anaesthesia.
> Excessive positive pressure ventilation may result in exacerbation of right-to-left shunt or further barotrauma in already damaged lungs.

Reference
Peiris K, Fell D. The prematurely born infant and anaesthesia. *Contin Educ Anaesth Crit Care Pain*. 2009; 9 (3): 73–77.

A 5-year-old boy presents for a myringotomy and grommet insertion as a day case. During your preoperative assessment, you notice that he has a nasal discharge.

a) List the features in the history (5 marks) and examination (6 marks) that would potentially cause an increased risk of airway complications.

b) Why would it be inappropriate to cancel the operation? (6 marks)

c) What social factors would prevent this child being treated as a day case? (3 marks)

September 2017

Chairman's Report

74% pass rate.

This question had also been used before and was thought to be moderately difficult. It had the highest correlation with overall performance. Candidates generally did better on this occasion then when it was last used, so it seems that knowledge of this important and frequently seen scenario has improved.

This is almost identical to the paediatric question from March 2014. Basing revision on past questions makes sense because it means that you will revise topics that the College considers important. The paediatric anaesthesia curriculum is not vast; it is inevitable that there will be themes that repeat.

18. PAIN MEDICINE

A 68-year-old woman attends the Pain Management Clinic with a two-year history of pain in her back and legs.

a) Describe the pharmacological (30%) and other treatment options (40%), with examples, available for this lady.

b) What factors would alert you to the need for further investigation or referral? (30%)

September 2011

Back pain is a common reason for attendance at pain clinics, and you should have a clear idea of what the underlying causes are, how to distinguish them, and how they can be managed. Part (a) of this question focuses on the management of musculoskeletal and radicular pain, whilst part (b) wants to ensure you know the features of serious spinal pathology, the 'red flags,' that should prompt further investigation.

There are three main causes of back pain:
> *Musculoskeletal: 95% (sacroiliac joint, facet joint, discogenic pain, ligamental injury, myofascial pain).*

>> *Features: dull, mechanical ache, lumbosacral and buttocks. Referred pain to legs is common but not below knee. Those aged 20–55 years most affected.*
> *Nerve root (radicular) pain: 4% (due to disc herniation, spinal stenosis and epidural adhesions).*

>> *Features: well localised, sharp electric shock pain, typically radiating below the knee. Exacerbated by coughing, straining, sneezing. Straight leg raise or femoral stretch test will reveal nerve root irritation. Neurological examination may show sensory, motor and reflex abnormalities.*
> *Serious spinal pathology: 1% (due to trauma, malignancy, inflammatory conditions, infection).*

a) Describe the pharmacological (30%) and other treatment options (40%), with examples, available for this lady.

Note that NICE guidance from 2016 does not support TENS or acupuncture for treatment of low back pain.

Pharmacological options:
> Paracetamol, but not to be used alone.
> NSAIDs – assess risks and benefits, consider need for gastric protection, lowest dose for shortest duration possible.
> Weak opioid for acute management if NSAIDs not tolerated, contraindicated or ineffective. Not to be used long-term.
> Amitriptyline, duloxetine, gabapentin or pregabalin only if neuropathic component.

Other treatment options:
> Self-management. Reassurance, information, advice to continue usual activities and exercise.
> Exercise, including group NHS classes.
> Manual therapy as part of an overall management package.

> Psychological therapy. Cognitive behavioural therapy to be used within a pain management programme.
> Pain management programme (PMP): all interventions combined into one package of care; education, exercise, relaxation techniques, goal setting, pacing, psychological therapy.
> Interventional treatments such as caudal epidural for early treatment of nerve root pain, facet joint injections or radiofrequency lesioning of lumbar medial branch.
> Spinal cord stimulation for radicular pain.
> Surgery: e.g. laminectomy for spinal stenosis or discectomy for nerve root pain.

b) What factors would alert you to the need for further investigation or referral? (30%)

This is asking you for the factors that might indicate to you that the patient has serious spinal pathology, the 'red flags.' If you can remember the possible causes of serious spinal pathology, then you will be able to list the symptoms and signs that would raise your suspicions.

> Her age (presentation under 20 or over 55 years old).
> History of significant trauma.
> Constant progressive thoracic pain.
> Past history of cancer, steroid therapy, intravenous drug abuse or HIV infection.
> Unexplained weight loss.
> Systemically unwell.
> Cauda equina syndrome (saddle anaesthesia, gait/sphincter disturbance).
> Structural deformity.
> Marked restriction of lumbar flexion.
> Non-mechanical pain.

References

Jackson M, Simpson K. Chronic back pain. *Contin Educ Anaesth Crit Care Pain*. 2006; 6 (4): 152–155.

National Institute for Health and Care Excellence. Neuropathic pain in adults: pharmacological management in non-specialist settings CG173. November 2013, updated February 2017.

National Institute for Health and Care Excellence. Low back pain and sciatica in over 16s: assessment and management NG59. November 2016.

a) Describe the anatomy of the coeliac plexus. (35%)

b) What are the indications for coeliac plexus block? (15%)

c) List the anatomical approaches used for coeliac plexus block. (10%)

d) Which specific complications are associated with coeliac plexus block? (40%)

March 2013

Chairman's Report

36.4% pass rate.

This question was the best discriminator of the paper and proved to be difficult. The anatomy of the coeliac plexus was almost universally answered poorly and one candidate misread the question and wrote an exposition on the cervical plexus! For two marks, any of the following approaches to the coeliac plexus were acceptable: Anterior (retro or transcrural), posterior, trans-aortic, transdiscal and paramedian. There were twelve specific complications of coeliac plexus block in the model answer and only eight were required for full marks.

Specific examples included: Retroperitoneal bleeding due to aorta or inferior vena cava injury by the needle: Paraplegia from injecting phenol into spinal cord blood supply; CNS damage; Intravascular injection into great vessels (should be prevented by checking the needle position with radio-opaque dye).

Generic answers such as local anaesthetic toxicity, painful injection, infection and bleeding were not accepted.

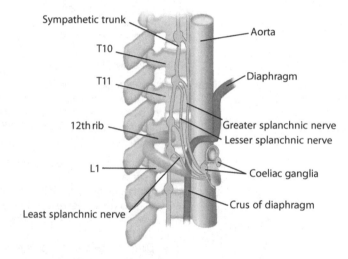

Coeliac plexus anatomy

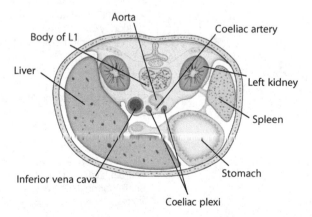

Cross-section of the coeliac plexi

a) Describe the anatomy of the coeliac plexus. (35%)

The coeliac plexus is a bilateral structure, made up of preganglionic sympathetic fibres from greater splanchnic (T5–10), lesser splanchnic (T10–11) and least splanchnic (T11–12) nerves. The nerves coalesce anteriorly to the body of T12 before entering the abdomen posterior to the diaphragmatic crura.

It is:
> Retroperitoneal.
> Anterolateral to the body of L1 bilaterally.
> Anterior to the aorta and crura of diaphragm.
> Either side of the origin of the coeliac artery.
> Medial to the inferior vena cava.
> Posterior to the stomach and pancreas

b) What are the indications for coeliac plexus block? (15%)

The coeliac plexus supplies the liver, gall bladder, spleen, stomach, pancreas, kidneys, adrenals, small intestine and large intestine proximal to splenic flexure. Any cause of intractable pain involving these organs can be managed with coeliac plexus block.

> Pancreatic cancer pain.
> Stomach cancer pain.
> Chronic pancreatitis pain.
> In theory, coeliac plexus block can be used for upper abdominal surgery but is not as there are superior alternatives without the associated risks.

c) List the anatomical approaches used for coeliac plexus block. (10%)

They haven't asked for a description of any of the approaches, no doubt to the utter relief of the candidates of the day, so make sure you stick to a list.

> Posterior approach.
> Anterior (retro or transcrural).
> Trans-aortic.
> Transdiscal.
> Paramedian.

d) Which specific complications are associated with coeliac plexus block? (40%)

You will not get any marks for listing 'bleeding' and 'nerve damage' as complications of blocks – you have got to specify which vessel and which nerves are at risk. Only 8 of the College's list of 12 complications were required for full marks for this section. Therefore, 4 would have been enough to be on target for half marks overall, a pass for a difficult question.

> Retroperitoneal bleeding due to aorta or inferior vena cava injury by the needle.
> Intravascular injection into great vessels (should be prevented by checking the needle position with radio-opaque dye).
> Paraplegia secondary to phenol injection into arterial supply of spinal cord.
> Direct spinal cord or nerve root damage.
> Retrocrural spread of phenol, causing spinal nerve root damage.
> Intrathecal or epidural injection.
> Visceral puncture, damage, abscess or cyst formation (stomach or kidney).
> Injection into psoas muscle with risk of cyst or abscess formation.
> Pneumothorax.
> Chylothorax.
> Thrombosis.
> Sexual dysfunction (phenol spread along sympathetic chain).
> Leg warmth.
> Hypotension (dilatation of upper abdominal vessels).

References

Menon R, Swanepoel A. Sympathetic blocks. *Contin Educ Anaesth Crit Care Pain*. 2010; 10 (3): 88–92.

Scott-Warren J, Bhaskar A. Cancer pain management: Part II: Interventional techniques. *Contin Educ Anaesth Crit Care Pain*. 2015; 15 (2): 68–72.

a) What are the complications of continuous epidural analgesia (CEA) in the ward setting? (40%)

b) How should patients be monitored throughout the period of CEA? (25%)

c) Outline the safety features that relate to equipment used for CEA. (35%)

September 2013

Chairman's Report

70.4% pass rate.

The question was based on the Best Practice in the management of epidural analgesia in the hospital setting (November 2010), published by the Faculty of Pain Medicine of the Royal College of Anaesthetists. Section (a) was divided into: complications of local anaesthetic, complications of opioids, human and organization factors (inadequate analgesia; drug administration errors; post dural puncture headache) and siting issues (infection). The safety features relating to equipment included both the pump and giving set. Some candidates focused on the giving set only. The pump should be configured specifically for epidural infusion and should be standardised as per MRHA, have alarms and be tamperproof.

This is an example of a question based entirely on a recent College publication. However, I think that any anaesthetist who regularly cares for patients with epidurals will be able to answer this question well, and this is reflected by the good pass rate.

a) What are the complications of continuous epidural analgesia (CEA) in the ward setting? (40%)

A systematic approach helps you think of all the complications more easily. If you don't divide up the complications under the same headings as the College, you wouldn't lose points as long as you still produce a coherent and comprehensive answer.

Opioid related:
> Pruritis.
> Respiratory depression or arrest.

Local anaesthetic related:
> High block with cardiovascular collapse or respiratory arrest.
> Hypotension.
> Urinary retention.
> Motor block.
> Pressure sores.
> Local anaesthetic toxicity.

Catheter related:
> Unexpected development of high block (e.g. catheter migration, intrathecal injection).
> Postdural puncture headache and subdural haematoma.
> Superficial infection around insertion site.
> Epidural haematoma or abscess.
> Meningitis.
> Spinal cord ischaemia.
> Permanent harm, e.g. paraplegia, nerve injury.

Human factors and organisational issues:
> Drug administration errors (especially wrong route).
> Inadequate analgesia.

b) How should patients be monitored throughout the period of CEA? (25%)

Before you launch into listing the observations detailed on your hospital's epidural charts, think about the organisational aspects of the manner in which patients with epidurals should be monitored.

> Trained nursing staff (able to deal with complications), acute pain team, 24-hour anaesthetic service, handover of ongoing CEAs, ongoing duty of care by the anaesthetist who sited the epidural (or the consultant under whose supervision they were working).

> Ward must be adequately staffed, patient close to nurses' station.
> Protocols with action plan in event of abnormal observations.
> More frequent physiological observations in first 12 hours and after top-ups/changes in infusion rate/periods of cardiovascular or respiratory instability.
> Heart rate.
> Blood pressure.
> Respiratory rate.
> Sedation score.
> Temperature.
> Pain score.
> Motor and sensory block.
> Pressure areas.
> Venous cannula patency.
> Epidural site.
> Pump: prescription and volume given.

c) Outline the safety features that relate to equipment used for CEA. (35%)

The Chairman's Report does not mention the epidural kit itself. I think that this is equipment used for CEA and so would have included it in my answer if I had sat this exam.

Equipment standardised throughout Trust, staff training.

NPSA 2009: recommendation that equipment for neuraxial and regional anaesthesia and analgesia techniques should not connect with intravenous Luer connectors or intravenous infusion spikes. Not yet achieved nationwide.

Pumps:
> Configured for epidural analgesia only in millilitres.
> Labelled as such.
> Preset limits for maximum infusion rate and bolus size.
> Lock-out time.
> Alarms (air, end of infusion, high pressure).
> Locked box (but able to see fluid without unlocking).
> Lock/code required for programming/bolus administration.
> Documented maintenance programme.

Epidural infusion system:
> Closed, no injection ports.
> Antibacterial filter.
> Labelled as epidural with yellow label.
> Yellow stripe to infusion system.
> Anti-siphon valve

Epidural kit:
> Needle: standardised, markings, Huber tip with blunt leading edge, stylet, wings.
> Syringe: low resistance.
> Connector: securely fastening to minimise risk of breaches in circuit.
> Catheter: blue tip, multiple fenestrations, blunt tip, standardised markings.

Reference

Faculty of Pain Medicine of the Royal College of Anaesthetists. *Best Practice in the Management of Epidural Analgesia in the Hospital Setting*. London: The Royal College of Anaesthetists; 2010.

A 68-year-old patient attends the Pain Management Clinic with a history of intractable low back pain.

a) What symptoms and signs would alert you to the need for urgent investigation and referral? (50%)

b) List recommended treatment options that may be considered (with examples) if a magnetic resonance imaging (MRI) scan has excluded significant pathology. (50%)

March 2014

Chairman's Report

68.9% pass rate.

Generally well answered. Most candidates understood the importance of 'red flags' in this clinical scenario. Some candidates ignored the result of the MRI scan and gave treatment options which referred to abnormal imaging (e.g. surgical approaches) and consequently detracted from their score. Reference to psychological and alternate/complementary therapies contributed to a high scoring answer.

a) What symptoms and signs would alert you to the need for urgent investigation and referral? (50%)

This question is very similar to that of March 2011, and section (a) is once again asking for the 'red flags,' just in a slightly different way.

b) List recommended treatment options that may be considered (with examples) if a magnetic resonance imaging (MRI) scan has excluded significant pathology. (50%)

Again, this is asking for the pharmacological and other treatment options, but with slightly different wording. This time, you are told that the MRI excludes significant pathology, so there will be no possibility that surgery will be a treatment option.

You are called to the emergency department to assess a 63-year-old man with known chronic respiratory disease. He has sustained unilateral fractures to his 9th, 10th and 11th ribs but has no other injuries. Paracetamol and codeine phosphate have not provided adequate pain relief.

a) What respiratory problems could result from inadequate pain relief in this patient? (5 marks)

b) How can the effectiveness of his pain relief be assessed? (8 marks)

c) What other methods are available to improve management of this patient's pain? (7 marks)

September 2014

Chairman's Report

43.7% pass rate.

Examiners expressed the view at SSD that this question was too easy so it is likely that the poor pass rate reflects the limited exposure of candidates to the clinical scenario. Many candidates were unable to suggest how the effectiveness of analgesic interventions could be assessed, and few offered regional techniques in their answer. It was surprising that a number suggested codeine/paracetamol compounds in their answer despite the question indicating that these agents had been unhelpful. This emphasises the need to read the question thoroughly.

This is a very straightforward question that merely requires a logical approach to a common pain problem. You will notice that I have done what the Chairman's Report said not to: I have included prescription of paracetamol and codeine in my answer because their question did not specify whether it is being given regularly or at what dose. In real life, I would check both of these things before working further along my plan of optimising analgesia.

a) What respiratory problems could result from inadequate pain relief in this patient? (5 marks)

> Respiratory depression due to pain.
> Basal atelectasis.
> V/Q mismatch.
> Poor oxygenation.
> Respiratory failure.
> Failure of secretion clearance.
> Pneumonia.

b) How can the effectiveness of his pain relief be assessed? (8 marks)

> Pain scores, either VAS (visual analogue scores) or matching face to pain.
> Intervals between assessment should be as short as 15 minutes until good pain control has been achieved and then less frequently.
> Assess pain at rest, on movement, deep breathing, coughing, on incentive spirometry, and ability to comply with respiratory physiotherapy.
> Other physiological parameters: heart rate, respiratory rate, blood pressure.
> Frequency of use of breakthrough pain medication.
> Involvement of pain team to facilitate regular assessment.

c) What other methods are available to improve management of this patient's pain? (7 marks)

Oral analgesia:
> Ensure paracetamol and codeine are administered regularly with the maximum appropriate codeine dose for the patient.
> Consider NSAIDs: must actively seek contraindications, limit duration and consider gastrointestinal protection.
> If codeine insufficient, change to a stronger opioid, e.g. oral morphine sulfate solution as required, and then to modified release oral morphine once total daily dose required is known.

Intravenous analgesia:
> PCA, either morphine or fentanyl. However, if the patient already has compromised respiratory function, beware of causing further deterioration.

Topical analgesia:
> Local anaesthesia patches.

Regional analgesia:
> Thoracic epidural: offers excellent analgesia without causing respiratory depression. However, might be limited by hypotensive effect and can usually only be managed in specific wards.
> Thoracic paravertebral block or catheter: requires anaesthetist skilled in such techniques. Catheter offers longer-lasting solution to pain. Avoids the hypotensive effect of epidural.
> Intercostal block or catheter: as above.
> Serratus anterior block or catheter: as above.

Surgical intervention:
> Operative fixation.

Reference

May L, Hillermann C, Patil S. Rib fracture management. *BJA Educ*. 2016; 16 (1): 26–32.

You are called to see a 25-year-old man who suffered a traumatic below knee amputation 24 hours ago. He is using patient controlled analgesia (PCA) with intravenous morphine and was comfortable until two hours ago, when he started to experience severe pain.

a) Why might his pain control have become inadequate? (5 marks)

b) How would you re-establish optimal pain control? (6 marks)

c) Which factors would suggest that this patient has phantom limb pain (PLP)? (3 marks)

d) What further pharmacological options are available for managing PLP? (6 marks)

March 2015

Chairman's Report

53.6% pass rate; 10.0% of candidates received a poor fail.

A strongly discriminatory question; weak candidates simply wrote 'neuropathic pain' as the answer and did not describe what they meant by the term. The specifics of managing phantom limb pain were not addressed by failing candidates in section (d).

Phantom limb pain occurs as a result of nerve damage, resulting in changes to the nervous system at multiple locations, causing dysfunctional transmission of sensory information and abnormal pain perception.

Peripheral nerves:
> *Upregulation of voltage gated sodium channels – spontaneous firing of damaged nerves peripherally or in dorsal root ganglion (DRG).*
> *Neuroma development in damaged nerves that are sensitive to chemical or mechanical stimuli.*
> *Neural injury due to amputation causes release of pro-inflammatory mediators that lower the activation thresholds of nociceptors.*

Spinal cord:
> *Aβ fibres from Rexed's laminae III and IV sprout into Rexed's laminae I and II due to the absence of input from C fibres from amputated limb – therefore, touch and pressure may be interpreted as pain. NMDA receptors are thought to have a critical role in this phenotypic change.*
> *Sympathetic nerves sprout into the dorsal root ganglion, again stimulating pain pathways.*

Somatosensory cortex:
> *Errors in cortical remapping of the homunculus – over-amplification of pain experience, touch being interpreted as pain, pain being felt when other structures touched.*

a) Why might his pain control have become inadequate? (5 marks)	*Imagine yourself being called to the ward to see this patient – what would your thought processes be? It has not stated where the pain is, so consider other causes.* > Failure of morphine delivery: check syringe full, pump working well, patient using pump well, cannula patent. > Acute pain: failure to manage acute pain due to e.g. development of infection, wound dehiscence, haematoma formation in stump. > Neuropathic pain: development of phantom limb pain. Phantom limb pain occurs as a result of nerve damage, resulting in changes to the nervous system at multiple locations, causing dysfunctional transmission of sensory information and abnormal pain perception. > Other pain source: major trauma victim – check for coexisting injuries.
b) How would you re-establish optimal pain control? (6 marks)	> Assessment of pain, degree of psychological distress and physiological effect. > Intravenous morphine titrated to effect, with oxygen saturations, respiratory rate, heart rate and blood pressure monitoring. > Increase PCA bolus dose and hourly limit if considered safe to do so.

> Multimodal approach: ensure regular paracetamol and NSAIDs, if appropriate. Consider gabapentinoid.
> Consideration of addition of ketamine ivi (up to 15 mg/h) if difficulty re-establishing control.
> Consideration of sciatic and femoral nerve blocks or even epidural if pain very severe and intractable.

c) Which factors would suggest that this patient has phantom limb pain (PLP)? (3 marks)

> Nature of pain: shooting, burning, cramping, aching.
> Location of pain: distal to stump, associated with the missing leg.
> Degree of pain: apparent disproportion between pain experienced and stimulus applied.

d) What further pharmacological options are available for managing PLP? (6 marks)

As per NICE CG173:

> Amitryptilline is first-line treatment, moving on to any of the other three if ineffective/not tolerated.
> Duloxetine.
> Gabapentin.
> Pregabalin.
> Capsaicin cream if oral treatment not tolerated.
> (Tramadol use restricted to acute rescue therapy).

References

National Institute for Health and Care Excellence. Neuropathic pain in adults: pharmacological management in non-specialist settings CG173. November 2013, updated February 2017.

Neil M. Pain after amputation. *BJA Educ*. 2016; 16 (3): 107–112.

a) How should you manage the perioperative opioid requirements of a patient who is having elective surgery and who takes regular opioids for non-malignant pain? (8 marks)

b) Give the conversion factors for oral tramadol, codeine and oxycodone to the equianalgesic oral morphine dose. (3 marks)

c) What are the perioperative implications of an existing spinal cord stimulator? (6 marks)

d) What additional perioperative precautions should be taken if the patient has an intrathecal drug delivery system fitted? (3 marks)

September 2015

Chairman's Report

25.0% pass rate.

It was anticipated that candidates would find this question difficult and this proved to be the case. Some candidates lost marks because they wrote exclusively about the drugs they would use to manage opioid requirements for this patient but did not mention more general measures such as involvement of the pain team. Very few candidates gave any information about management of transdermal pain patches in the perioperative period. There are differing opinions as to whether patches should be continued, particularly in the case of buprenorphine, but candidates were able to gain marks for either opinion provided they showed that they were aware of the potential problems of altered absorption and partial antagonism.

Difficult questions only require 10–11/20 in order to pass. It is interesting to see that the College recognises the varying opinions related to this topic and that marks would have been given for either stance.

a) How should you manage the perioperative opioid requirements of a patient who is having elective surgery and who takes regular opioids for non-malignant pain? (8 marks)

Perioperative = preoperative + intra-operative + immediately postoperative.

Preoperative:
> Ensure the patient's preoperative pain is fully managed. Delay non-urgent surgery if not yet fully optimised. Involve chronic pain team. May include use of non-opioids.
> Establish the reason for the patient's opioid analgesia use. This may have implications for the perioperative period, e.g. positioning limitations.
> Establish drug, dose, duration of use, route of administration.
> Formulate plan for postoperative pain relief depending on the nature of surgery, e.g. degree of pain likely to be involved, whether patient will be able to take medications via oral route, make calculations of equivalence if patient's condition will dictate conversion to intravenous analgesia postoperatively. Need to ensure usual 24-hour dose PLUS extra to manage the pain from surgery.
> Normal doses of oral slow release and immediate release opioids to be taken on day of surgery.

Intraoperative:
> The decision as to whether to continue opioid patches depends on the nature of surgery. For example, it may be appropriate to continue patch with non-opioid analgesics and immediate-release oral morphine for breakthrough if day case surgery with low predicted pain (e.g. minor orthopaedics), whereas if the patient is to have major surgery and need for intravenous morphine is predicted, it would be more appropriate to calculate the equivalent dose of intravenous morphine and include this in the overall predicted 24-hour morphine dose. Furthermore, transdermal absorption perioperatively may not be reliable and is certainly not titratable. Buprenorphine is a partial antagonist so may complicate top-up dosing with morphine. All staff should be made aware of the physical location of the patch (if it is left on) so that it may be removed in the case of narcosis.

> Awareness that larger doses of morphine intraoperatively will be required to achieve the same effect compared with opioid-naïve patients.
> Use of regional techniques, where feasible, to reduce overall opioid requirement.

Postoperative:
> Regular input from inpatient acute pain team.
> Higher bolus doses of morphine in PCA will need to be kept under review regularly as equivalence calculations are approximate: the patient is therefore at risk of both unrelieved pain and narcosis.
> Use pain scores to assess for unrelieved pain.
> Be aware of signs of withdrawal (adrenergic hyperactivity, generalized malaise, abdominal cramps, yawning, and perspiration).
> Be aware of signs of overdosing (sedation, low oxygen saturations, reduced respiratory rate, small pupillary size).
> In view of the risk of either overdosing or withdrawal, it may be appropriate to manage the patient in a higher dependency setting than would normally be dictated by the nature of surgery, or extended recovery may be required.
> If intravenous morphine is used, convert back to oral dosing as soon as is feasible (consider any change in renal function postoperatively and its impact on opioid clearance).

b) Give the conversion factors for oral tramadol, codeine and oxycodone to the equianalgesic oral morphine dose. (3 marks)

There is a useful webpage by the Faculty of Pain Medicine that details the conversion ratios for oral and transdermal opioids.

	Potency ratio with oral morphine	Equivalent does to 10 mg oral morphine
Tramadol	0.15	67 mg
Codeine	0.1	100 mg
Oxycodone	2	5 mg

c) What are the perioperative implications of an existing spinal cord stimulator? (6 marks)

Spinal cord stimulators (SCSs) are used for neuropathic pain, CRPS, and ischaemic pain due to angina or peripheral vascular disease. They achieve their effect through gate control theory and also modulation of release of other neurotransmitters. Leads are surgically placed in the dorsal epidural space (usually requires laminotomy) or percutaneously via Tuohy. During trial period, the pulse generator is left external to the body to check efficacy. The pulse generator can then be placed in a subcutaneous pocket (e.g. abdomen, gluteal) and the leads tunnelled subcutaneously to it.

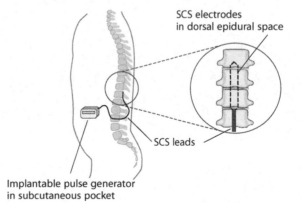

SCS electrodes in dorsal epidural space

SCS leads

Implantable pulse generator in subcutaneous pocket

Spinal cord stimulator

> Preoperatively, make contact with the team who manages the patient to check battery life and any other issues.
> Bipolar diathermy should be used wherever possible. If unipolar absolutely necessary, position the return plate to avoid electrical passage through the SCS.
> Neuraxial block likely to be contraindicated (risk of infection or direct lead damage). If considered essential, consult the pain team who manages the patient's SCS and perform under fluroscopic/ultrasound guidance to avoid the device.

d) What additional perioperative precautions should be taken if the patient has an intrathecal drug delivery system fitted? (3 marks)

Intrathecal drug delivery systems (ITDDs) deliver drugs to the dorsal horn: opioids, local anaesthetic, clonidine or ziconotide for refractory pain or baclofen for spasticity. The pump may be external or fully implanted with reservoir filling performed percutaneously. It may have a fixed rate or be programmable. It may be sited anywhere from thoracic level to the second sacral segment. Risks: dural granuloma formation, leg oedema, infection.

> Spinal anaesthesia by lumbar puncture should be avoided, although intrathecal bolus may be given via the device if it is at a suitable level. However, the system will be primed with the usual drug it delivers, beware delivering a large bolus along with the intended bolus.
> Meticulous aseptic technique when utilising the ITDD to avoid risk of infection.
> Epidural anaesthesia is feasible above or below the ITDD site.
> Opioid dosing as for opioid naïve patient (unless patient also takes oral opioids).
> No diathermy within 30 cm of pump or catheter.

References

Faculty of Pain Medicine. Dose equivalent and changing opioids. http://www.rcoa.ac.uk/faculty-of-pain-medicine/opioids-aware/structured-approach-to-prescribing/dose-equivalents-and-changing-opioids [Accessed 29th June 2017].

Lynch L. Intrathecal drug delivery systems. *Contin Educ Anaesth Crit Care Pain*. 2014; 14 (1): 27–31.

National Institute for Health and Care Excellence. Spinal cord stimulation for chronic pain of neuropathic or ischaemic origin. TA159. October 2008.

Raphael J, Mutagi H, Kapur S. Spinal cord stimulation and its anaesthetic implications. *Contin Educ Anaesth Crit Care Pain*. 2009; 9 (3): 78–81.

a) What are the <u>site of action</u> and the <u>intra and extracellular mechanisms of analgesic effect</u> within the spinal cord following the administration of <u>intrathecal</u> (IT) opioids? (6 marks)

b) List the principal side effects of IT opioids. (7 marks)

c) What factors may increase the risk of postoperative respiratory depression following administration of IT opioids? (7 marks)

March 2016

Chairman's Report

31.7% pass rate.

It was anticipated that candidates would find this question difficult, and this proved to be the case. Intrathecal opioids are used widely in anaesthetic practice, but candidates' knowledge of their use was poor. Advanced sciences are part of the intermediate curriculum so knowledge of applied pharmacology is expected. Some candidates failed to read part (b) of the question and gave the side effects of intravenous opioids or intrathecal local anaesthetic in their answer.

The examiners will often underline parts of the question so as to draw your attention to them. In this paper this was done in part (a) of question 3 about intrathecal opioids – What are the site of action and intra and extracellular mechanisms of analgesic effect within the spinal cord following the administration of intrathecal (IT) opioids? Despite this, some candidates wrote about the mechanism of action of local anaesthetics.

a) What are the <u>site of action</u> and the <u>intra and extracellular mechanisms of analgesic effect</u> within the spinal cord following the administration of <u>intrathecal</u> (IT) opioids? (6 marks)

> MOP (μ), DOP (δ) and KOP (κ) receptors are G protein linked receptors.
> Present in laminae I and II of dorsal horn.
> Found presynaptically on primary afferent C and Aδ fibres and postsynaptically to a lesser extent.
> Presynaptic stimulation causes inactivation of voltage sensitive calcium channels (VSCC) (KOP) or potassium channel opening (DOP and MOP), resulting in hyperpolarisation of the cell and so reduced release of excitatory neurotransmitters glutamate and substance P.
> Postsynaptic activation of opioid receptors causes potassium channel opening and indirect activation of descending inhibitory pathways from brainstem.
> Intrathecal opioids spread caudally (pumped upwards by effect of respiration and pulsation of brain with heartbeat) to cause central effects: stimulation of receptors in nucleus raphe magnus and periaqueductal grey (PAG) results in reduced GABAergic tone on the descending inhibitory pathways, thus allowing them to exert an antinociceptive effect at spinal level.
> Lipid soluble opioids may behave like local anaesthetics due to similar pKa, molecular weight, and partition coefficients.

b) List the principal side effects of IT opioids. (7 marks)

> Nausea and vomiting.
> Respiratory depression.
> Pruritis.
> Sedation.
> Delayed gastric emptying.
> Urinary retention.
> Sweating.

c) What factors may increase the risk of postoperative respiratory depression following administration of IT opioids? (7 marks)

> Hydrophilic opioid use: lipophilic opioids rapidly partition to receptor and non-receptor sites, i.e. epidural fat, myelin, white matter. CSF concentration reduces rapidly, and so the peak in plasma concentration occurs rapidly. Therefore, centrally mediated respiratory depression and that mediated by decreased sensitivity of peripheral chemoreceptors happens early. Hydrophilic opioids maintain a high CSF concentration for longer, allowing more drug to spread caudally with time, and for the peak plasma concentration to occur much later.
> Increasing age.
> Concomitant use of long-acting sedatives.
> Co-existing respiratory disease.
> Positive pressure ventilation.

References

Hindle A. Intrathecal opioids in the management of acute postoperative pain. *Contin Educ Anaesth Crit Care Pain*. 2008; 8 (3): 81–85.

McDonald J, Lambert G. Opioid receptors. *Contin Educ Anaesth Crit Care Pain*. 2005; 5 (1): 22–25.

a) List the signs and symptoms of complex regional pain syndrome (CRPS). (9 marks)

b) What other features, apart from signs and symptoms, are essential for the diagnosis of CRPS? (2 marks)

c) What are the available treatments for CRPS? (9 marks)

September 2016

Chairman's Report

75.2% pass rate.

This question had the greatest predictive value of the 12, which means that candidates who scored highly in this question tended to do well overall. Most marks were gained in part (c), which dealt with treatment options for complex regional pain syndrome. The signs and symptoms of the syndrome are based on the Budapest criteria, and knowledge of these appeared to be patchy.

There was a very similar question in 2008:
  a) *Describe the symptoms and signs of complex regional pain syndrome. (50%)*
  b) *How many symptoms and signs are required to make the diagnosis? (20%)*
  c) *What are the other pre-requisites for the diagnosis? (20%)*

a) List the signs and symptoms of complex regional pain syndrome (CRPS). (9 marks)

The symptoms and signs are virtually identical; I have underlined the differences.

Symptoms	Signs
Sensory: • Hyperaesethesia. • Allodynia.	**Sensory:** • Hyperalgesia (to pinprick). • Allodynia (to light touch or deep somatic pressure or joint. movement).
Vasomotor: • Temperature asymmetry. • Skin colour changes. • Skin colour asymmetry.	**Vasomotor:** • Temperature asymmetry. • Skin colour changes. • Skin colour asymmetry.
Sudomotor/Oedema: • Oedema. • Sweating changes. • Sweating asymmetry.	**Sudomotor/Oedema:** • Oedema. • Sweating changes. • Sweating asymmetry.
Motor/trophic: • Decreased range of motion. • Motor dysfunction (weakness, tremor, dystonia). • Trophic changes (hair, nail, skin).	**Motor/trophic:** • Decreased range of motion. • Motor dysfunction (weakness, tremor, dystonia). • Trophic changes (hair, nail, skin).

b) What other features, apart from signs and symptoms, are essential for the diagnosis of CRPS? (2 marks)

According to the Budapest criteria, there are four criteria that need to be satisfied for diagnosis. The first two are:

> *At least one symptom in at least three of the four symptom categories.*
> *At least one sign in at least two of the four sign categories.*

The remaining two criteria are the answers to section (b) of this question:

> Continuing pain disproportionate to inciting event.
> No other diagnosis that can explain symptoms and signs.

c) What are the available treatments for CRPS? (9 marks)

Prevention is ideal: there is evidence to suggest that good early pain control after injury may reduce incidence of CRPS. Also, a single, prospective, double-blinded study of vitamin C (an oxygen free radical antagonist) after wrist fracture (500 mg od, 50 days) showed reduced incidence of CRPS.

There are four management 'pillars'; start early and aggressively for best outcome:

1. Patient information and education:

   Outcome may be improved by full patient education about what CRPS is and how it is to be managed.

2. Physical and vocational rehabilitation:
   - Physiotherapy: desensitisation, gradual weight bearing, fine motor exercises, aerobic conditioning, TENS, hydrotherapy.
   - Oedema control strategies.
   - Occupational therapy: pacing prioritising planning, vocational support, relaxation techniques.
   - Multidisciplinary pain management.
   - Motor therapy: mirror visual feedback.

3. Pain relief (medication and procedures):
   - Start with amitryptiline, move on if not effective or not tolerated to duloxetine, gabapentin or pregabalin.
   - Tramadol for rescue only, not long term.
   - Consider capsacin cream for localised neuropathic pain or to avoid oral treatments.
   - Bisphosphonates: pamidronate 60 mg single intravenous dose for patients with CRPS less than six months' duration to help maintain bone integrity and function.
   - Spinal cord stimulation: NICE approved for pain persisting greater than six months.

4. Psychological interventions:
   - Cognitive behavioural therapy: ensure that fear does not reduce limb movement and use which can exacerbate disuse atrophy.
   - Possible psychiatric issues and other life stressors should be sought and dealt with.

Reference
Ganty P, Chawla R. Complex regional pain syndrome: recent updates. *Contin Educ Anaesth Crit Care Pain*. 2014; 14 (2): 79–84.

a) Define persistent postoperative pain. (Also known as chronic or persistent post-surgical pain) (3 marks)

b) Which surgical procedures are most commonly associated with persistent postoperative pain? (5 marks)

c) What are the risk factors for development of persistent postoperative pain? (8 marks)

d) What pathophysiological changes occur at spinal cord level during the transition from acute to persistent postoperative pain? (4 marks)

March 2017

Chairman's Report

37.4% pass rate.

This was adjudged to be a hard question and did indeed have a relatively low pass rate. In general, global knowledge of this syndrome was poor, but specifically, the last section on pathophysiology was particularly badly answered.

Hard questions need scores of 10–11/20 in order to pass.

a) Define persistent postoperative pain. (Also known as chronic or persistent post-surgical pain) (3 marks)

Persistent postoperative pain has been defined in different studies in different ways, contributing to difficulty in evaluating its true impact and extent. This is the IASP definition:

> Pain developing after surgical procedure lasting greater than two months.
> Other causes excluded, including preoperative cause.

b) Which surgical procedures are most commonly associated with persistent postoperative pain? (5 marks)

It is difficult to give a definitive list as different studies have assessed different operations, based on differing definitions. These procedures seem to feature most commonly.

> Inguinal hernia repair.
> Coronary artery bypass grafting (CABG).
> Thoracotomy.
> Femoral popliteal bypass.
> Hip and knee arthroplasty.
> Amputation.
> Mastectomy.
> Vasectomy.
> Caesarean section.

c) What are the risk factors for development of persistent postoperative pain? (8 marks)

Preoperative:
> Genetic susceptibility.
> Preoperative pain.
> Psychological factors: anxiety, fear of surgery, tendency to catastrophise.
> Poor social support.
> Age: increasing age reduces risk.
> Possibly female gender.

Intraoperative:
> Procedure that involves significant nerve and tissue damage.
> Specific procedures, see part (b).

Postoperative:
> Poor pain control postoperatively, days of poor control being worse than single episode of severe pain.
> Radiotherapy.
> Neurotoxic chemotherapy.

d) What pathophysiological changes occur at spinal cord level during the transition from acute to persistent postoperative pain? (4 marks)

> Repeated peripheral nerve stimulation or nerve damage causes increased sodium channel expression, resulting in reduced threshold for, or spontaneous, firing of peripheral nerves. This results in increased glutamate release from these first-order neurones at the dorsal horn. Glutamate receptor density of postsynaptic membranes on second-order neurones increases. Transmission occurs in previously inactive second-order neurones, neurones that do not normally transmit pain information, and transmission may persist beyond duration of initial input, 'central sensitisation.'

> Microglia, activated by nerve damage, release substances that further sensitise and excite neurones.

References

International Association for the Study of Pain. Pain Clinical Updates. 2011; 19 (1). https://www.iasp-pain.org/PublicationsNews/PainNewsletterList.aspx?navItemNumber=2059 [Accessed 5th January 2018].

Niraj G, Rowbotham D. Persistent postoperative pain: where are we now? *Br J Anaesth*. 2011; 107 (1): 25–29.

Werner M, Kongsgaard U. Defining persistent post-surgical pain: is an update required? *Br J Anaesth*. 2014; 113 (1): 1–4.

You are called to the emergency department to assess a 63-year-old man with known chronic obstructive pulmonary disease (COPD). He has sustained fractures to his 9th, 10th and 11th ribs but has no other injuries.

Paracetamol and codeine phosphate have not provided adequate pain relief.

a) What are the possible effects on the respiratory system of inadequate pain relief in this patient? (6 marks)

b) How can the effectiveness of his pain relief be monitored? (5 marks)

c) What methods, other than the drugs that have already been given, are available to improve management of this patient's pain? (9 marks)

September 2017

Chairman's Report

74.8% pass rate.

This was an easy question that covered a very common clinical scenario. It is reassuring to see such widespread appreciation of how to monitor and manage a common but potentially serious condition.

This is virtually identical to the question from September 2014. In part (c), I still think that it is important to state that oral analgesia should be given regularly and in appropriate doses.

19. OPHTHALMIC

A 76-year-old man is scheduled for elective cataract surgery under local anaesthesia.

a) Summarise the goals of local anaesthesia (LA) for this procedure. (15%)

b) Which LA techniques may be used for cataract surgery? (20%)

c) List the contraindications to the use of LA as the sole technique for the procedure. (25%)

d) Which details specific to an LA block should be documented in the anaesthetic record? (40%)

September 2013

Chairman's Report

81.5% pass rate.

This question was answered well and was also a good discriminator. The question was based on the document entitled 'Local Anaesthesia for Ophthalmic Surgery: joint guidelines from the Royal College of Anaesthetists and the Royal College of Ophthalmologists' (February 2012).

I wouldn't have liked to find a question on ophthalmology in my final. However, keeping an eye on the RCoA website in the months leading up to the exam should have alerted candidates to the publication of this guideline (a time lag like this is typical). Also, once the panic subsides, it's clear that even if the guideline hasn't been read, the points for parts (a) and (c) are readily achievable through application of common sense. For part (d), writing down the list of points you would record for any block would gain most of the points available – there is very little that is ophthalmic-specific in the answer I have given that comes directly from the guideline. After that, all you have to do is remember the names of some blocks that are specifically used in ophthalmic surgery.

a) Summarise the goals of local anaesthesia (LA) for this procedure. (15%)

> To provide pain-free surgery.
> To facilitate the surgical procedure.
> To minimise the risk of systemic and local complications.
> To reduce the risk of surgical complications.

b) Which LA techniques may be used for cataract surgery? (20%)

> Topical.
> Subconjunctival.
> Sub-Tenon's.
> Peribulbar (extraconal).
> Retrobulbar (intraconal).

c) List the contraindications to the use of LA as the sole technique for the procedure. (25%)

> Patient refusal.
> Allergy to LA.
> Localised sepsis.
> Inability to cooperate due to anxiety, confusion, learning difficulties.
> Inability to lie flat and still due to musculoskeletal, respiratory or cardiac conditions, or significant cough.
> Inability to tolerate ocular manipulation without blepharospasm.
> Grossly abnormal coagulation.

d) Which details specific to an LA block should be documented in the anaesthetic record? (40%)

The name, job role and GMC number of the person performing the block.

The exact technique employed, including the following:

> Asepsis.
> Entry site/s.
> Length and type of needle/cannula.
> Volume and concentration of LA agent and adjuvant.
> Requirement for supplemental LA.
> Use of oculo-compression.
> Use of systemic analgesia or sedation.
> Quality of block.
> Complications.

Monitoring techniques, frequency and recordings should be noted.

Details of any complications, discussions, interventions or advice offered.

References

Anker R, Kaur N. Regional anaesthesia for ophthalmic surgery. *BJA Educ*. 2017; 17 (7): 221–227.

Royal College of Anaesthetists and the Royal College of Ophthalmologists. *Local Anaesthesia for Ophthalmic Surgery: Joint Guidelines from the Royal College of Anaesthetists and the Royal College of Ophthalmologists*. London 2012.

20. PLASTICS AND BURNS

You are asked to assess a 24-year-old male who has been admitted to the emergency department with 30% burns from a house fire.

a) What would lead you to suspect significant inhalational injury? (40%)

b) Which investigations would you use to assess the severity of the inhalational injury and what are the likely findings? (30%)

c) List the indications for early tracheal intubation to secure the airway. (20%)

d) How do burn injuries influence the use of suxamethonium? (10%)

March 2013

Chairman's Report

64.2% pass rate.

Section (a) required details of the history (burn received in enclosed space/delayed escape), general observations, features of upper and lower airway injury and harm from noxious gases.

a) What would lead you to suspect significant inhalational injury? (40%)

History:
> Fire in enclosed space.
> Flames/fumes/smoke/steam/superheated gases and liquids.
> Delayed escape.
> Loss of consciousness at scene due to drugs/alcohol/head injury/hypoxia/carbon monoxide poisoning/cyanide poisoning.

Symptoms and signs:
> Voice change, stridor, hoarseness.
> Cough.
> Burns to face, lips, tongue, pharynx.
> Soot in sputum, nose, mouth.
> Crackles on chest auscultation consistent with pulmonary oedema.
> Respiratory distress, increased respiratory rate, cyanosis, reduced oxygen saturations.
> Reduced level of consciousness, agitation.

b) Which investigations would you use to assess the severity of the inhalational injury and what are the likely findings? (30%)

It hasn't said whether this is to assess the awake or anaesthetised patient, so I have included both to be on the safe side.

> Arterial blood gas analysis: hypoxaemia, raised carboxyhaemaglobin level, lactic acidosis.
> Venous blood gas: decreased arteriovenous oxygen difference (due to inability to utilise oxygen following carbon monoxide and cyanide poisoning).
> Chest X-ray: may be normal, may show atelectasis, pulmonary oedema, ARDS.
> Fibreoptic laryngoscopy (awake patient): laryngeal oedema, mucosal pallor or erythema and ulceration.
> Bronchoscopy (anaesthetised patient): carbonaceous deposits, mucosal pallor or erythema and ulceration.

c) List the indications for early tracheal intubation to secure the airway. (20%)

> Stridor (indicating impending airway obstruction) or actual airway obstruction.
> Respiratory distress causing inadequate gas exchange.
> Hypoxaemia or hypercapnia.
> Full-thickness neck burns.
> Oropharyngeal oedema.
> Low GCS.
> Cardiac arrest.
> Imminent transfer required and risk of deterioration en route.

Facial swelling and oedema are likely to be significant. Use uncut tube to accommodate this swelling and ensure that tube fixation is monitored to ensure that the swelling does not cause the tube to migrate up and out of the airway.

d) How do burn injuries influence the use of suxamethonium? (10%)

Suxamethonium can be used within the first 24 hours following a significant burn (unless the patient is already hyperkalaemic from rhabdomyolysis) and then not for a year. This is due to upregulation of nicotinic receptors with the consequent risk of hyperkalaemia.

There is conflicting evidence about how rapidly nicotinic receptors are upregulated, with evidence to suggest that it is safe to use suxamethonium up to six days post-burns. However, what is stated is generally accepted guidance.

References

Bishop S, Maguire S. Anaesthesia and intensive care for major burns. *Contin Educ Anaesth Crit Care Pain*. 2012; 12 (3): 118–122.

Gill P, Martin R. Smoke inhalation injury. *Contin Educ Anaesth Crit Care Pain*. 2015; 15 (3): 143–148.

You are asked to assess a 24-year-old male who has been admitted to the emergency department with 30% burns from a house fire.

a) What clinical features would lead you to suspect significant inhalational injury? (10 marks)

b) List the indications for early tracheal intubation to secure the airway. (4 marks)

c) Which investigations would you use to assess the severity of the inhalational injury (3 marks) and what are the likely findings? (3 marks)

March 2017

Chairman's Report

57.9% pass rate.

This is an important topic that candidates should be expected to know. Some candidates placed too much emphasis on history when answering part (a), which actually asked for clinical features, and also tended to repeat their answer to part (a) when answering part (b).

a) What clinical features would lead you to suspect significant inhalational injury? (10 marks)

They have tweaked the wording of this question to ask for 'clinical features,' and so candidates have been criticised for including too much detail about the history. However, I would still have answered this question in the same way as I answered part (a) of the last question, as details of the nature of the injury are so useful in assessing overall risk.

b) List the indications for early tracheal intubation to secure the airway. (4 marks)

c) Which investigations would you use to assess the severity of the inhalational injury (3 marks) and what are the likely findings? (3 marks)

Parts (b) and (c) are as for the previous question, although in a different order. If you look at the curriculum, these questions cover a large proportion of what you are required to know about for burns. A question from October 2008 covers much of the rest of the required learning.

21. VASCULAR SURGERY

A 79-year-old patient presents with a leaking abdominal aortic aneurysm. The vascular surgery/radiology team decide to undertake an endovascular aneurysm repair (EVAR) procedure.

a) What are the main preoperative anaesthetic considerations for this procedure? (55%)

b) Describe options for providing anaesthesia for this case and give the advantages/disadvantages of each. (45%)

March 2012

Chairman's Report

54.1% pass rate.

Many candidates missed the point of the question and launched into the detailed anaesthetic management, not mentioning many of the organizational issues. It appeared from the answers that many candidates had not seen elective or emergency EVAR.

It really is easier to describe something that you have seen rather than just read about. Look at the exam syllabus and try to address your blind spots by arranging to go to some specific lists either in your own hospital or elsewhere within your School of Anaesthesia. However, even if you have never seen an EVAR, many of the issues associated with management of a patient with ruptured aneurysm for open repair are relevant here.

a) What are the main preoperative anaesthetic considerations for this procedure? (55%)

Patient assessment:
> Rapid patient assessment. Limited time for investigations due to urgency of surgery.
> Airway and past anaesthetic assessment as standard.
> Respiratory assessment: patients with aortic aneurysms are commonly smokers or ex-smokers. Lung disease may impact on best choices for anaesthesia. Assess symptoms (cough, shortness of breath, exercise tolerance) and signs (saturations, auscultation).
> Cardiovascular assessment: patient likely to have longstanding hypertension and possibly coronary artery disease. Take history of past issues and check for current symptomatology. Also assess cardiovascular stability from the point of view of leaking aneurysm, which will impact on choices for anaesthesia.
> Ask about history of diabetes mellitus and chronic kidney disease. Diabetes should be controlled intraoperatively with variable rate insulin infusion. Chronic kidney disease is associated with long-standing hypertension, so there is increased likelihood in these patients. EVAR involves significant contrast dose risking deterioration in function.
> Assess preoperative functioning. This information is relevant when considering postoperative management in the intensive care unit.
> If patient was known to have an aneurysm, they may already have undergone preoperative assessment and investigation, which can help guide the current situation.

> Medications and allergies.
> Time of last meal.
> Blood tests: two samples for cross-match, full blood count, coagulation, arterial blood gas, make use of near-patient testing for speed of results.

Patient management:
> A/B: Oxygen 15 l/min non-rebreathe bag.
> C: Two large-bore cannulae to be sited but fluid administration is to be restricted to that necessary to maintain cerebration. Raising blood pressure could change the leaking aneurysm into a ruptured aneurysm.
> D: small increments of morphine titrated against pain. However, do not give if patient is obtunded or blood pressure is critically low.

Organisation, communication, staffing:
> Contact consultant on call and other members of on-call team for assistance.
> Contact theatres: possibility of converting to open procedure, need for staffing.
> Discuss with ODP: check their familiarity with radiology suite. Ensure anaesthetic machine, drugs, difficult airway trolley are in location and ready for use.
> Liaise with radiology suite: radiographer to ensure preparations are being made to receive the patient.
> Contact blood bank to request blood products – institute major haemorrhage protocol if necessary.
> Discuss with vascular surgical colleagues – establish surgical plan.
> Ensure porters available for blood product access and to help transfer to radiology.
> Discuss with intensive care consultant regarding postoperative care.
> Explain plans and prognosis with the patient and the patient's family.

b) Describe options for providing anaesthesia for this case and give the advantages/ disadvantages of each. (45%)

Whatever the choice of anaesthesia, all patients will need:

> *Full monitoring.*
> *IABP (right radial for ease of access once c-arm is in place and in case of need for surgical access via the left radial artery).*
> *Consideration of central line (depends on comorbidities, cardiovascular stability, time permitting – difficult to get access after procedure starts due to c-arm).*
> *Avoidance of nephrotoxins.*
> *Large volumes of fluid to avoid contrast-induced nephropathy (CIN) (aim to limit amount of contrast used if possible).*
> *Urinary catheter.*
> *Heparin 5000u on exposure of arteries (depends on degree of leak – this would be omitted if patient was coagulopathic).*
> *Availability of emergency drugs.*

As with any operation, you have got to be able to discuss the options for anaesthesia and weigh up the advantages and disadvantages of each.

Advantages	Disadvantages
Local anaesthesia +/– sedation	
Preservation of cardiovascular stability.	Need to lie still for a long period.
Avoids affecting respiratory mechanics in patients with respiratory comorbidity.	Does not deal with ischaemic pain caused by periods of arterial occlusion.
Good postoperative pain control.	Respiratory or cardiac comorbidities may make lying flat problematic.
If patient fully awake, they can cooperate with periods of cessation of breathing.	Does not facilitate conversion to open procedure.
	Sedation may cause dysphoria.
Neuraxial block +/– sedation	
Reduced pain from ischaemia compared to local anaesthesia.	Restlessness due to prolonged immobility on a narrow table remains a problem.
Good postoperative analgesia.	Risk of neuraxial procedure in a patient who may already have deranged coagulation from blood loss. Patient will be anticoagulated postoperatively, so need careful timing of removal of epidural catheter.
If patient fully awake, they can cooperate with periods of cessation of breathing.	Spinal may not offer sufficient duration of anaesthesia and is associated with more cardiovascular side effects than epidural.
	Does not facilitate conversion to open procedure.
	Sedation may cause dysphoria.
General anaesthesia	
Permits conversion to open procedure.	Potential for cardiovascular instability in already compromised patient.
Maximally comfortable for patient intraoperatively.	Does not offer any inherent postoperative analgesia (although little is required for EVAR).
Can control breathing of intubated, ventilated patient.	
Secured airway – in all other situations, patient at risk of aspiration if becomes obtunded.	

Reference

Nataraj V, Mortimer A. Endovascular abdominal aortic aneurysm repair. *Contin Educ Anaesth Crit Care Pain*. 2004; 4 (3): 91–94.

A 56-year-old man is listed for carotid endarterectomy 10 days after suffering a cerebrovascular accident.

a) What are the advantages (4 marks) and disadvantages (4 marks) of performing the procedure under regional anaesthesia?

b) What local or regional anaesthetic techniques may be used? (3 marks)

c) How can his risk of perioperative cerebrovascular accident be minimised? (6 marks)

d) Following this procedure, what other specific postoperative complications may occur? (3 marks)

March 2016

Chairman's Report

53.9% pass rate.

This question had one of the highest correlations with overall performance; i.e. candidates who did well in this question performed well in the SAQ overall. As mentioned above, some candidates did not read the question properly* but fortunately did not lose too many marks as a result.

*Failure to answer the question asked.

It is very important, even when pressed for time, to read the question carefully and answer what is asked. For example, in question 4 of this exam about carotid endarterectomy, part (c) asked for factors that would reduce the risk of perioperative cerebrovascular accident, and part (d) asked candidates to identify other specific postoperative complications. Unfortunately, some candidates mentioned the different forms of cerebrovascular accident that may occur postoperatively in their answer to part (d), so could not be given marks and wasted valuable time.

Carotid endarterectomy improves outcomes (reduces risk of fatal or disabling stroke) of symptomatic patients, with greater than 50% carotid stenosis compared with the best medical management (reduction in arterial pressure, antiplatelet drugs, statins or diet to reduce serum cholesterol, stopping smoking, controlling diabetes and reducing alcohol intake). Neurologically stable patients who have had a transient ischaemic attack or stroke should ideally have carotid endarterectomy within two weeks if stenosis is 50%–99%. ECST-2 (European Carotid Surgery Trial) should help determine which of medical or surgical management of asymptomatic patients is the better option, and ACST-2 (Asymptomatic Carotid Surgery Trial) aims to determine whether stent or carotid endarterectomy is best for asymptomatic patients. Once again, the question wants proof of your understanding about the advantages and disadvantages of the various possible anaesthetic techniques.

A very brief description of the surgical approach to carotid endarterectomy:

> *Exposure of carotid.*
> *Cross-clamping above and below the area of stenosis (heparin given immediately prior to this).*
> *Vertical incision.*
> *Cerebral blood flow reduced whilst cross-clamp on, dependent on the collateral flow via Circle of Willis. Ipsilateral blood flow can be improved with a shunt from below to above cross-clamps. Some surgeons use shunts routinely, some only in anaesthetised patients (as neurological status cannot be monitored), some only if perfusion appears inadequate.*
> *Atheroma removed, defect closed by primary closure or using a patch (synthetic or autologous vein graft). Using a patch reduces the risk of re-stenosis.*

a) What are the advantages (4 marks) and disadvantages (4 marks) of performing the procedure under <u>regional anaesthesia</u>?

Advantages	Disadvantages
An awake patient provides their own real neurological monitoring.	Risks associated with blocks; intravascular/epidural/subarachnoid injection, local anaesthetic toxicity, phrenic nerve damage etc.
Monitoring in the early postoperative period improved as not recovering from general anaesthetic.	Risk of need to convert to GA with restricted airway access intraoperatively.
Lower need for shunt with its attendant risks; particulate or bubble embolisation, arterial wall dissection, kinking, thrombosis.	Needs cooperative patient; surgery may be prolonged, claustrophobia from drapes, overheating, full bladder.
Artery is closed at normal patient blood pressure; may reduce postoperative haematoma. Possibly more stable blood pressure throughout.	Potential for patient movement causing surgical difficulty.
Avoids airway instrumentation, general anaesthetic, and its associated risks (everything from sore throat to failed intubation and, more specifically in this situation, the cardiovascular instability caused by induction and intubation).	Potential for patient stress/pain causing myocardial ischaemia.

b) What local or regional anaesthetic techniques may be used? (3 marks)

Just a list required – there are only 3 points for this answer.

> Local anaesthetic infiltration.
> Superficial cervical plexus block.
> Deep cervical plexus block.
> Combined superficial and deep cervical plexus blocks.
> Cervical epidural, although this is now never used due to its burden of adverse effects: high block, hypotension.

c) How can his risk of perioperative cerebrovascular accident be minimised? (6 marks)

The question has not actually asked what types of cerebrovascular accident there are, but addressing each in turn seems a natural way of approaching this question.

Embolic (biggest risk):
> Avoid shunt use where possible, or meticulous surgical technique to avoid thromboembolism or air embolism when using shunt.
> Meticulous surgical technique to avoid dislodgement of atheroma.
> Perioperative administration of antiplatelets, usually dual antiplatelet therapy (DAPT).
> Heparin before cross-clamping.

Ischaemic:
> Use of a shunt if collateral circulation is inadequate during cross-clamp.
> Pharmacological management of perioperative hypotension.

Haemorrhagic:
> Pharmacological management of perioperative hypertension.

d) Following this procedure, what other <u>specific</u> postoperative complications may occur? (3 marks)

Three marks, three complications. You wouldn't even need all that detail on cerebral hyperperfusion syndrome; I have just included it here as an explanation.

> Postoperative haematoma, which may ultimately compromise airway.
> Haemodynamic instability secondary to impaired carotid baroreceptor reflexes resulting in periods of hyper- or hypotension, which may precipitate cardiovascular events.
> Cerebral hyperperfusion syndrome, occurs from immediately postoperatively until a month later. Chronic hypoperfusion results in areas of impaired autoregulation. Increased microvascular permeability occurs on reperfusion of previously underperfused areas of brain,

increasing vulnerability to oedema: ischaemia-reperfusion injury. Extreme hypertension resulting from impaired carotid baroreceptor function postoperatively, in combination with the previous changes, may result in oedema and haemorrhage. Result: hypertensive encephalopathy, severe headache, variable neurological deficits, seizures, cerebral oedema, cerebral haemorrhage.

Reference

Ladak N, Thompson J. General or local anaesthesia for carotid endarterectomy? *Contin Educ Anaesth Crit Care Pain*. 2012; 12 (2): 92–96.

A 79-year-old man with a 6-cm infra-renal abdominal aortic aneurysm is to undergo an endovascular aneurysm repair (EVAR). He is known to have chronic obstructive pulmonary disease.

a) What are the advantages of an EVAR compared to an open repair of the aneurysm for this patient? (8 marks)

b) List the risk factors for acute kidney injury (AKI) during any EVAR procedure. (6 marks)

c) Describe perioperative measures to prevent AKI following EVAR. (6 marks)

September 2016

Chairman's Report

57.2% pass rate.

There were no major themes that emerged in the answers to this question. It was presumably easier to answer for those who had had the chance to see the procedure during their training.

a) What are the advantages of an EVAR compared to an open repair of the aneurysm for this patient? (8 marks)

They are specifically asking about <u>this patient</u>. *The issues to focus on are that the patient is elderly, that he has chronic obstructive pulmonary disease and that the aneurysm is infra-renal.*

> Open repair may be optimal in younger patients with few comorbidities as although the intraoperative risks are higher, there are fewer long-term problems with the graft, e.g. endoleak. This gentleman is elderly and has comorbidities that mean that the risk of long-term problems is less of an issue when compared to the intraoperative risks to him of an open repair.
> In view of the patient's age, he is likely to have other comorbidities, including cardiovascular and renal disease, increasing the need for a minimally invasive technique with fewer perioperative complications and less metabolic and haemodynamic stress.
> EVAR offers potential for avoidance of intubation, effects of positive pressure ventilation on diseased lungs, risk of pneumonia – EVAR may be done under neuraxial technique or even local anaesthetic to groins.
> Avoids presence of large abdominal wound, the pain of which can cause difficulty achieving deep breathing and adequate cough postoperatively, thus increasing the risk of respiratory complications.
> Reduces the possible need for opioid analgesia postoperatively with its respiratory depressant effect.
> Infra-renal aneurysms tend to be technically the most straightforward AAA to be done by EVAR; thus, operating time for an awake technique should be tolerable.
> Early ambulation (next day) facilitated, helping to maintain muscle strength and reducing risks of deep vein thrombosis, deconditioning and pneumonia in vulnerable individual.
> Reduced risk of large blood loss and coagulopathy, important in a patient with limited reserve to tolerate it.

b) List the risk factors for acute kidney injury (AKI) during any EVAR procedure. (6 marks)

We've moved on from the specific patient to more general issues. This often happens in final SAQ questions and is a common source of error when candidates fail to notice the shift in focus. Read the questions carefully, underline key words.

> Advancing age.
> Pre-existing renal impairment.
> Diabetes mellitus.
> Cardiac failure.
> Perioperative dehydration.
> Nephrotoxic drugs: ACE inhibitors, angiotensin II receptor antagonists, aminoglycosides, diuretics.
> High contrast load: including high cumulative contrast load from preoperative investigations, for example CT angiography.

> Surgical complications: embolisation of atheromatous plaque into renal arteries, obstruction of renal arteries by stent.

c) Describe perioperative measures to prevent AKI following EVAR. (6 marks)

> Avoid perioperative dehydration: minimise preoperative starvation time, cardiac output monitoring to guide fluid replacement intraoperatively (and possibly postoperatively), start fluids pre-procedure, ensuring full circulation at that point, monitor urine output. Monitor blood loss and replace, as indicated by near patient testing.
> Avoid perioperative hypotension: management of fluid status as earlier, with use of vasopressor if indicated.
> Avoid nephrotoxic drugs perioperatively where possible. NSAIDs not a suitable choice for pain control.
> Limitation of contrast load, especially in patients with pre-existing chronic kidney disease or risk of acute kidney injury. Scheduling of surgery so that kidneys have a week to recover from any preoperative contrast. Some centres use sodium bicarbonate or *N*-acetylcysteine, although evidence is currently lacking.
> Glucose control: maintain normal range in diabetic patients, use variable rate insulin infusion in type I diabetes.
> Minimise surgical complications with meticulous technique.

Reference

Webb S, Allen S. Perioperative renal protection. *Contin Educ Anaesth Crit Care Pain*. 2008; 8 (5): 176–180.

22. ANATOMY

a) List the nuclei of the vagus nerve. (10%)

b) Describe the immediate relations of the right vagus nerve in the neck at C6 (15%) and thorax at T4. (15%)

c) List the branches of the vagus nerve. (30%)

d) Which clinical situations commonly produce vagal reflex bradycardia? (30%)

March 2014

Chairman's Report

44.4% pass rate.

As in past years, knowledge of anatomy proved generally very poor. Candidates performed better in sections (c) and (d), which were most clinically orientated. Anatomical knowledge is clearly relevant to the invasive procedures undertaken in anaesthetic practice and possibly vital to the interpretation of images generated by ultrasound devices. Candidates must understand that relevant anatomy will be tested throughout all parts of the Final FRCA examination and should not write the subject off. This question failed to discriminate between generally strong and generally weak candidates due to widely distributed ignorance of the subject matter within the cohort, as was seen with question 8.*

Question 8 was the one that directly preceded this, concerning propofol TCI. Parts (a) to (c) are pure book-work. However, 30% of the marks could have been gained by applying clinical knowledge.

a) List the nuclei of the vagus nerve. (10%)

> Dorsal (vagal) nucleus.
> Nucleus ambiguus.
> Solitary nucleus (nucleus of the tractus solitarius).
> Spinal trigeminal nucleus: fibres supplying sensation to the pharynx and larynx are carried by the vagus to the spinal nucleus of the trigeminal nerve.

b) Describe the immediate relations of the right vagus nerve in the neck at C6 (15%) and thorax at T4. (15%)

Cross-sections at T4 and C6 are important areas of anatomy to revise for every stage of the exam.

C6:

> Lies within the carotid sheath with carotid artery anteromedially, internal jugular vein anterolaterally.
> Anteriorly: omohyoid and thyroid gland.
> Posteriorly: longus coli, anterior scalene, phrenic nerve.
> Medially: sympathetic trunk.
> Laterally: sternocleidomastoid.

T4:

> Anteriorly: phrenic nerve, superior vena cava.
> Posteriorly: oesophagus and right lung.
> Medially: trachea.
> Laterally: azygos vein and right lung.

c) List the branches of the vagus nerve. (30%)

Jugular fossa:
> Meningeal branch.
> Auricular nerve.

Neck:
> Pharyngeal nerve.
> Superior laryngeal nerve.
> Right recurrent laryngeal nerve.
> Cardiac branches.

Thorax:
> Oesophageal branches.
> Pericardial branches.
> Left recurrent laryngeal nerve.
> Branches to cardiac plexus.
> Branches to pulmonary plexus.

Abdomen:
> Gastric branches.
> Hepatic branch.
> Coeliac branches.

d) Which clinical situations commonly produce vagal reflex bradycardia? (30%)

> Central afferent pathway triggered by stress or pain.
> Oculocardiac reflex caused by traction on extra-ocular muscles during surgery.
> Trigeminocardiac reflex during maxillofacial surgery.
> Stimulation of larynx during intubation, laryngoscopy or with suctioning.
> Peritoneal stretch during laparoscopic surgery.
> Manipulation of abdominal and pelvic organs.
> Cervical or anal dilatation during surgery or examination.

Reference

Ellis H, Feldman S, Lawson S. *Anatomy for Anaesthetists*. 7th edition. Oxford: Blackwell Science; 1997.

23. APPLIED CLINICAL PHARMACOLOGY

a) What are the indications for anti-platelet drugs in clinical practice? (25%)

b) List the agents currently in clinical use and their underlying mechanisms of action. (50%)

c) How may active bleeding be managed following administration of one of these agents? (25%)

March 2013

Chairman's Report

66.1% pass rate.

This was a straightforward question that is very topical. This was reflected by a good pass rate.

a) What are the indications for anti-platelet drugs in clinical practice? (25%)

> Primary prevention in patients at risk of thrombotic cardiovascular events.
> Primary prevention in patients at risk of thrombotic cerebrovascular events.
> Secondary prevention of thrombotic events in patients who have had myocardial infarction, any percutaneous coronary intervention including coronary stent or bypass surgery.
> Secondary prevention of thrombotic events in patients who have transient ischaemic attacks or thrombotic stroke.
> Anticoagulation of e.g. haemofiltration circuits when heparin cannot be used.
> Side effect of a drug's intended use, e.g. antipyretics, analgesics.

b) List the agents currently in clinical use and their underlying mechanisms of action. (50%)

What follows is an incredibly simplified version of platelet activation. I have focused on the chemicals that antiplatelet medications act upon to achieve their effect:

> *The intact endothelium releases chemicals such as prostacyclin and nitric oxide, which keep platelets in their inactive form. Inactive platelets maintain calcium efflux via a cAMP-driven pump.*
> *Exposed collagen or von Willebrand's Factor (due to damage to the endothelium) or thrombin in the blood (due to activation of the coagulation pathways) activates platelets.*
> *The activated platelets release ADP from granules and make thromboxane A_2 via the COX pathway.*
> *ADP and thromboxane A_2 go on to activate other platelets: ADP reduces cAMP, thus inactivating the outward pump of calcium, allowing a conformational change in the platelets, resulting in degranulation, and thromboxane A_2 activates other platelets' GPIIb/IIa receptors.*
> *The glycoprotein IIb/IIIa receptors on the surfaces of activated platelets change from resting to active.*

> Activated GPIIb/IIIa receptors will bind fibrinogen at both ends, thus linking activated platelets together, or bind to von Willebrand Factor exposed in the damaged endothelium, thus anchoring the platelet plug in place.

Agent	Mechanism of action
Aspirin	Irreversible nonselective cyclo-oxygenase inhibitor, stopping thromboxane A_2 production.
Thienopyridines (clopidogrel, ticlodipine)	Irreversible inhibition of P2Y12 ADP receptor.
Glycoprotein IIb/IIIa receptor inhibitors (tirofiban, abciximab)	Prevents GPIIb/IIa fibrin cross-linking with other activated platelets or von Willebrand Factor cross-linking to the subendothelium.
Dipyridamole	1. Phosphodiesterase inhibitor. Increases the presence of cAMP by reducing its breakdown by phosphodiesterase, increasing the tendency of platelets to remain in the inactive state. 2. Blocks thromboxane A2 receptors.
Prostacyclin	Binds to platelet G-protein coupled receptor, increasing cAMP production by adenylate cyclase, helping maintain platelets in their inactive state.

c) How may active bleeding be managed following administration of one of these agents? (25%)

How do you manage any bleeding? Make sure you cover the basics before launching in with platelet transfusions.

> I would assess and manage the patient simultaneously, following an ABC approach, to include administration of oxygen, assessment of adequacy of ventilation with definitive management as indicated, and large-bore cannulation.
> Discontinue further antiplatelet administration if risk/benefit assessment makes this appropriate.
> Pressure, tourniquet use, surgical or radiological management of the source of bleeding.
> Early consultation with a haematologist for guidance. Activate Major Haemorrhage Protocol if appropriate.
> Point-of-care and laboratory tests of full blood count and coagulation to guide administration of blood, fresh frozen plasma, cryoprecipitate and coagulation factor concentrates.
> May need large volumes of platelet transfusions as infused platelets will become inactivated by the presence of the antiplatelet drug.
> Consideration of tranexamic acid.

Reference
Smart S, Aragola S, Hutton P. Antiplatelet agents and anaesthesia. *Contin Educ Anaesth Crit Care Pain*. 2007; 7 (5): 157–161.

An adult patient is to receive a target controlled infusion (TCI) of propofol.

a) Detail how TCI devices ensure a steady-state blood concentration. (50%)

b) What additional pharmacokinetic data is required to allow effect-site targeting? (20%)

c) What are the advantages of a TCI device compared to a manual propofol infusion regime? (30%)

March 2014

Chairman's Report

17.5% pass rate.

This was the most poorly answered question of the paper. The written answers reflected a 'black-box' mentality from the majority of candidates, with little real understanding of how infusion devices work or of the underlying pharmacokinetics. In particular, effect site targeting was poorly understood. This question failed to discriminate between generally strong and generally weak candidates due to widely distributed ignorance of the subject matter within the cohort. It is of some consolation that a few candidates could reproduce the recommendations of the Safe Anaesthesia Liaison Group regarding total intravenous anaesthesia even though such details were not asked for. Given that the administration of TCI propofol is used nationwide, the poor performance observed must reflect a paucity of formal teaching of the subject within Schools of Anaesthesia.

If you were thinking you could leave pharmacology behind now that you have done your primary, think again! Remember the three compartment model?

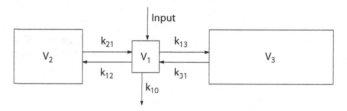

Three-compartment model

a) Detail how TCI devices ensure a steady state blood concentration. (50%)

> TCI devices and programmes rely on the concept of a three-compartmental model of the way in which a specific drug behaves within the body.
> V_1, the central compartment, is the plasma into which the drug is injected and any tissues that behave like plasma in respect to that particular drug. To achieve a particular drug concentration rapidly, a bolus is given that is equal to the desired concentration multiplied by this volume of distribution ($Cp \times V_1$).
> Drug leaves this central compartment down its concentration gradient initially to vessel-rich tissues (V_2) and then to tissues with poorer blood supplies (V_3). There are therefore two superimposed reducing infusion rates that allow for this loss from the central compartment.
> Once equilibrium has occurred between all three compartments, the only loss of drug from the central compartment is via metabolism (to inactive metabolites) and elimination from the body. The final steady-state infusion rate therefore matches this removal rate.
> The sizes of the different compartments and the rate constants between them depend upon the model and drug being used. The size of the compartments, according to these models, depends on certain patient characteristics such as height, weight and age, which will require inputting into the administration device being used.
> In summary, a steady-state blood concentration is achieved by a bolus dose followed by three superimposed infusion rates, two that exponentially reduce and one that is constant to match elimination.

b) What additional pharmacokinetic data is required to allow effect-site targeting? (20%)

> Targeting the effect-site concentration aims to eliminate the hysteresis observed between plasma concentration and actual drug effect that takes place in the brain.
> The effect-site compartment volume is negligibly small and so the rate constant determining movement of drug to effect site (K_{eo}) is one way only, from plasma to effect site, unlike the rate constants determining movement between other compartments. K_{eo} is not known and must be determined through experiment.
> Peak drug effect will occur when the curve of the declining plasma concentration of the drug after bolus injection crosses the curve of the rising effect-site concentration. Different, hypothetical, K_{eo} values are used to plot effect-site concentration curves, and the one that results in a concentration matching plasma concentration at peak observed drug effect is then determined as the actual K_{eo}.

c) What are the advantages of a TCI device compared to a manual propofol infusion regime? (30%)

> Bolus dose and infusion rate determined by computer model based on patient and drug characteristics, not guess-work.
> Theoretically, can achieve steady state more rapidly. If a propofol infusion is initiated at a fixed rate, it takes 5 half-lives to reach steady state.
> Theoretically, correct dosing therefore reduces risk of awareness, on one hand, and excessive cardiovascular and respiratory effects on the other.
> Changing infusion rate with TCI results in pause or bolus as well, to achieve desired effect more rapidly – not so with manual.
> Using TCI is less labour-intensive than repeatedly checking and changing the rate manually.
> More rapid wake-up at end of surgery by avoiding excessive dosing during the preceding infusion.

Reference

Absalom A, Mani V, De Smet T, Struys M. Pharmacokinetic models for propofol – defining and illuminating the devil in the detail. *Br J Anaesth*. 2009; 10 (1): 26–37.

a) Outline the mechanisms of spontaneous recovery from neuromuscular blockade following the administration of rocuronium. (2 marks)

b) Which classes of drugs can be used to antagonise the action of rocuronium (2 marks) and how do they work? (5 marks)

c) What are the advantages and disadvantages of these antagonist drugs? (11 marks)

March 2015

Chairman's Report

52.7% pass rate; 10.9% of candidates received a poor fail.

The pass rate is disappointing as these agents are 'meat and drink' to the profession. The mechanisms by which the action of rocuronium spontaneously degrades were poorly understood. Sugammadex may not be readily available in some Trusts but it is reasonable to expect specialist trainee anaesthetists to understand its pharmacology and clinical usage.

a) Outline the mechanisms of spontaneous recovery from neuromuscular blockade following the administration of rocuronium. (2 marks)

> After the administration of rocuronium, there is a dynamic association and dissociation of the rocuronium with the nicotinic receptors.
> Redistribution of the drug occurs down its concentration gradient into the plasma, once plasma levels start to decrease.
> The reduction in plasma concentration is driven by metabolism in the liver and excretion in the bile.

b) Which classes of drugs can be used to antagonise the action of rocuronium (2 marks) and how do they work? (5 marks)

Reversible acetylcholinesterase inhibitors: neostigmine.

Neostigmine hydrolyses acetylcholinesterase by forming a carbamylated enzyme complex with the esteratic site, thus increasing amount of acetylcholine at neuromuscular junction and competing with residual rocuronium.

Cyclodextrins: sugammadex.

Sugammadex has a ring-like structure with a hydrophilic outer surface and lipophilic inner surface that encapsulates the lipophilic rocuronium.

c) What are the advantages and disadvantages of these antagonist drugs? (11 marks)

	Cyclodextrin	Reversible acetylcholinesterase inhibitor
Advantages	• With appropriate dosing, reverses from full paralysis with rocuronium, useful in 'can't intubate, can't oxygenate'(CICO) situations. • Effective for rocuronium and vecuronium for routine reversal. • In typical circumstances, no risk of recurarisation due to irreversible encapsulation of neuromuscular blocking drug. • No significant cardiovascular effects. • May be used to temporarily reverse neuromuscular block intraoperatively. • Facilitates rapid turnover of cases that require full paralysis but are of short duration such as airway or laparoscopic surgery. • Facilitates reversal of neuromuscular blockade in patients with myotonic dystrophy for whom neostigmine should be avoided.	• Cheap. • Familiar.
Disadvantages	• Flucloxacillin and fusidic acid may displace neuromuscular blocking drug from sugammadex, potentiating block. • Sugammadex will encapsulate progesterone, reducing the efficacy of hormonal contraceptives. • Cost. • Potential for allergic reactions. • Not effective against benzylisoquinoliniums.	• Unwanted muscarinic receptor action causing bradycardia, gut stimulation (possibly with implications on anastomotic integrity), secretions, bronchospasm, urinary retention. • Co-administration of glycopyrolate to mitigate muscarininc effects results in dry mouth, tachycardia. • No use in CICO when neuromuscular blocking drug has just been given. • Observer error in train-of-four monitoring may lead to overestimation of level of reversibility, resulting in ineffective administration or premature administration with the possibility of recurarisation.

Reference

Khirwadkar R, Hunter J. Neuromuscular physiology and pharmacology: an update. *Contin Ed Anaesth Crit Care Pain*. 2012; 12 (5): 237–244.

a) In a patient with diabetes mellitus, what clinical features may indicate autonomic involvement? (4 marks)

b) What are the other microvascular (3 marks) and macrovascular (3 marks) complications of diabetes mellitus?

c) List the classes of oral hypoglycaemic agents that are available. (5 marks) Describe their mechanisms of action. (5 marks)

September 2016

Chairman's Report

38.4% pass rate.

Knowledge of the complications of diabetes was comprehensive and probably reflects the fact that we all see a great many diabetic patients in our everyday practice. Marks were lost in section (c) as very few candidates knew about any oral hypoglycaemic drugs other than sulphonylureas and biguanides. The other classes of drugs are now quite frequently used and should therefore be known about, particularly given the aforementioned increasing prevalence of type 2 diabetes in our surgical and intensive care populations. It is important to remember that applied basic sciences such as pharmacology form part of the syllabus for this exam.

a) In a patient with diabetes mellitus, what clinical features may indicate autonomic involvement? (4 marks)

> Cardiovascular: resting tachycardia, arrhythmias, orthostatic hypotension.
> Gastrointestinal: bloating after meals, constipation and diarrhoea.
> Sweating: gustatory sweating or reduced ability to sweat.
> Genitourinary: impotence, loss of bladder control.

b) What are the other microvascular (3 marks) and macrovascular (3 marks) complications of diabetes mellitus?

Microvascular:
> Retinopathy.
> Nephropathy.
> Neuropathy; sensory and motor polyneuropathy in glove and stocking distribution, and autonomic neuropathy.
> Microvascular cardiac disease.

Macrovascular:
> Coronary artery disease.
> Cerebrovascular disease.
> Hypertension.
> Peripheral vascular disease.

c) List the classes of oral hypoglycaemic agents that are available. (5 marks) Describe their mechanisms of action. (5 marks)

This question asks about oral hypoglycaemics, but don't forget to learn about the injectable hypoglycaemic class of drugs, GLP-1 analogues.

Drug class	Mechanism of action
Biguanides e.g. metformin.	Decrease hepatic gluconeogenesis, improved peripheral insulin sensitivity.
Thiazolidinediones e.g. pioglitazone.	Improved peripheral insulin sensitivity, increasing peripheral glucose uptake.
Sulphonylureas e.g. gliclazide.	Stimulate pancreatic insulin secretion.
Meglitinides e.g. repaglinide.	Stimulate pancreatic insulin secretion.
Alpha glucosidase inhibitors e.g. acarbose.	Slow digestion of carbohydrate in gut, decreasing glucose absorption.
SGLT-2 (sodium-glucose-co-transporter) inhibitors e.g. canagliflozin.	Inhibits glucose reabsorption in the kidney.
DPP 4 inhibitors (gliptins) e.g. sitagliptin.	Inhibit breakdown of endogenous GLP-1 by DPP 4, allowing GLP-1 to stimulate insulin secretion and inhibit glucagon release after meals.

References

Association of Anaesthetists of Great Britain and Ireland. Peri-operative management of the surgical patient with diabetes. *Anaesth*. 2015; 70: 1427–1440.

Nicholson G, Hall G. Diabetes and adult surgical inpatients. *Contin Educ Anaesth Crit Care Pain*. 2011; 11 (6): 234–238.

a) List the patient-related (7 marks) and anaesthetic-related (3 marks) risk factors for postoperative nausea and vomiting (PONV) in adult patients.

b) What are the unwanted effects of PONV in adults? (6 marks)

c) Which non-pharmacological interventions have been shown to be effective in reducing PONV in adults? (2 marks)

d) Briefly explain the proposed mechanisms of action of 5HT3 antagonists such as ondansetron when used as anti-emetics. (2 marks)

March 2017

Chairman's Report

68.3% pass rate.

This was one of the two easy questions and the pass rate was the second highest overall, as might be expected given the frequency with which PONV occurs. Despite this, many candidates had insufficient knowledge of risk factors for PONV and of the non-pharmacological methods that may be used to reduce it. Candidates who scored well had a sensible structured approach to this common problem.

A score of 14/20 is required to pass an easy question. Postoperative nausea and vomiting were the basis of a question in 2008.

a) List the patient-related (7 marks) and anaesthetic-related (3 marks) risk factors for postoperative nausea and vomiting (PONV) in adult patients.

Patient factors:
> Female gender.
> History of postoperative nausea and vomiting.
> History of motion sickness.
> Non-smoker.
> Other possible risk factors include anxiety, ASA 1 or 2 status, history of migraine, and age (children less affected under three years of age, then risk declines through adulthood).

Anaesthetic factors:
> Volatile use.
> Nitrous oxide use.
> Intra- and postoperative opioid use.
> Increased duration of anaesthesia.

b) What are the unwanted effects of PONV in adults? (6 marks)

> Reduced patient satisfaction.
> Delayed discharge from PACU.
> Delayed discharge from hospital/unexpected hospital stay in day case patients (with the implications of cost, inconvenience, poor bed usage).
> Delayed return to oral intake (especially important in diabetic patients).
> Suture dehiscence.
> Aspiration of gastric contents.
> Dehydration, electrolyte imbalance, metabolic alkalosis.
> Oesophageal rupture.

c) Which non-pharmacological interventions have been shown to be effective in reducing PONV in adults? (2 marks)

> Avoidance of general anaesthesia (no anaesthesia/regional anaesthesia).
> Acupressure, acupuncture.
> Aromatherapy.
> Avoidance of dehydration (avoid excessive starvation period).

d) Briefly explain the proposed mechanisms of action of 5HT3 antagonists such as ondansetron when used as anti-emetics. (2 marks)

Make sure you relearn the vomiting pathways. It makes remembering the mechanisms of action of the drugs more straightforward.

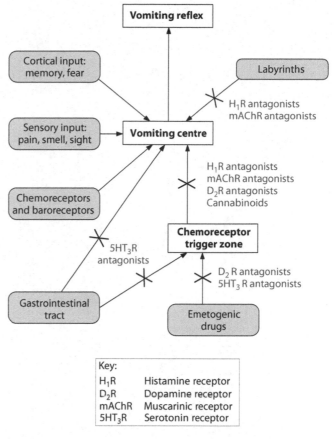

Vomiting pathways

> Enterochromaffin cells in the small intestine release 5-hydroxytryptamine (5HT) in response to stimulation by drugs. 5HT stimulates the vagus, fibres of which terminate in the chemoreceptor trigger zone (CRTZ) and the vomiting centre.
> There are also $5HT_3$ receptors in the CRTZ.
> Ondansetron blocks $5HT_3$ receptors.

Reference

Pierre S, Whelan R. Nausea and vomiting after surgery. *Contin Educ Anaesth Crit Care Pain* 2013; 13 (1): 28–32.

24. APPLIED PHYSIOLOGY AND BIOCHEMISTRY

a) What factors determine how long oxygen saturation is maintained in an apnoeic patient? (30%)

b) How may pre-oxygenation be performed and its progress assessed? (30%)

c) What are the clinical advantages and disadvantages of pre-oxygenating a fit adult? (40%)

March 2012

Chairman's Report

50.5% pass rate

This question was featured in the past and was poorly answered. Section (a) focused on the physiology. Key words such as FRC, oxygen consumption, carbon dioxide production, alveolar ventilation, alveolar gas equation and wash-in all too often were missing. Section (b) concentrated on the techniques of effective preoxygenation and again was poorly answered.

This question is almost identical to one that featured in 2008, four years before. It's fair game, as it's pretty central to our practice!

a) What factors determine how long oxygen saturation is maintained in an apnoeic patient? (30%)

This depends upon the balance between how quickly the oxygen is being used, how much of a reservoir there is to use, and whether there is a way to keep topping up that reservoir. The reservoir is the product of the functional residual capacity and its oxygen content.

Remember the alveolar gas equation?

$$PAO_2 = PiO_2 - PaCO_2/RQ$$

It demonstrates that increasing PiO_2 increases PAO_2 and how a raised $PaCO_2$ has a negative impact on PAO_2.

Reservoir available – product of the functional residual capacity (FRC) and its oxygen content:

Size of FRC dependent on:
> Posture (FRC is less when supine, can be improved by head-up tilt).
> Anaesthesia (reduces FRC).
> Encroachment on FRC (obesity, pregnancy, ascites, bowel obstruction, kyphoscoliosis).
> Age (lower FRC per unit weight in children).

Oxygen content dependent on:
> Fraction of inspired oxygen preceding apnoea (the alveolar gas equation determines that breathing 100% oxygen increases the available reservoir by a factor of nearly 5, compared to room air).

> Lung disease (shunt reduces effectiveness of preoxygenation).
> $PaCO_2$ (according to the alveolar gas equation, an elevated $PaCO_2$ results in a reduced PAO_2).

Rate of oxygen consumption:

Increased in:
> Sepsis.
> Thyrotoxicosis.
> Pregnancy.
> Critical illness.
> Fasciculations secondary to suxamethonium.
> Childhood – greater oxygen consumption per unit weight.

Patency of airway:

At normal steady state, oxygen is removed from the lungs at the rate of its consumption (approximately 250 ml/min in a textbook adult). Carbon dioxide delivery to the lungs is 80% of this, as determined by a respiratory quotient of 0.8. After apnoea, oxygen removal from the lungs persists at the same rate. However, as the partial pressure of carbon dioxide in the alveoli starts to rise, the concentration gradient between blood and alveoli reduces, negatively impacting on further movement of carbon dioxide into the lungs. Lung volume consequently falls. If the airway is patent, this results in apnoeic mass movement of gas (oxygen, if anaesthetic mask is still firmly held in place) into the lungs, significantly extending the time to desaturation (although not addressing acidosis and hypercapnia).

b) How may pre-oxygenation be performed and its progress assessed? (30%)

> Explanation to and consent from patient, improves compliance.
> Head-up tilt to increase the size of FRC.
> Tight-fitting mask (anaesthetic machine circuit) avoids entrainment of room air.
> 100% FiO_2.
> Gas flow to exceed patient's minute ventilation to ensure gas in circuit remains 100% oxygen whilst the patient is still breathing, and high-flow oxygen facilitates apnoeic mass movement after cessation of breathing.
> Five minutes.
> Tidal breathing.
> Monitor fraction of expired oxygen (F_EO_2), to target greater than 0.9.

c) What are the clinical advantages and disadvantages of pre-oxygenating a fit adult? (40%)

Advantages	Disadvantages
Difficult to predict difficult intubation, therefore provides a margin of safety in unpredicted difficulties.	Risk of respiratory incident during induction in fit patients is low, so may be unnecessary.
Cannot predict severe laryngospasm.	Prolongs induction by five minutes.
	Intolerance of tight-fitting mask, sense of claustrophobia.
	Increases alveolar collapse at induction resulting in risk of atelectasis and postoperative hypoxia.

Reference
Sirian R, Wills J. Physiology of apnoea and the benefits of preoxygenation. *Contin Educ Anaesth Crit Care Pain*. 2009; 9 (4): 105–108.

a) Outline the major changes in the cardiovascular system of elderly patients. (35%)

b) What are the perioperative implications of each change? (65%)

September 2012

Chairman's Report

46.9% pass rate.

This question was set to explore the knowledge of both the physiological and pathological changes that occur as a result of ageing. Many of the answers were insufficiently detailed and not systematic. It is acceptable to structure your answers in tabulated form if the sections of a question are linked. In this case the answers to (a) and (b) were associated.

For example:

a) Cardiovascular change	b) Anaesthetic implication
Increased systemic vascular resistance Hypertension Left ventricular hypertrophy	Cardiovascular instability May need to obtund pressor responses Antihypertensive medication
Beta receptor down-regulation	Reduced responsiveness to catecholamines and sympathomimetic agents
Etc…	

Other cardiovascular changes include reduced autonomic responsiveness, reduced cardiac output secondary to reduced stroke volume, degeneration of SA/AV nodes and conducting system, increased incidence of valvular heart disease and ischaemic heart disease. Similar questions in future might feature changes of the respiratory or central nervous systems of the elderly.

You should be able to rattle through a systems-based approach to the physiological and anatomical differences between paediatric and adult patients. Similarly, you should be able to list the major systems-based changos that occur with ageing.

a) Outline the major changes in the cardiovascular system of elderly patients. (35%)

b) What are the perioperative implications of each change? (65%)

a) Cardiovascular change	b) Anaesthetic implication
Reduced arterial elasticity and arteriosclerosis causing raised systemic vascular resistance, longstanding hypertension and consequent left ventricular hypertrophy.	Cardiovascular instability. Excessive pressor responses, may need obtunding. Need to maintain blood pressure at usual levels to ensure cerebral perfusion. Antihypertensive medication may result in electrolyte imbalance or perioperative hypotension. Diastolic dysfunction, reduced ability to cope with fluid load.
Loss of atrial pacemaker cells.	Lower intrinsic heart rate. In conjunction with reduced ability to increase stroke volume, there is less ability to respond to reduced blood pressure caused by vasodilatation caused by anaesthetic agents.
Loss of cells of the atrioventricular node and conduction pathways.	Susceptible to arrhythmias.
Increased risk of valvular disease.	Depends on valve and problem with valve: issues include reduced ability to cope with fluid loads or losses; fixed cardiac output state which may contraindicate neuraxial techniques.
Decreased beta receptor function and numbers.	Impaired response to catecholamines and sympathomimetics, hypotension more difficult to treat.
Reduced carotid baroreceptor response to hypotension.	Impaired response to hypotension.
Increased risk of ischaemic heart disease.	Increased risk of perioperative acute coronary syndrome.

Reference

Murray D, Dodds C. Perioperative care of the elderly. *Contin Educ Anaesth Crit Care Pain*. 2004; 4 (6): 193–196.

a) List the causes of primary hyperparathyroidism. (10%)

b) Which biochemical abnormalities are seen in primary hyperparathyroidism? (15%)

c) What are the systemic effects of hyperparathyroidism? (20%)

d) What important factors must the anaesthetist consider before, during and after anaesthesia for parathyroidectomy? (55%)

September 2012

Chairman's Report

46.1% pass rate.

Knowledge of the causes and clinical features of primary hyperparathyroidism was generally adequate. However candidates appeared to have little idea of the anaesthetic issues and often wrote generic answers with little or no focus on the specifics of parathyroid surgery. It was a common misconception that parathyroid adenomas are large and will obstruct the airway. Hardly any candidates mentioned gland localization techniques (methylene blue), and a significant number did not include hypocalcaemia as an important postoperative problem. Many failed to mention optimal patient positioning and the fact that the surgeon may wish to use a peripheral nerve stimulator.

There are four parathyroid glands, located at the poles of the thyroid gland. However, there is great variation in their location. They are small, 3 × 6 × 2 mm. Blood supply is from the inferior thyroid artery. Their secretion is inhibited by high parathyroid hormone and calcium levels and stimulated by high phosphate levels.

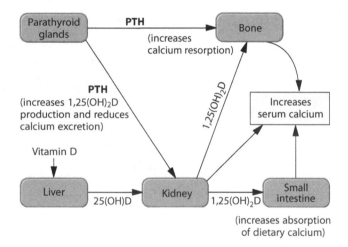

Key:
PTH — Parathyroid hormone
25(OH)D — Hydroxycholecalciferol
1,25(OH)$_2$D — Dihydroxycholecalciferol

Calcium regulation

a) List the causes of primary hyperparathyroidism. (10%)

> Parathyroid adenoma.
> Gland hyperplasia.
> Parathyroid cancer.

Secondary hyperparathyroidism occurs in chronic kidney disease: the failing kidney does not excrete phosphate efficiently and does not hydroxylate vitamin D, reducing calcium absorption from the gastrointestinal tract. After a prolonged period of secondary hyperparathyroidism, tertiary hyperparathyroidism may develop. Here, even once calcium and phosphate levels return to normal (for example after a renal transplant), the parathyroid glands continue to oversecrete.

b) Which biochemical abnormalities are seen in primary hyperparathyroidism? (15%)

> Elevated parathyroid hormone.
> Elevated calcium.
> Reduced phosphate.
> Elevated alkaline phosphatase.

c) What are the systemic effects of hyperparathyroidism? (20%)

'Stones, bones, abdominal groans, psychic moans'.

Renal: stones, impaired concentrating ability, polyuria, renal failure.

Skeletal: bone resorption, pain, fractures, osteitis fibrosis cystica.

Gastrointestinal: calcium-induced gastric hypersecretion, peptic ulceration, acute and chronic pancreatitis, nonspecific abdominal pain.

Central nervous system: nonspecific symptoms, weakness, deterioration in memory and cerebration.

Cardiovascular: conduction defects, hypertension.

d) What important factors must the anaesthetist consider before, during and after anaesthesia for parathyroidectomy? (55%)

Parathyroidectomy may be performed for primary or tertiary hyperparathyroidism.

Preoperative:
> Consider underlying cause and associated issues: coexistent endocrine disease, chronic kidney disease, recent transplant.
> Consider the impact of hyperparathyroidism: calcium level (may need correction preoperatively, pamidronate and fluids), renal function, cardiac rhythm (check ECG).

Intraoperative:
> Anaesthesia: surgical field near airway. Reinforced tube or LMA. Can be performed with regional anaesthetic technique; bilateral superficial cervical plexus blocks with supplementation.
> Position: supine, head-up tilt, sandbag under shoulders, head ring. Care with positioning; risk of osteoporosis and pathological fractures.
> Warming: potentially long surgery especially if checking with frozen sections for completeness of adenoma resection or on-table parathyroid hormone assays.
> Methylene Blue to identify glands: risk of anaphylaxis, interference with oxygen saturations monitoring.
> Recurrent laryngeal nerve monitoring: short-acting muscle relaxant for intubation. Consider remifentanil infusion thereafter.

Postoperative:
> Hypocalcaemia: check at 6 hours and 24 hours. May need oral or intravenous supplementation.
> Recurrent laryngeal nerve palsy: voice change, difficulty breathing.
> Incomplete resection.
> Analgesia: requirements low with local anaesthetic use. NSAIDs may be contraindicated due to comorbidities.

Reference
Malhotra S, Sodhi V. Anaesthesia for thyroid and parathyroid surgery. *Contin Educ Anaesth Crit Care Pain*. 2007; 7 (2): 55–58.

A 56-year-old man is listed for elective surgery. He received an orthotopic heart transplant 12 years before.

a) What key alterations in cardiac physiology and function must be considered when planning general anaesthesia? (50%)

b) What are the implications of the patient's immunosuppressant therapy for perioperative care? (30%)

c) What long-term health issues may occur in this type of patient? (20%)

March 2013

27% pass rate.

It is not uncommon to have a patient presenting for surgery that has received a transplanted organ and is on immunosuppressive therapy. A similar question was asked in October 2001. This question proved to be the most difficult question on the paper. A majority of the candidates demonstrated poor understanding of the physiology of a transplanted heart and the side effects of immunosuppressive therapy of relevance to the anaesthetist.

> Increased infection risk – may need antibiotic prophylaxis/strict asepsis.
> Common agents cause a degree of chronic kidney disease.
> Avoid NSAIDs – enhanced side effects.
> Important to maintain stable plasma levels – ensure drugs taken/given.
> IV steroid cover may be required.
> Cyclosporine enhances and azothioprine reduces aminosteroid NMB action.

a) What key alterations in cardiac physiology and function must be considered when planning general anaesthesia? (50%)

> Cardiac allograft vasculopathy: immunologically and non-immunologically (hyperlipidaemia, hypertension, hyperglycaemia) mediated. Heart is denervated so may present at a late stage with e.g. arrhythmias or left ventricular dysfunction. Must maintain coronary perfusion pressure and consider myocardial oxygen demand perioperatively. Patients are followed up with echo (function), endomyocardial biopsy (rejection) and surveillance angiogram (coronary artery disease).
> Permanent pacemaker: the heart rate is dependent on donor sinoatrial node activity. Surgical disruption to blood supply during transplantation may cause persistent bradycardia necessitating pacemaker insertion.
> Conduction abnormalities: due to surgical disruption to blood supply to atrioventricular node or other conduction pathways. Detection of intraoperative ischaemia may therefore be difficult.
> Loss of autonomic innervation:
  • Loss of vagal tone. Resting heart rate is 90–100/minute due to ongoing effect of circulating catecholamines.
  • The heart rate response to intraoperative triggers such as laryngoscopy, pain, or light anaesthesia is lost.
  • Loss of baroreceptor reflex: if systemic vascular resistance drops due to anaesthetic drugs, there is no compensatory heart rate increase. Starling's law therefore determines cardiac output – it is therefore important to maintain preload.
> Denervation effects on pharmacology:
  • Heart is denervated. Atropine, glycopyrrolate, neostigmine and suxamethonium have no effect on heart rate.
  • Denervation supersensitivity to adrenaline, noradrenaline, adenosine.

b) What are the implications of the patient's immunosuppressant therapy for perioperative care? (30%)

Common combination = antimetabolite (azathioprine, mycofenolate mofetil) + antiproliferative (tacrolimus, cyclosporin) + steroid.

Important to maintain consistent plasma levels in perioperative period to avoid rejection:

> Consider period of starvation, suitable intravenous formulations not always available.
> Postoperative nausea and vomiting, or ileus will impact on absorption.
> Discuss with transplant centre.

Specific issues with certain drugs:

> Cyclosporin is nephrotoxic. Many antibiotics and amiodarone increase concentrations, therefore increasing the risk of renal damage. Cyclosporin plus other nephrotoxins (NSAIDs, aminoglycosides) increases the risk of nephrotoxicity. Chronic kidney disease impacts on choice of drugs (neuromuscular blocking agents, opioids).
> Cyclosporin causes elevated blood pressure.
> Tacrolimus and steroids are diabetogenic.
> Steroids cause hypertension, thinning of skin, raised BMI – all of which have perioperative implications.
> Steroid cover for major surgery may be necessary.

Susceptibility to infection:

> Strict asepsis, remove unnecessary lines as soon as possible.
> High index of suspicion of infection in unusual sites with unusual organisms.
> Prompt microbiological advice if infection suspected/discuss need for prophylaxis.

c) What long-term health issues may occur in this type of patient? (20%)

> Cardiac allograft vasculopathy.
> Rejection causing reduction in graft function.
> Chronic kidney disease due to immunosuppression.
> Malignancy (squamous cell carcinoma, lymphoma) due to immunosuppression.
> Hypertension due to immunosuppression and its consequent organ damage, e.g. heart, kidneys.
> Effects of systemic disease that caused the need for transplant in the first place (atherosclerosis, sarcoid, amyloid, diabetes).
> Effects of diabetes caused by steroids or tacrolimus.

Reference

Morgan-Hughes N, Hood G. Anaesthesia for a patient with a cardiac transplant. *BJA CEPD Rev*. 2002; 2 (3): 74–78.

a) Outline the production and circulation of cerebrospinal fluid (CSF) and how intracranial pressure affects production and absorption. (5 marks)

b) How does the biochemistry of CSF differ from plasma? (4 marks)

c) List the indications for lumbar puncture. (6 marks)

d) Which factors predispose to the development of a post-dural puncture headache after lumbar puncture? (5 marks)

September 2015

Chairman's Report

For example, in question 1 of this exam about CSF, part (d) asked for factors predisposing to the development of a post-dural puncture headache after lumbar puncture. Unfortunately, many candidates talked about the factors that increase the risk of accidental dural puncture and, whilst the information they gave on that topic was correct, it was not what was asked for so they could not be given any marks.

50.9% pass rate.

This was one of the easy questions in the paper, so we would have expected the pass rate to have been a little higher. As mentioned above, some candidates did not answer the question asked in part (d) so lost marks.

a) Outline the production and circulation of cerebrospinal fluid (CSF) and how intracranial pressure affects production and absorption. (5 marks)

> Choroid plexuses (tufts of capillaries) secrete sodium into the lateral and 4th ventricles creating osmotic pressure that draws water with it thus creating CSF.
> Production rate of 500 ml/day, but constant reabsorption means volume present is only approximately 150 ml.
> Circulation of CSF occurs throughout the ventricles and down the spinal canal. It enters the subarachnoid space via the foramina of Luschka and Magendie.
> Absorption is via arachnoid granulations, outpouchings of the arachnoid through the dura that exist in close proximity to venous sinuses. CSF pressure is higher than venous pressure, favouring reabsorption of the CSF into the venous system.
> Small increases in ICP can be 'buffered' by movement of CSF out of the ventricles and down to the spinal cord.
> Production is opposed if intracranial pressure rises, causing CSF hydrostatic pressure to oppose the osmotic pressure generated by sodium secretion.
> Reabsorption is dependent on pressure gradient from CSF to venous system so the rate of reabsorption is increased if intracranial pressure rises.

b) How does the biochemistry of CSF differ from plasma? (4 marks)

I would hope that a description of the differences would suffice here, rather than actual values. I don't think I would be prepared to give brain space to memorising the actual values.

> Osmolarity of CSF and serum is equal.
> CSF sodium levels are higher than plasma due to active secretion. Chloride is also higher as it accompanies sodium to maintain electrical neutrality.
> All other ions found in plasma are also found in the CSF but at a lower level.
> CSF glucose is approximately two-thirds of the level of plasma or more.
> CSF protein content is very low in disease-free state.

c) List the indications for lumbar puncture. (6 marks)

It's easy to just list our specialty's encounters with lumbar puncture, but, just as with indications for arterial cannulation, try to think of reasons why other specialties may need to access the subarachnoid space.

Diagnosis
> Central nervous system (CNS) infections such as meningitis or encephalitis due to viral, bacterial, fungal or mycobacterial causes.
> Subarachnoid haemorrhage.
> CNS diseases such as Guillain–Barré, multiple sclerosis.
> Carcinomatous meningitis.
> Intrathecal administration of contrast media for myelography or cisternography.

Therapy
> Intrathecal administration of chemotherapy or antibiotics.
> Therapeutic relief of idiopathic intracranial hypertension or for spinal drain insertion.

Anaesthesia
> Spinal anaesthesia.

d) Which factors predispose to the development of a post-dural puncture headache after lumbar puncture? (5 marks)

> Multiple punctures.
> Larger-gauge needle.
> Use of traumatic, cutting needle rather than pencil-point.
> Age: increased incidence in young adults (20–40 years), lower incidence in older adults, lower perceived rate in children but probably due to failure to report.
> Gender: more common in women.
> Increased incidence in pregnancy.
> Lower body mass index.

References

Aitkenhead A, Moppet I, Thompson J. *Smith and Aitkenhead's Textbook of Anaesthesia*. 6th Edition. Churchill Livingstone; 2013.

Turnbull D, Shepherd D. Post-dural puncture headache: pathogenesis, prevention and treatment. *Br J Anaesth*. 2003; 91 (5): 718–729.

Wrobel M, Volk T. Post-dural puncture headache. *Anesth Pain*. 2012; 1 (4): 273–274.

a) List the effects of cigarette smoking on the cardiovascular system and on oxygen delivery, outlining the pathophysiological mechanisms involved. (12 marks)

b) List the effects of cigarette smoking on the respiratory system, other than those you have outlined above, that are relevant to the conduct of general anaesthesia. (4 marks)

c) What advice would you give a smoker 24 hours before a scheduled procedure under general anaesthesia and why? (4 marks)

September 2015

Chairman's Report

55.5% pass rate.

The relevance of this question to everyday practice makes the fact that it was well answered all the more pleasing. Candidates who lost marks generally did so because they did not know the pathophysiological mechanisms involved in the difficulties caused by smoking. Remember that applied physiology is also part of the syllabus.

a) List the effects of cigarette smoking on the cardiovascular system and on oxygen delivery, outlining the pathophysiological mechanisms involved. (12 marks)

Cardiovascular:
> Hypertension: raised circulating catecholamine levels and accelerated atherosclerosis formation increase left ventricular afterload, resulting in left ventricular hypertrophy, diastolic dysfunction and, ultimately, heart failure.
> Tachycardia: raised circulating catecholamine levels due to stimulation of nicotinic receptors.
> Peripheral vascular disease: accelerated atherosclerosis formation.
> Ischaemic heart disease: accelerated atherosclerosis formation and prothrombotic state (due to carbon monoxide, nicotine and other chemicals in cigarette smoke causing polycythaemia, enhanced platelet action, increased fibrinogen levels).
> Heart failure: subsequent to infarction, ischaemia and cardiac muscle damage.

Oxygen delivery:
> Airway conditions related to smoking that result in reduced oxygen availability within the alveolus and reduced effective gas exchange. Hypoxic hypoxia.
> Carboxyhaemoglobin formation: haemoglobin has a 250-fold increased affinity for carbon monoxide compared to oxygen, thus reducing oxygen carriage. Anaemic hypoxia.
> Shift of oxygen dissociation curve to left: carbon monoxide shifts the dissociation curve reducing the ability of hemoglobin to release oxygen. Anaemic hypoxia.
> Inhibition of cytochrome oxidase by carbon monoxide, reducing oxygen-dependent synthesis of ATP in mitochondria. Histotoxic hypoxia.

The combined effect is reduced oxygen delivery to the myocardium during a time of increased need, resulting in increased risk of ischaemia, which further promotes carboxyhaemoglobin formation, further reducing myocardial oxygen delivery, increasing the risk of perioperative ischaemia and infarction.

b) List the effects of cigarette smoking on the respiratory system, other than those you have outlined above, that are relevant to the conduct of general anaesthesia. (4 marks)

> Pre-existing airways disease as a result of smoking such as cancer, chronic obstructive pulmonary disease.
> Increased upper airway irritability: breath-holding, laryngospasm at induction and instrumentation.
> Increased lower airway reactivity, bronchospasm, mucus secretion.
> Impaired mucociliary transport and secretion clearance: risk of atelectasis, postoperative pneumonia, shunt.
> Accelerated rate of FEV_1 reduction with age: significantly reduced level predictive of postoperative respiratory complications.
> Increased closing capacity.
> Increased risk of pulmonary embolism due to hypercoagulability: thromboembolic preventative measures to be taken.

c) What advice would you give a smoker 24 hours before a scheduled procedure under general anaesthesia and why? (4 marks)

To stop smoking for the remaining 24 hours preoperatively and, ideally, to stop thereafter:

> Circulating catecholamine levels return to normal within 1 hour and carboxyhaemoglobin clearance occurs within 24 hours, thus massively improving oxygen delivery to all tissues including the myocardium, reducing the risk of perioperative ischaemic event. As oxygen carriage improves, physiological reserve to cope with perioperative periods of inadvertent hypoxia improves.

> Postoperatively, ongoing smoking is known to be associated with poor tissue healing, including wounds, anastomoses, flaps. Blood hypercoagulability will start to improve as carbon monoxide levels fall, reducing risk of postoperative thrombotic events.

Reference

Moppett I, Curran J. Smoking and the surgical patient. *CEPD Rev*. 2001; 1 (4): 122–124.

a) What physiological factors determine the rate of fall in arterial oxygen saturation in an apnoeic patient (3 marks), and which patient groups are most likely to show a rapid fall? (4 marks)

b) How may oxygenation, prior to intubation, be optimised during a rapid sequence induction (8 marks), and how can its progress be measured? (1 mark)

c) What are the possible respiratory complications of prolonged delivery of 100% oxygen? (4 marks)

March 2016

Chairman's Report

44.4% pass rate.

Again the pass rate for this question was low. The physiology surrounding oxygenation and the practice of preoxygenation should be well understood by candidates as this subject is very relevant to every day clinical practice. As mentioned above applied physiology is part of the syllabus, yet many candidates had no knowledge of the physiology in part (a). Part (b) was also poorly answered, with candidates failing to give sufficient detail about how to effectively preoxygenate a patient.

This question requires the same knowledge as that from March 2012 and the question four years before that in 2008.

a) What physiological factors determine the rate of fall in arterial oxygen saturation in an apnoeic patient (3 marks), and which patient groups are most likely to show a rapid fall? (4 marks)

This is essentially the same as part (a) of the question from March 2012. The organisation of the answer is just a bit different. When two separate questions appear together like this, be really careful to answer both parts.

1. Reservoir available (size of the functional residual capacity, FRC, and its oxygen content).
2. Rate of oxygen consumption.
3. Patency of airway.

At normal steady state, oxygen is removed from the lungs at the rate of its consumption (approximately 250 ml/min in a textbook adult). Carbon dioxide delivery to the lungs is 80% of this, as determined by a respiratory quotient of 0.8. After apnoea, oxygen removal from the lungs persists at the same rate. However, as the partial pressure of carbon dioxide in the alveoli starts to rise, the concentration gradient between blood and alveoli reduces, negatively impacting on further movement of carbon dioxide into the lungs. Lung volume consequently falls. If the airway is patent, this results in apnoeic mass movement of gas (oxygen, if anaesthetic mask is still firmly held in place) into the lungs, significantly extending the time to desaturation (although not addressing acidosis and hypercapnoea).

Patients most likely to show a rapid fall in oxygen consumption:

Patients with low FRC:
> Poor positioning prior to induction (FRC is less when supine, FRC can be improved by head-up tilt).
> Encroachment on FRC (obesity, pregnancy, ascites, bowel obstruction, kyphoscoliosis).
> Age (lower FRC per unit weight in children).

Patients with reduced oxygen content of FRC:
> Lung disease causing shunt reduces effectiveness of preoxygenation.
> Lung disease causing elevated $PaCO_2$ (according to the alveolar gas equation, an elevated $PaCO_2$ results in a reduced PAO_2).

Patients with increased rate of oxygen consumption:
> Sepsis.
> Thyrotoxicosis.
> Pregnancy.
> Critical illness.

> Fasciculations secondary to suxamethonium.
> Childhood – greater oxygen consumption per unit weight.

b) How may oxygenation, prior to intubation, be optimised during a rapid sequence induction (8 marks), and how can its progress be measured? (1 mark)

This differs from part (b) of the March 2012 question in that it is asking about how oxygenation can <u>continue</u> to be optimised even after preoxygenation has been completed. It really is so important to read the question, underlining bits if necessary.

> Explanation to and consent from patient will assist compliance.
> Head-up tilt to increase the size of FRC.
> Manage any issues that are reversibly causing an impact on FRC, e.g. aspirate gastric contents in a patient with small bowel obstruction, use of non-invasive ventilation to recruit areas of atelectasis.
> Tight-fitting mask (anaesthetic machine circuit) to ensure no entrainment of room air.
> 100% FiO_2.
> Gas flow to exceed patient's minute ventilation to ensure gas in circuit remains 100% oxygen whilst patient is still breathing, and high flow facilitates apnoeic mass movement after cessation of breathing.
> 5 minutes.
> Tidal breathing.
> Keep mask in situ and maintain airway patency until ready to intubate.
> High-flow transnasal humidified oxygenation after mask removal may help maintain oxygenation by apnoeic mass movement and maintenance of airway patency through positive airway pressure. Research into the use of such methods instead of standard preoxygenation techniques is ongoing.
> Standard nasal cannulae delivering high-flow oxygen may help maintain oxygenation by mass movement after mask removal. They can be fixed into place before starting preoxygenation as long as they do not negatively affect the seal of the face mask.
> Progress can be measured by monitoring the fraction of expired oxygen (F_EO_2), aiming for greater than 0.9.

c) What are the possible respiratory complications of prolonged delivery of 100% oxygen? (4 marks)

> Oxygen leaves the lung and enters the blood, driven by a concentration gradient that is generated by the body's constant utilisation of oxygen. When breathing room air, the collapse of alveoli is prevented by the ongoing presence of nitrogen within them; nitrogen is in equilibrium with its concentration in blood. However, if breathing 100% oxygen, alveolar collapse occurs as oxygen leaves. This results in <u>atelectasis</u>.
> Areas of perfused lung that are no longer being ventilated results in <u>shunt</u>.
> Hypoxic pulmonary vasoconstriction works to reduce perfusion to unventilated portions of the lung. However, this results in <u>raised pulmonary vascular resistance</u> and risk of right heart dysfunction and alveolar capillary leak in susceptible patients.
> Atelectatic areas of lung are at risk of development of <u>pneumonia</u>.
> Efforts to re-recruit atelectatic lungs may result in <u>volu- and barotrauma</u>.
> Patients with type 2 respiratory failure may be dependent on a degree of hypoxaemia to maintain respiratory drive. Loss of this drive due to prolonged administration of 100% oxygen may result in hypoventilation, raised arterial carbon dioxide and consequent obtundation.

Reference

Patel A, Nouraei S. Transnasal Humidified Rapid-Insufflation Ventilatory Exchange (THRIVE): a physiological method of increasing apnoea time in patients with difficult airways. *Anaesthesia*. 2015; 70: 323–329.

a) Define pulmonary hypertension. (2 marks)

b) What are the causes of pulmonary hypertension? (5 marks)

c) What are the specific anaesthetic goals when anaesthetising a patient with pulmonary hypertension? (7 marks)

d) What pharmacological treatments are available for this condition? (6 marks)

September 2017

52.7% pass rate.

This was one of the questions that the examiners thought would prove difficult, so it is good to see a respectable pass rate. Part (b) of the question asked for causes of pulmonary hypertension and some candidates displayed a poor understanding of cardiac physiology in answering this, seemingly confusing the right and left sides of the heart. In part (c) where candidates were asked about anaesthetic goals when anaesthetizing a patient with pulmonary hypertension, some gave very generic answers related to cardiac disease in general, rather than outlining specific goals for this condition.

The examiners thought this was a difficult question and so only 10–11/20 would have been required to pass.

a) Define pulmonary hypertension. (2 marks)

Mean pulmonary artery pressure of 25 mm Hg or greater at rest or 30 mm Hg on exercising.

b) What are the causes of pulmonary hypertension? (5 marks)

> Pulmonary arterial hypertension:
  • Idiopathic (may be familial, abnormal genes have been identified).
  • Associated with systemic disease such as connective tissue diseases, HIV, chronic haemolytic anaemia.
  • Drug and toxin associated.
  • Persistent pulmonary hypertension of the newborn.
> Left heart disease.
> Chronic lung disease.
> Chronic thromboembolic disease.
> Other unclear underlying cause.

c) What are the specific anaesthetic goals when anaesthetising a patient with pulmonary hypertension? (7 marks)

Chronic pulmonary hypertension results in hypertrophy of the right heart. It therefore requires better perfusion due to the increased muscle bulk but actually gets less, resulting in ischaemia. Coronary perfusion occurs in diastole and is dependent on aortic root pressure and so is compromised by tachycardia, poor left ventricular output and reduced systemic afterload. Reduced right ventricular output and deviation of the interventricular septum due to overfilling of the right ventricle may result in reduced left heart filling and consequent reduced output. A rise in pulmonary vascular resistance may result in acute right heart failure.

Avoidance of increased pulmonary vascular resistance. Triggers include the following:
> Hypoxaemia.
> Hypercarbia.
> Hypothermia.
> Pain.
> Acidaemia.
> High airway pressures and PEEP.
> Use of nitrous oxide.

Avoidance of reduction in systemic vascular resistance (coronary perfusion being dependent on perfusion pressure at aortic root):
> Invasive blood pressure monitoring starting prior to induction to facilitate rapid response to a decrease in blood pressure: aim to maintain BP at preoperative values.

> Cardiostable induction using increased opioid dose, reduced induction agent dose.
> Use of vasoconstrictor to mitigate vasodilatory effects of commonly used anaesthetic agents.

Avoidance of reduction in preload:
> Treat blood loss rapidly.
> Appropriate fluid loading in response to vasodilatory effects of general or neuraxial anaesthetic techniques.
> Consideration of cardiac output monitoring to guide fluid administration.

Maintenance of sinus rhythm, normal rate:
> Avoidance of causes of tachycardia: pain, light anaesthesia, drugs.
> Avoidance of bradycardia: prompt management of reflex bradycardia due to vagal stimulation, beware of effect of loss of thoracic sympathetic stimulation associated with high spinal blockade.

d) What pharmacological treatments are available for this condition? (6 marks)

Treatment of underlying condition:
> Long-term anticoagulation with warfarin to reduce thromboembolic risk.
> Inhaled beta-2-agonists and steroid treatment as part of the management of chronic lung disease.
> Diuretics and angiotensin-converting-enzyme inhibitor or angiotensin receptor blocker as part of the management of left heart disease.

General treatment for patients with pulmonary hypertension:
> Warfarin or direct oral anticoagulants (abnormal vasculature may predispose to clots in the pulmonary vessels causing further deterioration).
> Diuretics to reduce fluid retention associated with right heart failure.
> Oxygen to raise oxygen saturations and cause pulmonary vasodilatation.

Targeted treatment to cause pulmonary vasodilatation in idiopathic pulmonary arterial hypertension:
> Calcium channel blockers.
> Endothelin receptor antagonists.
> Phosphodiesterase 5 inhibitors.
> Prostaglandins.
> Soluble guanylate cyclase stimulators.

References

Elliot C, Kiely D. Pulmonary hypertension. *Contin Educ Anaesth Crit Care Pain*. 2006; 6 (1): 17–22.

Pilkington S, Taboada D, Martinez G. Pulmonary hypertension and its management in patients undergoing non-cardiac surgery. *Anaesthesia*. 2015; 70: 56–70.

25. PHYSICS AND CLINICAL MEASUREMENT

a) What types of infusion control devices are used in clinical settings? (15%)

b) What are the general (35%) and specific (20%) characteristics of pumps used for target controlled infusion (TCI) anaesthesia?

c) What precautions should be undertaken to guarantee drug delivery when administering total intravenous anaesthesia (TIVA)? (30%)

September 2011

a) What types of infusion control devices are used in clinical settings? (15%)

Non-electrical:
> Manually adjustable clamps, e.g. roller clamp on standard fluid administration set.
> Elastomeric pumps.

Electrical:
> Volumetric pumps.
> Syringe drivers.

b) What are the general (35%) and specific (20%) characteristics of pumps used for target controlled infusion (TCI) anaesthesia?

General:
> Mains and rechargeable battery powered with alarm if threat of power loss.
> Clear user interface, control buttons and screen.
> Clamp or other fixing device to position pump close to the level of the patient.
> Short- and long-term accuracy in infusion rate.
> Able to deliver a bolus with accuracy of volume.
> Able to be purged.
> High-pressure detection with alarm in the event of occlusion.
> Minimal post-occlusion bolus ('back-off' facility).
> Alarm/notification of user in event of incorrectly inserted syringe.
> Alarm in the event of infusion nearing end.
> Ability to program small variations in flow rate over a wide range of rates.
> Secure fitting of syringe into driver mechanism.

Specific:
> Programmed with TCI algorithms (some only programmed for a specific drug, others have a range of algorithms).
> Ability to input patient's weight and age.
> Screen that clearly shows the drug and algorithm in use as well as other key information such as effect site or plasma concentration.
> Specific syringe compatibilities (some only work with specific syringes, e.g. the Diprifusor with propofol in pre-prepared syringes with magnetic strip).

c) What precautions should be undertaken to guarantee drug delivery when administering total intravenous anaesthesia (TIVA)? (30%)

A large chunk of the marks were for this part of the question. Guaranteeing drug delivery in TIVA was the focus of a Safe Anaesthesia Liaison Group publication in 2009. However, even if you hadn't read the report, if you have used TIVA, have attended M&M meetings and structure your answer, you should be able to pick up many of the points.

Organisational:
> Pumps should undergo regular maintenance checks.
> Staff should be trained in pump use.
> Anaesthetist should have adequate training in TIVA prior to using TIVA solo.
> Pumps to be plugged in to charge when not in use.
> Pumps should be standardised within each trust.

Prior to use:
> Check that the pump is functioning and has run self-check.
> Correct entry of patient data.
> Correct drug in syringe, correctly drawn up (check with second person) and correct algorithm entered.
> Syringe intact and correctly seated in the mechanism to avoid siphoning.
> Priming of line to minimise 'backlash' and to eliminate air bubbles.
> Dedicated line/multilumen connector with low compliance tubing – anti-reflux valve in any other line, correctly orientated. Monitor for disconnections.

During use:
> Cannula visible at all times to check for disconnection/extravasation.
> Pump at similar height to the patient to minimise risk of siphoning or under-delivery of drug.
> Keep pump plugged in when possible.
> Intermittent check that the expected volume of drug has been infused.
> Respond appropriately to pump alarms.

References

Keay S, Callander C. The safe use of infusion devices. *Contin Educ Anaesth Crit Care Pain*. 2004; 4 (3): 81–85.

Safe Anaesthesia Liaison Group. Guaranteeing drug delivery in total intravenous anaesthesia. 2009. https://www.rcoa.ac.uk/system/files/CSQ-PS-2-Safety-notification-TIVA.pdf [Accessed 20th December 2017].

a) How may ultrasound techniques be used in anaesthetic and critical care practice? (40%)

b) What information can echocardiography provide in a haemodynamically unstable patient? (45%)

c) What is the Doppler effect? How may this be used in echocardiography? (15%)

September 2011

The College LOVES ultrasound. There are four questions based on its use over the 13 papers that this book covers.

a) How may ultrasound techniques be used in anaesthetic and critical care practice? (40%)

> Airway:
  • Check for anterior vessels prior to percutaneous tracheostomy.
> Respiratory:
  • Locate pleural effusions to guide insertion of pleural drains.
  • Identify areas of consolidation or oedema.
> Cardiovascular:
  • Identification of vessels for cannulation, both peripheral and central.
  • Transoesophageal/thoracic echo: to guide fluid management, assess ejection fraction, detect air embolism, assess valvular function, detect tamponade or even complete echocardiographic assessment of the heart.
  • Oesophageal Doppler: optimise filling, inotrope and vasopressor use.
  • Identification of pericardial effusion.
  • FAST (focused assessment with sonography for trauma) scanning: assessment of bleeding in thorax or abdomen.
> Neurological:
  • Identification of nerves for peripheral nerve blocks.
  • Identification of epidural space.
  • Transcranial Doppler ultrasonography.
> Gastrointestinal:
  • To guide insertion of abdominal drain.
  • Identification of ascites for drainage.

b) What information can echocardiography provide in a haemodynamically unstable patient? (45%)

> Preload assessment:
  • Reduced left ventricular end-diastolic area (LVED) and left ventricular end-systolic area (LVES) indicate reduced preload.
  • 'Kissing' papillary muscles in systole indicates hypovolaemia.
> Assessment of systemic vascular resistance:
  • Normal LVED and reduced LVES indicate reduced systemic vascular resistance as seen in anaphylaxis or sepsis.
> Myocardial function:
  • Contractility and thickening of myocardium during systole indicate left ventricular systolic function.
  • Regional wall motion abnormalities may indicate ischaemia.
  • Assessment of right heart function.
> Specific diagnoses:
  • Left ventricular outflow tract obstruction.
  • Cardiac tamponade.
  • Valvular disease, or paravalvular leak or valve malfunction following replacement.
  • Endocarditis.
  • Aortic dissection.
  • Trauma: pericardial collection, myocardial contusion, mediastinal haematoma, aortic dissection/transection, pleural collections.
  • Thromboembolic disease: right ventricular dilatation and dysfunction. Rarely, thrombus may be seen in the right ventricle or pulmonary arteries.

c) What is the Doppler effect? How may this be used in echocardiography? (15%)

Two questions in one, make sure you answer both parts.

The Doppler effect is the change in perceived frequency of a sound wave when the source is moving in relation to the observer. The frequency, and therefore pitch, increases as the distance between observer and source reduces.

$$V = \frac{\Delta F.c}{2F_0.cos\theta}$$

V = velocity of object

ΔF = frequency shift $(F_R - F_0)$

c = speed of sound in blood

F_0 = frequency of emitted sound

θ = angle between sound and object

Ultrasound provides the image of the structure of the heart itself, but Doppler provides the information about all moving aspects of the echocardiography study:

> Valve function, direction of flow, turbulent flow due to stenosis.
> Cardiac output.
> Dynamic obstructions.
> Coronary artery flow.

References

Cross M, Plunkett E. *Physics, Pharmacology and Physiology for Anaesthetists Key Concepts for the FRCA*. Cambridge: Cambridge Medicine; 2008.
Roscoe A, Strang T. Echocardiography in intensive care. *Contin Educ Anaesth Crit Care Pain*. 2008; 8 (2): 46–49.

a) How may ultrasound techniques be used in anaesthetic and critical care practice? (30%)

b) What information can echocardiography provide in a haemodynamically unstable patient? (50%)

c) What is the Doppler effect? How may this be used in clinical practice? (20%)

March 2012

Chairman's Report

66.5% pass rate.

In general, candidates demonstrated sound clinical knowledge but had greater difficulty in explaining the Doppler effect and how the principle is applied. This question was used in the September 2011 paper.

This question is very similar to that from just six months earlier. Parts (a) and (b) are identical except that the weighting of points for each has changed. This time, part (c) is asking about all clinical applications of Doppler, not just about its use in echocardiography.

c) What is the Doppler effect? How may this be used in clinical practice? (20%)

First part of this answer is as it was last time. The second part of the question highlights the importance of being observant in your day-to-day practice.

> Echocardiography: flow across valves, cardiac output, dynamic obstructions, coronary artery flow.
> Fetal wellbeing: umbilical artery flow, fetal heart rate.
> Transcranial Doppler: cerebral perfusion.
> Oesophageal Doppler: blood velocity in descending aorta to indicate cardiac output and guide fluid and vasopressor use.
> Peripheral pulses and blood pressure: assessment of patients with peripheral vascular disease.

a) Outline the principles of capnography using infrared light absorption. (30%)

b) What diagnostic information can be gained from capnography in anaesthetic practice? (40%)

c) In which clinical situations and locations should continuous capnography be available for use? (30%)

March 2012

Chairman's Report

60.8% pass rate.

a) Outline the principles of capnography using infrared light absorption. (30%)

> Molecules containing dissimilar atoms absorb infrared light, resulting in molecular vibration.
> A small proportion of the patient's expired gas is diverted to the capnography sample chamber.
> Infrared (generated by a heated wire) is filtered to the appropriate wavelength and passed through the sample chamber and a reference chamber.
> The chamber windows are made of crystal, as glass will absorb infrared, thus affecting overall absorption.
> The proportion of infrared absorbed by the carbon dioxide depends on the Beer-Lambert law, i.e. the concentration of the carbon dioxide present in the chamber (the variable being measured) and the path length (which is the distance within the chamber and is therefore fixed).
> The remaining radiation is focused onto a photodetector and an electronic monitor displays the exhaled carbon dioxide concentration and waveform.
> Modern capnographs use a disc of rotating filters in order to measure the concentration of volatile agents as well.

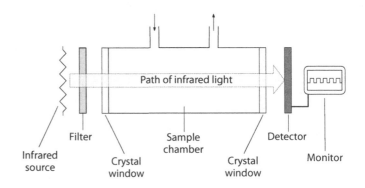

Capnograph monitor

b) What diagnostic information can be gained from capnography in anaesthetic practice? (40%)

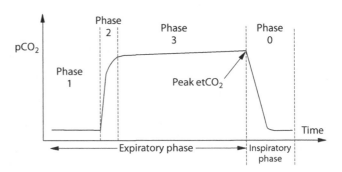

Capnograph waveform

Information is gained from the absolute value of end-tidal carbon dioxide (etCO$_2$) and the waveform.

	Value of etCO$_2$	Waveform
Ventilatory sufficiency	High if underventilated, low if overventilated.	Normal waveform, but height proportional to value of etCO$_2$. Rate will be demonstrated by the number of waveforms per unit time.
Respiratory disease, ranging from stable chronic obstructive pulmonary disease to acute bronchospasm under anaesthesia	May be normal or elevated.	Gradually upsloping phase 3, failure to achieve plateau.
Acute reduction or loss of cardiac output	Rapidly reducing etCO$_2$ value.	Normal morphology but waveform rapidly reducing in size with sequential breaths.
Soda lime exhaustion or inadequate fresh gas flow rate	Elevated etCO$_2$.	Baseline not returning to zero between breaths.
Disconnection of breathing system/accidental extubation/dislodgement of tracheostomy tube	No etCO$_2$.	Sudden loss of trace.
Inadequate paralysis	If inadequate paralysis interferes with effective ventilation, etCO$_2$ will rise.	Clefts in the plateau phase of the trace. Extra, small waveforms interspersed in the overall trace.
Incorrect tube placement	Reducing value of etCO$_2$, if any at all.	It is possible that there may be approximately three smaller-than-usual waveforms after oesophageal intubation (as carbon dioxide present in the stomach is expelled), or there may be no trace at all.
Malignant hyperthermia	Rapidly rising etCO$_2$ value.	Morphology of the trace will remain normal, but the height of the waveform will rise with successive breaths.

c) In which clinical situations and locations should continuous capnography be available for use? (30%)

This question featured a year after the updated statement from the AAGBI concerning when and where capnography should be used. The AAGBI's statement quoted NAP4 (then recently published), which stated that 80% of deaths from airway complications in the ICU and 50% of deaths from airway complications in ED were caused by absence of or failure of proper use of capnography.

> All anaesthetised patients, regardless of the airway device used or the location of the patient.
> All intubated patients, regardless of location.
> All patients undergoing moderate or deep sedation.
> All patients undergoing advanced life support.
> Continuous capnography should be available wherever patients are recovered from anaesthesia and moderate or deep sedation.

References

Association of Anaesthetists of Great Britain and Ireland. The use of capnography outside the operating theatre. Updated Statement from the Association of Anesthetists of Great Britain and Ireland. 2011.

Cook T, Woodall N, Frerk C (eds.). *4th National Audit Project of the Royal College of Anaesthetists and the Difficult Airway Society. Major Complications of Airway Management in the United Kingdom*. London: The Royal College of Anaesthetists and Association of Anaesthetists of Great Britain and Ireland; 2011.

Kerslake I, Kelly F. Uses of capnography in the critical care unit. *BJA Educ*. 2017; 17 (5): 178–183.

Langton J, Hutton A. Respiratory gas analysis. *Contin Educ Anaesth Crit Care Pain*. 2009; 9 (1): 19–23.

a) What are the advantages (15%) and disadvantages (20%) of low-flow anaesthesia?

b) Describe how a circle system should be checked before each anaesthetic? (45%)

c) What other components of the anaesthetic work-station must be checked before each anaesthetic? (20%)

March 2013

Chairman's Report

35.3% pass rate.

The answers to this question were very disappointing. Candidates should have far better knowledge of a breathing system that most would use every day. There is no excuse for the apparent ignorance of a safety checking system that should be performed many times a week, particularly when the Association of Anaesthetists of Great Britain and Ireland have recently published a safety guideline on checking anaesthetic equipment (2012). These new guidelines emphasise that checks of equipment should be undertaken before each operating session and then a shorter set of checks before each case.

35% of the marks for this question relate to science knowledge. Anyone who has ensured that they have kept up to date with important guidelines issued during the years leading up to this exam could have gained the remaining 65%.

a) What are the advantages (15%) and disadvantages (20%) of low-flow anaesthesia?

Advantages:
> Economy (reduced volatile use).
> Heat and moisture conservation (less relevant when HME used).
> Pollution reduction (chlorine-containing volatiles cause ozone destruction).

Disadvantages:
> Carbon dioxide absorber required.
> Gas analysis required (increasing difference between inspired gas concentrations and rotameter levels as anaesthesia continues).
> Leak-free circle system required (so not suitable for mask anaesthesia or if LMA poorly fitting or if uncuffed tube with large leak).
> Slow response to changed setting on vaporiser.
> Accumulation of unwanted gases:
  • Substances exhaled by patient: alcohol, methane, carbon monoxide, acetone, therefore contraindicated in intoxication, diabetic ketoacidosis, carbon monoxide poisoning.
  • Products of reaction with absorbents, e.g. carbon monoxide production resulting from reaction of desflurane and dry baralyme.

b) Describe how a circle system should be checked before each anaesthetic? (45%)

A circle system comprises: the fresh gas supply; the carbon dioxide absorption canister; the reservoir bag; unidirectional inspiratory and expiratory valves; and the pressure relief valve.

> Visual inspection: ensure correct configuration and assembly, no foreign material in tubing, no leaks in reservoir bag.
> Manually check: 'push & twist' all connections.
> Pressure leak test: between 20 and 60 cm H_2O, occlude patient end and squeeze reservoir bag, ensuring no leak.
> Carbon dioxide absorber: inspect contents, ensure adequate supply and ensure the colour indicates sufficient absorption capacity.
> Correct gas outlet selected.
> Two-bag test (after ventilator and vaporisers checked):
  • Attach a second bag on patient end (ensure angle piece and filter attached).
  • Set fresh gas flow to 5 l/min and manually ventilate – check whole breathing system patent and unidirectional valves are moving appropriately.

- Check function of APL by squeezing both bags together.
- Turn on ventilator. Turn off fresh gas flow. Turn on and off each vaporiser in turn – there should be no loss of volume.

c) What other components of the <u>anaesthetic work-station</u> must be checked before each anaesthetic? (20%)

> Breathing system:
  - System patent, leak-free, two-bag test.
  - Vaporisers correctly fitted, filled, leak free, plugged in if necessary.
  - Alternative systems (Bain, T-piece) checked.
  - Correct gas outlet selected.
> Ventilator: functioning and correctly configured.
> Airway equipment: full range required, working, with spares.
> Suction: clean, functioning.

Reference

Association of Anaesthetists of Great Britain and Ireland. Checking Anaesthetic Equipment 2012. *Anaesthesia*. 2012; 67: 660–668.

a) What are the indications for arterial cannulation? (35%)

b) How may an invasive arterial pressure measuring system be calibrated? (20%)

c) Outline the sources of error when measuring invasive arterial pressure. (45%)

March 2013

Chairman's Report

35.8% pass rate.

This question was poorly answered and therefore had a high failure rate despite a low pass mark being set. Many candidates wrongly interpreted the question as 'indications for intra-aortic balloon pump.' The indications for arterial cannulation were for measurement (continuous blood pressure; cardiac output; blood gases), diagnostic (angiography) and therapeutic purposes (thrombolysis, vasodilators chemotherapy, EVAR, ECMO, stenting, renal replacement therapy). Many candidates focused on aspects of measurement only. All transducers are calibrated in the factory, but calibration is carried out in the clinical environment using static and dynamic testing methods; a short description was all that was required. Sources of error included transducer drift, the causes of damping/resonance and incorrect transducer height. There appeared to be a lack of understanding of the physical principles of transducers and confusion between damping and resonance. The ODP might well calibrate the transducer for you, but this fact was not included in the model answer as it is important that anaesthetists understand the methods and principles of calibration even if they do not carry them out themselves.

A 'low' pass mark implies that this would have been viewed as a difficult question. The pass mark for these is 10–11/20. I think that it is unsurprising that anaesthetists did not come up with the range of indications for arterial cannulation as listed in the Chairman's Report. However, the answers to sections (b) and (c) would be straightforward to those who re-revised the primary syllabus.

a) What are the indications for arterial cannulation? (35%)

Measurement:
> Blood pressure monitoring (in ICU; on transfers; for patients who have arrhythmias, are on inotropes, or who are critically ill).
> Arterial blood gas analysis.
> Cardiac output monitoring.

Diagnostic:
> Angiography.

Therapeutic:
> Thrombolysis.
> Vasodilator administration.
> Chemotherapy administration.
> EVAR.
> ECMO.
> Stenting.
> Embolisation.
> Renal replacement therapy.

b) How may an invasive arterial pressure measuring system be calibrated? (20%)

Calibration: to set or check the graduations by comparison with a standard. I don't believe we truly calibrate the system clinically, but we do zero it, level it and then check that it gives roughly the same reading as noninvasive blood pressure monitoring.

The transducer will have been calibrated at the time of manufacture.

Before clinical use:

> Zero: aseptic technique, turn stopcock 'off' to patient, open cap to air, press 'zero' on IABP module, check the trace is at zero and the monitor states zero, replace cap, open three-way tap between patient and transducer. Atmospheric pressure is therefore set as zero and blood pressure is measured against that pressure.
> Level: once zeroed, the transducer must be placed level with the heart in order to ensure that the hydrostatic pressure of blood is not included in the blood pressure recording (4th intercostal space midaxillary line).
> Calibrate clinically: compare invasive with noninvasive blood pressure. Invasive systolic blood pressure is usually 5–10 mm Hg higher than NIBP, diastolic BP usually 5–10 mm Hg lower, mean should be the same.

c) Outline the sources of error when measuring invasive arterial pressure. (45%)

> Failure to zero.
> Failure to keep level with heart (a 10 cm error in positioning height will lead to a 7.4 mm Hg error in blood pressure recording).
> Transducer drift (repeated exposure of the transducer to pressure causes distortion of the materials with which it is made, causing sensed value to gradually drift away from actual value).
> Resonance. All objects have a natural frequency, a frequency at which the object will readily oscillate if force is applied to it at a frequency close to the natural frequency. This is resonance. If the natural frequency of the invasive blood pressure measuring system was similar to the frequencies of the sine waves that make up the arterial pressure waveform, then the system would resonate, causing the output of the system to be greater than it should be. So, the natural frequency of the measuring system is intentionally made higher than the frequencies of the waveforms that make up the arterial pulse. It is important that a short, rigid-walled cannula is used and that the tubing does not exceed 120 cm in length in order to maintain the high natural frequency of the measuring system.
> Over- or underdamping. Damping is a decrease in the amplitude of an oscillation as a result of energy losses within a system. Overly compliant tubing, air bubbles in the column of fluid between patient and transducer, clots in the cannula and an excess of three-way-taps will all result in overdamping. An underdamped system records an erroneously low systolic blood pressure and high diastolic pressure, although mean arterial pressure remains less affected. An underdamped system is unlikely to occur if the correct equipment is utilised in assembling an invasive blood pressure monitoring system.

Reference

Jones A, Pratt O. Physical principles of intra-arterial blood pressure measurement. *Anaesthesia Tutorial of the Week*. 2009; 137.

a) What are the indications for insertion of an implantable cardiac defibrillator (ICD)? (20%)

b) How might surgical diathermy affect the ICD? (20%)

c) A patient with an ICD is listed for elective surgery; what preparations are necessary preoperatively, intra-operatively and postoperatively? (45%)

d) How does the management differ if this patient requires emergency surgery? (15%)

March 2014

Chairman's Report

67.1% pass rate.

Generally well answered. Indications for a pacemaker are part of core knowledge incorporating many conditions which have a bearing on the management of anaesthesia. For section (c), some candidates gave generalized answers and failed to focus on the specifics of how the risk of an ICD working inappropriately, or failing to work when necessary, would influence anaesthetic practice. In an emergency situation, deactivation of the ICD would be a reasonable 'balance of risks' action.

a) What are the indications for insertion of an implantable cardiac defibrillator (ICD)? (20%)

> Patients with a history of serious ventricular arrhythmia who:
  • Have survived cardiac arrest.
  • Have had significant haemodynamic compromise or syncope.
  • Have left ventricular ejection fraction (LVEF) less than 35% but no worse than class III New York Heart Association function.
> Patients with familial conditions predisposing them to ventricular arrhythmia or following surgical correction of congenital heart disease.
> In conjunction with cardiac resynchronization therapy for selected patients with LVEF less than 35%.

b) How might surgical diathermy affect the ICD? (20%)

> Damage to and, therefore, malfunction of device.
> Sensing of diathermy by ICD as arrhythmia, resulting in inappropriate shock delivery.
> Energy induction in cardiac leads, resulting in tip heating and tissue damage. Scar development around the lead tips can cause changes in resistance and failure of the device to work.

c) A patient with an ICD is listed for elective surgery; what preparations are necessary preoperatively, intraoperatively and postoperatively? (45%)

They've given you the classification they want, make sure you follow it.

Preoperatively:
> Patient history and examination focusing on cardiac conditions and symptoms.
> Check electrolytes – increased risk of arrhythmia if abnormal.
> Device registration card:
  • Manufacturer, model number, serial number.
  • Implanting hospital, follow-up hospital.
  • Date of and reason for implant.
> ICD check within the last three months:
  Extent of any heart failure.
  • Battery life, leads, sensing, correct functioning.
> Discussion with surgeon regarding need for use of diathermy or any other possible risk of interference that may be interpreted as arrhythmia by ICD.
> Reprogramme ICD component to 'monitor only' mode – patient to have ECG monitoring from the time of ICD deactivation.
> Diathermy may be interpreted as cardiac activity by pacemaker, resulting in risk of asystole in a pacemaker-dependent patient. Pacemaker can be switched to fixed mode to avoid this.

Intraoperatively:
> Ensure availability of cardio-pulmonary resuscitation, temporary external/ transvenous pacing and external defibrillation equipment. Attach remote pads before surgery starts if this would be problematic to do

intraoperatively. Anterior–posterior positioning recommended to minimise current passage through device.

> Ensure availability of appropriate cardiac personnel especially cardiac physiologist.
> ECG monitoring throughout.
> Avoid diathermy use if possible. If diathermy needed, ideally use bipolar, keeping the cables away from the ICD as much as possible. If monopolar essential, ensure the return electrode is anatomically positioned so that the current pathway between the diathermy electrode and return electrode is as far away from the ICD (and leads) as possible. Limit use to short bursts.

Postoperatively:
> Patient to remain fully monitored in a high-observation area until ICD reactivated and checked for functionality.

d) How does the management differ if this patient requires emergency surgery? (15%)

> If the emergency surgery is during normal working hours with usual staffing, aim to follow the same approach as for elective surgery.
> If out-of-hours, or time not permitting, a clinical magnet secured over the implant site with surgical tape will deactivate shock mode. Any subsequent VT/VF will need to be treated using external defibrillation (although magnet can be removed and functionality should return within a number of seconds if problems with external defibrillation). The pacemaker component would be put into a fixed mode.

References

Medicines and Healthcare Products Regulatory Agency. Perioperative management of pacemakers/ICDs: Guidelines for the perioperative management of patients with implantable pacemakers or implantable cardioverter defibrillators, where the use of surgical diathermy/electrocautery is anticipated. 2006.

National Institute for Health and Care Excellence. Implantable cardioverter defibrillators and cardiac resynchronisation therapy for arrhythmias and heart failure [TA314]. June 2014.

Thomas H, Turley A, Plummer C. *British Heart Rhythm Society Guidelines for the Management of Patients with Cardiac Implantable Electronic Devices (CIEDs) Around the Time of Surgery*. British Heart Rhythm Society. 2016.

a) Outline the basic principles of ultrasound signal and image generation. (6 marks)

b) How may physical factors influence the image quality of an ultrasound device? (6 marks)

c) Which two needling techniques are commonly used in ultrasound-guided nerve blocks and what are the advantages and disadvantages of each? (8 marks)

September 2014

Chairman's Report

5.7% pass rate.

The very poor scores for this question were surprising given the widespread use of ultrasound imaging in current clinical practice. Eight marks were attainable for discussing two types of needling technique, hence this question was deemed to be moderately difficult and not hard. Despite this, many candidates failed to score more than five marks. A 'black box' approach was evident in the written answers and examiners questioned whether the candidates had any knowledge of the factors which affect the generation of a good quality ultrasound image. Previous reports from the SAQ Group Chair have emphasised that knowledge acquired in preparation for the Primary FRCA examination can be tested in any element of the Final FRCA process. This advice seems to have been largely ignored. The question was of moderate discriminatory value as ignorance of the topic was widespread within the candidate cohort.

This was deemed a moderate question and so a score of 12–13/20 would have been required to pass.

a) Outline the <u>basic</u> principles of ultrasound signal and image generation. (6 marks)

> The transducer contains a piezoelectric crystal. This means that current applied across it causes it to expand and contract as the polarity of the voltage changes.
> Ultrasound wave emission is therefore stimulated in the range of 2.5–15 MHz.
> The ultrasound wave is reflected at interfaces between structures of different acoustic impedance.
> The transducer is an emitter and receiver all-in-one: when the sound wave returns, it causes squeezing and stretching of the crystal, which generates a voltage change across the surface, thus transducing sound waves back into an electrical current, resulting in image generation.

b) How may physical factors influence the image quality of an ultrasound device? (6 marks)

> Attenuation: loss of energy of the ultrasound beam as it interacts with the tissues through which it passes. This affects higher-frequency ultrasound more than low. Attenuation occurs due to:
> • Divergence of the ultrasound beam.
> • Refraction: when the ultrasound beam hits an interface at an angle that is not 90°, the path of the ongoing beam deviates, resulting in artefact.
> • Scattering: when the ultrasound beam hits an object that is the same size or smaller than its own wavelength.
> • Absorption: resulting in heat generation.
> • Reflection: ultrasound bounces back at the interface of tissues with different acoustic impedances. Acoustic impedance is determined by the product of tissue density and the velocity of ultrasound within it. Reflection is the mechanism by which an ultrasound image is generated, but if reflection occurs at more superficial interfaces, then that part of the beam does not progress to deeper structures, where it would contribute to image generation. Acoustic shadowing is the absence of image of a tissue deep to a highly reflective surface such as an interface with bone, whereas post-cystic enhancement is the enhanced signal received from structures deep to fluid-filled spaces as the ultrasound passes readily through the fluid.

> Resolution: the ability to distinguish between two structural points. Includes lateral, axial and temporal resolution. Higher-frequency ultrasound waves improve axial resolution and focusing the ultrasound beam improves lateral resolution.
> Anisotropy: the image of tissues is dependent on the angle to the ultrasound beam at which they are viewed, with better resolution when the emitted and received ultrasound beams follow the same trajectory but in reverse. The image quality of a structure becomes poorer and disappears altogether as the angle between probe and skin becomes more acute.

c) Which two needling techniques are commonly used in ultrasound-guided nerve blocks and what are the advantages and disadvantages of each? (8 marks)

Long axis, in-plane:

Advantages:
- Needle visualised along full length.
- Good visualisation of needle tip near nerve.

Disadvantages:
- Difficult to keep full length of needle in view.
- Longer distance from skin to nerve, increased potential for pain (and possibly damage) as the needle passes through more structures.

Short axis, out-of-plane:

Advantages:
> Uses familiar entry points, comparable to non-ultrasound-guided nerve block techniques.
> Shortest skin–nerve distance.
> Less painful as the needle doesn't pass through muscle.

Disadvantages:
> Needle only seen as a bright dot when in the ultrasound beam.
> May be more difficult to visualise the proximity of the needle tip to the nerve.

References

Carty S, Nichols B. Ultrasound-guided regional anaesthesia. *Contin Educ Anaesth Crit Care Pain*. 2007; 7 (1): 20–24.

Ng A, Swanevelder J. Resolution in ultrasound imaging. *Contin Educ Anaesth Crit Care Pain*. 2011; 11 (5): 186–192.

a) Outline the basic physical principles involved in formation of an ultrasound image. (6 marks)

b) What patient factors (3 marks) and acoustic artefacts (4 marks) may influence the ultrasound image quality?

c) Which two needling techniques are commonly used in ultrasound-guided nerve blocks? (2 marks). List the advantages and disadvantages of one of these techniques. (5 marks)

September 2017

58.9% pass rate.

This question was used in a recent paper and was reused with only slight modification this time. The pass rate was significantly better on this occasion and it is good to see improved understanding of a technique that is a key component of modern anaesthesia. However, most marks were scored in part (c), the clinical application of ultrasound, with candidates still demonstrating a lack of knowledge of the basic scientific principles involved in generation of an image.

This question focuses on the same topics as the one on ultrasound in September 2014. The only difference is with part (b). It requires the same knowledge as part (b) from the previous question, but a slightly different approach is needed as it is asking about acoustic artefacts rather than the physical principles underlying image quality generation.

b) What patient factors (3 marks) and acoustic artefacts (4 marks) may influence the ultrasound image quality?

Patient factors:
> Obesity: increased distance of fat results in greater attenuation of ultrasound beam.
> Positioning: optimum imaging for some techniques requires specific patient positioning which may not be feasible, e.g. arm abduction for axillary nerve block, left lateral positioning during cardiac echo.
> Ability to comply with the study: patient will need to remain still to ensure best possible image generation, may not be feasible due to dementia, tremor, delirium.
> Previous surgical or traumatic disruption of the tissue to be imaged.

Acoustic artefacts:
> Contact artefact: where the probe is not in contact with the skin (via ultrasound gel), the image will be lost.
> Acoustic shadowing: much of the ultrasound beam is reflected back at interfaces between lesser and highly attenuating tissues. Tissues deep to these will therefore not be seen.
> Post-cystic enhancement: ultrasound passes readily through fluid filled structures, resulting in enhancement of structures deep to them.
> Lateral shadowing: when ultrasound beam hits the curved edges of a rounded structure, the beam is refracted and so does not bounce back to the ultrasound probe. Imaging of these parts of the structure is therefore lost.
> Reverberation artefact: reflection of the ultrasound beam from a highly reflective interface back to the probe, back to the interface, back to the probe, resulting in multiple representations of the same structure.
> Insufficient resolution: use of an ultrasound wavelength that is greater than the size of the structures being imaged may result in failure of the image to demonstrate the separation of those structures.
> Scattering: use of an ultrasound frequency of similar size or smaller than the structure being imaged will result in scattering of the reflected ultrasound beam rather than reflection of it back to the probe.
> Refraction: when the ultrasound beam hits an interface at an angle that is not 90°, the path of the ongoing beam deviates resulting in artefact.
> Anisotropy: the image of tissues is dependent on the angle to the ultrasound beam at which they are viewed, with better resolution when the emitted and received ultrasound beams follow the same trajectory but in reverse. The image quality of a structure becomes poorer and disappears altogether as the angle between the probe and the skin becomes more acute.

26. STATISTICAL BASIS OF TRIAL MANAGEMENT

A recent meta-analysis of studies of the utility of the Mallampati score in the prediction of a difficult airway found that it had a sensitivity of 60% and a specificity of 70%.

a) Outline what is meant by meta-analysis and the factors that ensure a high-quality conclusion from the process. (10 marks)

b) Explain what is meant by sensitivity and specificity as applied to the interpretation of the Mallampati data given above. (6 marks)

c) Rank the levels of scientific proof used to grade medical evidence. (4 marks)

September 2014

Chairman's Report

72.8% pass rate.

It was anticipated that candidates would find this subject matter to be difficult. Surprisingly, the question generated the highest overall pass rate, and the majority of candidates scored in excess of the pass mark. Weak candidates were unable to indicate how a high-quality conclusion can be ensured from a meta-analysis or to interpret the data for Mallampati studies in a meaningful way.

The CEACCP/BJA Education journals have a number of reasonably concise articles on statistics, addressing key concepts and definitions.

a) Outline what is meant by meta-analysis and the factors that ensure a high-quality conclusion from the process. (10 marks)

Meta-analysis: a quantitative* systematic review of data from all available primary studies that are similar in nature, in order to reach a valid statistical conclusion to a question.

Factors required for a high-quality conclusion:

> Clearly defined question as the basis of the analysis.
> Clear and reproducible methodology.
> Comprehensive search of all available electronic databases based on appropriate search terms, ensuring non-English studies are included.
> Clear and valid criteria for inclusion or exclusion of studies from the analysis, ensuring only studies of sufficient quality included.
> Consider publication bias to avoid risk of over-representation of studies with a positive outcome.

A systematic review is a qualitative review of all of the data of available similar studies.

Make sure you answer this question 'as applied to the interpretation of the Mallampati data given above' – read all questions carefully.

b) Explain what is meant by sensitivity and specificity as applied to the interpretation of the Mallampati data given above. (6 marks)

The sensitivity of a clinical test refers to the ability of the test to correctly identify those patients with the disease or issue in question.

The meta-analysis states that the Mallampati test has a sensitivity of 60%, which means that 60% of the people who have a difficult airway will be predicted as difficult by the Mallampati test.

$$\text{Sensitivity} = \frac{\text{True positives}}{\text{True positives} + \text{False negatives}}$$

The specificity of a clinical test refers to the ability of the test to correctly identify those patients without the disease or issue in question. The meta-analysis states that the Mallampati test has a specificity of 70%, which means that 70% of the patients assessed as having a straightforward airway will indeed have a straightforward airway.

$$\text{Specificity} = \frac{\text{True negatives}}{\text{True negatives} + \text{False positives}}$$

c) Rank the levels of scientific proof used to grade medical evidence. (4 marks)

1. Meta-analyses, randomised controlled trials (RCTs), or systematic reviews of RCTs.
2. Systematic reviews of, or individual, analytical non-RCTs such as case-control or cohort studies.
3. Non-analytic studies (for example, case reports, case series studies).
4. Expert opinion, formal consensus.

A grading code is then added after assessing the degree to which potential sources of bias have been eliminated.

References

Lalkhen A, McCluskey A. Statistics V: Introduction to clinical trials and systematic reviews. *Contin Educ Anaesth Crit Care Pain*. 2008; 8 (4): 143–146.

Lalkhen A, McCluskey A. Clinical tests: sensitivity and specificity. *Contin Educ Anaesth Crit Care Pain*. 2008; 8 (6): 221–223.

National Institute for Health and Clinical Excellence. Methods for development of NICE public health guidance. 2006.

INDEX

pulmonary thrombo-embolism, 168–169
refeeding syndrome, 172
renal replacement therapy, 177, 195
toxic megacolon, laparotomy to excise, 172
tricyclic antidepressant overdose, 176
ventilator associated pneumonia, 185–186
Internal mammary artery (IMA), 38
Interscalene block, 144, 148
Intra-aortic balloon pump (IABP), 44–45
Intra-arterial (IA) drug injection, 58–59
Intracranial pressure (ICP), 4
Intraoperative awareness, 56
Intrathecal drug delivery systems (ITDDs), 258
Intrathecal (IT) opioids, 259–260
Intrauterine fetal death (IUFD), 201–202, 221
Intravenous drug administration errors, 60–61

J

Jehovah's Witness, 125, 211
Jugular venous pressure (JVP), 5

K

Knee replacement, total, 128–130, 137

L

Laparoscopy
cholecystectomy, 131–132
Nissen fundoplication, 81–82, 93
Laser resection (endobronchial tumour), 32–33
Left ventricular ejection fraction (LVEF), 320
Lithium, 114
Liver disease, chronic, 121–122
Local anaesthesia (LA), 142, 144, 267
Low-flow anaesthesia, 316
Lumbar puncture, 300–301

M

Magnetic resonance imaging (MRI) scan, 115–116, 251
Major haemorrhage, 159–161
Mallampati score, 325
Mandatory level 1 care (MEOWS), 201
Massive blood transfusion, 160–161
Maxillo-facial surgery, see Head, neck,
maxillo-facial and dental surgery
Mean arterial pressure (MAP), 5, 15, 191
Meningococcal septicaemia, 225–226, 236
MEN syndrome, see Multiple endocrine neoplastic
syndrome
Meta-analysis, 325
Mid-face fractures, 99–101
Minimally invasive direct coronary artery bypass
(MIDCAB), 38
Mitral stenosis, 207–208
Monroe–Kelly doctrine, 4, 14

Morphine
intravenous, 254
oral dose, 257
MRI, see Magnetic resonance imaging
Multiple endocrine neoplastic (MEN) syndrome, 83
Myotonic dystrophy, 131–132

N

National Institute for Health and Clinical Excellence, 156
National Patient Safety Agency's 'Right Patient, Right
Blood' guideline, 124
National Poisons Information Service (NPIS), 176
Near-drowning, 162
Neck of femur fracture, 149–151, 155, 158
Neck surgery, see Head, neck, maxillo-facial and
dental surgery
Neuromuscular blocking drug (NMBD), 64
Neurosurgery, neuroradiology and neurocritical care,
1–21
acromegaly, 6, 8, 17
advantages of regional anaesthetic technique for
cystoscopy, 3
antiplatelet therapy, 12
clinical problems, 2–3
drug-eluting stent, 12
dual antiplatelet therapy, 12
Guillain–Barré syndrome, 18–20
obstructive sleep apnoea, 8
pituitary adenoma, 17
posterior fossa tumour excision, 10–11
raised intracranial pressure, 4–5
secondary brain injury, 14–15
stereotactic brain biopsy, 12–13
suxamethonium contraindicated, 3, 16
transection of spinal cord at first thoracic vertebral
level, 16
transection of spinal cord at fourth thoracic vertebra, 1
transection of spinal cord at sixth cervical vertebral
level, 21
trans-sphenoidal hypophysectomy, 6, 17
traumatic brain injury, 14–15
venous air embolism, 10, 11
'Never event,' 69–70
Nissen fundoplication, laparoscopic, 81–82, 93
Non-theatre, 111–116
coronary care unit, 111–112
electro-convulsive therapy, 113–114
magnetic resonance imaging scan, 115–116
severe depression, 113
urgent DC cardioversion, 111

O

Obstetrics, 197–221
airway-related morbidity and mortality, reduction of,
216–217

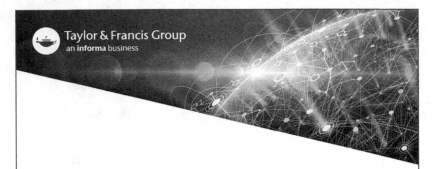

Printed in the United States
by Baker & Taylor Publisher Services